Curing the Incurable

With

Holistic Medicine

Curing the Incurable

With

Holistic Medicine:

The Da Vinci Secret Revealed

Discover the Hidden Causes of Incurable Diseases

George J Georgiou, Ph.D.,N.D.,DSc (AM)

World Health Solutions Press

For Reasons of Legality
The author of this book, George Georgiou, does not advocate the use of any particular form of healthcare but believes that the facts, figures, and knowledge presented herein should he available to every person concerned with improving his or her state of health. Although the author has attempted to give a profound understanding of the topics discussed and to ensure accuracy and completeness of any information that originates from any other source than his own, he and the publisher assume no responsibility for errors, inaccuracies, omissions, or any inconsistency herein. Any slights of people or organizations are unintentional. This hook is not intended to replace the advice and treatment of a physician who specializes in the treatment of diseases. Any use of the information set forth herein is entirely at the reader's discretion. The author and publisher are not responsible for any adverse effects or consequences resulting from the use of any of the preparations or procedures described in this book. The statements made herein are for educational and theoretical purposes only and are mainly based upon George Georgiou's own opinion and theories. You should always consult with a healthcare practitioner before taking any dietary, nutritional, herbal or homeopathic supplement, or beginning or stopping any therapy. The author is not intending to provide any medical advice, or offer a substitute thereof, and makes no warranty, expressed or implied, with respect to any product, device or therapy whatsoever. Except as otherwise noted, no statement in this book has been reviewed or approved by the United States Food & Drug Administration or the Federal Trade Commission or any other European commissions. Readers should use their own judgment or consult a holistic medical expert or their personal physicians for specific applications to their individual problems.

ISBN-13: 978-9963-8401-1-3

Published by World Health Solutions Press, Cyprus
Printed by Lightning Source Inc, UK, Europe & USA

First edition, Curing the Incurable With Holistic Medicine, November 2009

Cover Design and Artwork by Katerina Alexandrou

Table of Contents:

Introduction   xvi

PART A
Chapter 1 – Curing the Incurable

A personal odyssey in search of a return to health   1
My life story   2
Health deteriorates   2
Erratic performance and behaviour   3
Seeking help from natural medicine   5
Regaining my health   6
My diverse and evolving clinical practice   7
Success breeds success ...... and jealousy   9
Hassled and arrested   10
Seeing reputable results   16

Chapter 2 – The Holistic Model of Health

What is holistic medicine?   18
The medical model of disease   23
Let's whip out the gut   24
Why the blinkers?   26
Nutrition and health   28
Man and the environment   30
Energetic man   32
The psycho-emotional person   33
Holistic Medicine – the whole iceberg   35

Chapter 3 – Finding the Causes of Your Disease

Introduction   37
The IDEL Diagnostic Programme   40
Potential causative factors   42
Complete health history   42
Iridology   43
Structural problems – spine and feet   47
VEGA testing and Autonomic Response Testing (ART)   50
Heart Rate Variability Testing (HRV)   56

Digital Infrared Thermal Imaging (DITI) 58
Thermography detects hidden inflammation 59
Tooth and scar foci 61
Tooth foci 61
Scar foci 63
Digital homeopathy 63
Homeopathic sarcodes and isodes 65
Orthomolecular Nutrition 65
Nutritional testing for Metabolic Typing® 68
Live Blood Analysis 72
Biological Terrain Analysis (BTA) 76
Hair Tissue Mineral Analysis (HTMA) 78
Urine Indican Test (Obermeyer Test) 81
Breath testing for digestive problems 82
Final comments on the IDEL Diagnostic methodology 84

Chapter 4 – Detoxification: The Essence of Life

We are all toxic 85
Benefits of detoxification 87
Sources of toxins 88
Toxic from birth 93
North Americans are also toxic 97
Europeans of all age groups are toxic 98
Cosmetic beautify but they also poison 99
Mercury is everywhere 100
Mercury in amalgam fillings 101
Mercury in vaccines 102
Toxicity and fertility threat 104
Regulatory agencies react slowly 105
The toxic onslaught in a nutshell 107
Toxins vs nutrients: The uneven battle 108
New 21st century theory of disease 109
Signs and symptoms of chemical poisoning 110
Ways to address toxicity 111
The DaVinci Centre Detoxification Diet 113
The 15-Day Alkaline Detoxification Diet (15-DADD) 113
What will I be eating during the 15-DADD? 114
Lots of food and calories 116
Detoxification symptoms – "The Healing Crisis" 117
Phases of detoxification 118
Supplements that help the detoxification pathways 121

The good news! 122
Before starting the detox programme 122
Preparing for the detox 124
Major detoxification centres of the body 127
Food enzymes and detoxification 128
The infamous coffee enema – the detox secret! 129
How does the coffee enema work? 130
Preparing the coffee enema formula 132
Instructions for a coffee enema 133
What position should you use? 134
Administering your first enema 134
Other detoxification techniques 135
Skin brushing 135
Detox breathing exercise 136
Detox visualization 137
Epsom salt bath 138
Cider vinegar bath 138
Sauna or steam bath 139
Deeper cleansing 139
The Theory of Autointoxication 139
Constipation 140
Nature needs some help and urgently 142
Colon hydrotherapy 144
Indications for colon hydrotherapy 144
So what is colon hydrotherapy? 145
Heavy metal detoxification 146
Lung and lymphatic system 147
Detoxification exercises 148
Kidney and blood cleanse 149
Killing uninvited guests 150
The herbal parasite cleanse 152
The Liver and Gallbladder Flush 153
Gallstones 154
The pathogenesis of gallstones 155
Gallstones affect many millions of people 155
Removing gallstones without resorting to surgery? 156
Preparations for the gallbladder flush 159
Helpful hints 163
Infrared heat therapy 163
The sauna experience 164
Ionic footbath therapy 167

PART B
Chapter 5 – Systemic Candidiasis

Elimination using the DaVinci Candida Protocol — 169
What is Candida? — 170
What is the role of Candida? — 174
How do you get it? — 174
Why is it a serious problem? — 176
Toxic waste – acetaldehyde — 176
Effects on immunity — 177
What are the signs of Candida infection? — 182
How do you know you have it? — 185
Signs and symptoms — 185
Laboratory tests — 186
Biodemal screening — 187
Autonomic Response Testing (ART) — 188
The secrets to success — 188
The DaVinci Candida Protocol (DCP) — 189
Phase I – Starving the Candida — 191
Phase II – Killing the Candida — 192
Phase III – Repopulating the friendly bacteria — 192
Phase IV – Using isopathic remedies — 193
Phase V – Balancing the body chemistry — 194
Herxheimer reactions — 195
Case studies — 196

Chapter 6 – Parasites: The Uninvited Guests

What is a parasite? — 199
Nasty consequences — 201
So who are these uninvited guests? — 202
Categories of parasites — 202
Worms — 202
Roundworms — 202
Pinworms — 203
Tapeworms — 204
Hookworms — 206
Guinea worms — 207
Heartworms — 208
Warning signs of parasitic infestation — 209
Children — 211
Treatment: eliminating parasites — 212

Ozone and parasites 212
Dr. Hulda Clark's parasite cleanse 213
Homeopathics for parasitic infestation 216
Additional remedies 216
Shore up the defences 217
Specific recommendations for pregnant women 218

Chapter 7 – Killing Ourselves With Toxic Chemicals

Xenobiotics 222
Low-dose exposure 223
We are all toxic 224
Toxins in newborns 224
Toxins in the North Pole 225
Toxins in wildLife 226
Toxic contamination through the generations 226
Perfluorochemicals (PFCs) 228
Harmful health effects of PFCs 229
Phthalates 231
Harmful effects of phthalates 232
Phenols, bisphenyl A and nonylphenol 234
Harmful health effects of phenols 235
Polybrominated flame retardants (BFRs) 237
Harmful health effects of BFRs 239
Mercury: 'The Big One' 239
The mercury cycles 240
Many forms of mercury 241
Mercury in surprising places 242
The chemistry of methyl mercury 243
Mercury: crossing all barriers 245
Mercury and the central nervous system 246
The transport of mercury vapour around the body 247
Mercury and the autoimmune system 248
The effects of mercury on glutamate 248
Mercury and yeast infections 249
The mechanisms of mercury toxicity in the CNS 250
Mercury attacking the tissues 251
Methyl mercury and the foetal brain 251
Mercury toxicity in fish 252
Guidelines for minimizing mercury exposure from fish 253
Widespread health problems from mercury exposure 255
Dental amalgams – a closer look 257

Denying the truth about the dangers of amalgam toxicity 257
The nuts and bolts of mercury vapour inhalation 259
The effects of mercury on reproductive health 263
A unisex society! 264
Obesity and toxicity 265
Diagnosis of heavy metal toxicity 266
Hair Tissue Mineral Analysis (HTMA) 266
Urine and faeces testing 268
What can we do to protect ourselves? 268
Treating heavy metal toxicity using conventional chelators 268
Natural heavy metal chelators – do they work? 269
Research on HMD® 270
Independent Mercury trial using HMD® 273
Liver and kidney serum test results using HMD® 274
Natural heavy metal chelation protocol 275
Further research 286

Chapter 8 – The Dangers of Modern Dentistry

Dental mercury poisoning in focus 277
Removing amalgams safely 280
Patient protection protocol 280
What to expect following the safe removal of amalgams 284
Root canals and dental foci 287
What can be done? 295
Focal infection theory 298
Mechanisms of focal infection 299
Neural focal interference 304
So how can this be redressed? 305
Teeth and acupuncture meridians 307
Symptoms of dead teeth 309
Allergy to dental materials used to restore teeth 310
Electrogalvanism 311
Dental implants – bone graft and metallic incompatibility 312
Dental braces and nickel 314
Children at risk 317
Soladey tooth brush – no toothpaste! 318

Chapter 9 – Bioenergetic and Informational Medicine

A little history 323

How does the body work energetically? 325
Informational medicine 329
Visual Medicine – seeing the effects on water 331
The Human Bioenergetic System 332
The Vegetative Reflex Test using VEGA 335
Bioresonance therapy 337
Infrared Electric Light Sauna Therapy 341
Homeopathy 342
Low Intensity Lazer Therapy (LILT) 346
Orgone Accumulator 349
Ionizing footbath 352
Digital Infrared Thermal Imaging (DITI) or Thermography 355
Dr. Rife technology 360
Autonomic Response Testing (ART) 366
Su Jok Therapy 368
PAPIMI 372
Matrix Regeneration Therapy (MRT) 382

Chapter 10 – Healing the soul

Introduction 385
Hellinger's soul healing constellation workshops 386
The Family System or soul 387
Systemic Entanglements 389
Resolution of systemic entanglements 392
Opening up to love 395
The Constellation process 397
Acknowledging and Accepting What Is 400
The Intrinsic Order – the Orders of Love in family 403
Physical illness and disease 404

Chapter 11 – Viewing Cancer Holistically: Thinking Outside the Box

Cancer is multidimensional 405
Cancer is not a disease! 407
Chemotherapy and radiation – is this the solution? 408
Cancer and mitochondrial dysfunction 417
Cancer and anaerobic respiration 418
Reoxygenation of cancer cells 420
Steps in the development of a cancer cell 421
Reversing acid pH in cancer cells 424

Trophoblastic Theory forgotten   428
Treating cancer with systemic enzymes   431
Nutrition and cancer   432
Vitamin C and cancer   435
Laetrile or vitamin B17   436
Halting metastasis   439
Shark cartilage   439
Other causes of cancer   442
Constipation   442
Diseased teeth and cancer   444
Inflammation and cancer   445
Modified Citrus Pectin (MCP)   459
The DaVinci Cancer Programme   451

PART C
Chapter 12 – Patient's Case Histories

Case 1   456
Case 2   465
Case 3   475
Case 4   484
Case 5   492
Case 6   499
Case 7   507
Case 8   517
Case 9   527
Case 10   537
Case 11   542
Case 12   546
Case 13   552
Case 14   560
Case 15   567

Appendix A   576
Appendix B   578

Summary and Concluding Remarks   582
Clinical Consultations   584
DaVinci College of Holistic Medicine   584
About the Author   585

Dedications and Acknowledgments

I dedicate this book to all the courageous patients who helped to shape my career and who gave me the opportunity to learn by experimentation and trial and error – I am eternally grateful to all.

I also dedicate this book to my beloved family and children who have been patient with me while I was burning the midnight oil. A special remembrance to my beloved, deceased father for giving me the love and encouragement to persevere, be determined and not look back. My mother gave me the courage and strength to face up to the difficulties in life.

I would also like to thank all the people that helped during the writing of this text: Di Stoddard, one of the most meticulous proof readers that I have ever met who waded through the material in fine detail; also to Dr. Graham Hutt who read the script and made helpful comments of encouragement; to Dr. Hisham who has been a proponent of holistic medicine and has began the translation of this text into Arabic; to Steven Victor who read the chapter on Hellinger Soul Healing and made useful observations; to Katerina, the talented graphic designer who designed the front cover of this book; and to all the other reviewers who wrote their commentary on the back cover – all are "gurus" in their own right!

Many thanks of gratitude also go to the many teachers and mentors, too many to mention here by name, who have taught me what I know, as well as the many authors of the many books that I voraciously devoured while studying all these topics. All these scientists and researchers have laid the groundwork for this book in holistic medicine.

Last, I would like to prostrate to the Higher Powers that have always been there to help when the going got tough and always responded with love and care when asked.

INTRODUCTION

When I began writing this book my main intention was to share the model of Holistic Medicine with the layperson, in order to shed some insight into the pathogenesis of disease. As I progressed through the complexity of topics, I realized that there were a number of doctors and practitioners that were also interested in learning more about holistic medicine, but they wanted to know the scientific sources of the various diagnostic and healing modalities. I therefore began to pay particular attention to referencing material with scientific studies which are more for the benefit of the health practitioners and scientists, not so much the layperson.

There are more than 750 scientific references quoted in total. Maybe this scientific basis will help those who feel that holistic medicine is all "quackery" or "non-scientific" or not "evidence-based" to change their attitude – holistic medicine is as scientific as any other type of medicine. Many of the scientists quoted are Nobel Prize winners, and some have actually been awarded two Nobel prizes for their work, a rare honour for any scientist.

Holistic Medicine is the only way to cure complex, degenerative, chronic diseases that have multiple causes – the practitioner must be able to view the person on all levels, physical, biochemical, nutritional, environmental, energetic, psychological, emotional and spiritual to be able to stand any chance at healing the whole person. Simply viewing the body on any one of these levels will not achieve a total healing at all these levels – the person being treated is made up of all these levels, and often there are imbalances and dysfunctions found on every single level that needs addressing. These imbalances need to be identified and removed before the practitioner can begin repairing and rebuilding the damaged components. This is the essence of this book, based upon my own experience as a Holistic practitioner.

I will be the first to admit that the book is far from comprehensive – there are so many other details that we are all constantly learning about that it is impossible to include everything in one book. Hopefully, it will be a starting point for many doctors, natural medicine practitioners and the layperson to begin understanding that we need to undergo a paradigm shift from viewing the body mechanistically with simple working parts that need to be removed or suppressed with drugs, to a more lateral view of the person with all their levels and their complexities. Holistic Medicine is the only hope that we have of getting the person back to normal functioning, while practicing what Hippocrates taught us so many years ago:

Primum, Non Nocere – First, Do No Harm!

The title of the book: "Curing the Incurable with Holistic Medicine: The DaVinci Secret Revealed" needs a little explanation. First, the word "curing" is not the same as treating. We can all be "treated" for certain symptoms with either drugs or natural remedies for a long time without necessarily seeing any benefit or cure. Second, the word "incurable" is used in the context of what orthodox medicine believes is "incurable" – most if not all the case examples given in the last chapter are those that the medical profession think are "incurable," not that they are obdurately incurable – it requires a more multi-modal approach to cure, not the symptom-suppression approach that is often practiced by today's modern medicine.

The "DaVinci Secret Revealed" is based on the working model of the DaVinci Holistic Health Centre in Larnaca, Cyprus that all these diagnostic and healing modalities have been duly tested and tried, with numerous people seeing the benefits and regaining their health and quality of life. There are obviously many other diagnostic and treatment modalities that are used by many other health practitioners around the world – the holistic health model presented here is but one small portion of all these, however, it is one that has worked successfully for hundreds of patients suffering all types of health issues.

There are off course people who have reached such a point in life where the degeneration has reached a critical mass that nothing can help them to cure, but we can always give these people hope and help them to better the quality of their life, however long that may be. Preparing a person to "meet their Angels" is also another important part of the work of Holistic Medicine, as is healing of the soul which often encumbers the healing process. There is so much to talk about in Preventive Medicine too, but I have not really addressed this in any meaningful way as that is another book that needs to be written.

Regarding the books layout, it is divided into three parts. Part A provides the main reasons why I entered the field of Holistic Medicine and my experiences and adventures in this. Another chapter then follows, that provides a working definition of what I call Holistic Medicine and explains its philosophy, while contrasting it with the conventional medical approach. It also provides an overview of the failed state of conventional medicine as well as an overview of the reasons why that medical model is inconsistent and precarious. In this section, I also present the main thrust of my diagnostic and therapeutic methodology – a programme I have conveniently named "IDEL Diagnostic Programme," which is the acronym for "**ID**entify" and "**EL**iminate" the causative factors of disease.

Part B contains a series of chapters on nutrition, detoxification, Candida, parasites, xenobiotics and heavy metals, the dangers of dentistry, bioenergetic and informational medicine, healing the soul and holistic cancer treatments, all based on the Holistic Healing Model that I practice daily.

Part C includes 15 case histories and testimonials of patients from the DaVinci Holistic Health Centre in Larnaca, Cyprus. Some of the cases presented are indeed very special and they have no precedence in medical history as they are generally considered "incurable."

Finally, I present my concluding remarks. But first, I would like to introduce myself and give a little background information as to how I have come to my present standpoint with regard to the treatment of supposedly incurable disease.

The story begins with my own illness ....

PART A

Chapter One

CURING THE INCURABLE

A Personal Odyssey in Search of a Return to Health

Holistic Medicine is a topic very dear to my heart and probably ended up saving my life, not to mention greatly increasing its quality, and making me feel human again.

Following a 7-year period of chronic and at that time unexplainable illness, my great suffering became a powerful motive to find answers, and get to the root causes of my debilitating symptoms. I developed a burning desire to feel perfectly healthy again: to completely heal myself; and took matters into my own hands, engaging in a lifelong mission to pursue learning in the health sciences, which has now been ongoing for the last 25 years, and still continues to this day. I travelled to various parts of the world and obtained degrees and diplomas in a wide range of natural therapies and have studied and trained in numerous diagnostic and therapeutic techniques

After these long and intriguing years of training and application of these new therapeutic techniques I have fulfilled my dream and passion: to feel healthy and be able to remain healthy. Much of this process took place in parallel with my professional work in Cyprus.

I have also devoted myself to using this Holistic Medical Model in clinical practice, having tried and tested it with many hundreds of patients of all types – from migraines to metastatic cancers, and seeing its effectiveness again and again. Treating chronic diseases has now become the mainstay of my clinical practice as there is a great need for this type of work in today's sick and degenerating society.   I now wish to share this knowledge base with chronically ill people everywhere, which is one reason why I am writing this book.

1

My Life Story

When I arrived in Cyprus back in 1983 after completing undergraduate and postgraduate studies in the UK, I started my career as a teacher of biology, having completed an initial combined honours degree in biology/psychology. Upon completion of my postgraduate studies in clinical psychology I began seeing my first patients. It struck me that many of my patients were facing deep sexual issues that were proving intractable with my psychological training. That was the impetus for me to study human sexuality in depth, and completed a Doctorate degree in Clinical Sexology in the USA and became the first professional sexologist in the history of Cyprus.

Health Deteriorates

Despite all my knowledge in biology and the workings of the human body, at the age of 30 my health was a shambles. I could just about manage to crawl out of bed with excruciating pain in my body and band-type headaches that would last most of the day. I would have a painful breakfast, drag myself to my office, see patients for a couple of hours then back to bed for 2-3 hours before seeing a few more patients in the afternoon. Painkillers and anti-inflammatories were my main support to get through the day.

By evening I was too tired to do anything and it required a concerted effort just to hold a conversation. I tended to avoid company for this reason and became a recluse – living life close to my devoted family and trying to enjoy the small moments of watching my children develop. I absolutely hated the way I was, as by nature I am a "Type A" personality who loves to be on the go, researching new things – I generally have a very inquisitive mind and like people.

Upon deeper reflection, my health saga began a few years earlier at the age of 27, while I was serving in the National Guard of Cyprus after arriving from the UK, where I used to live. After a few months in quite adverse, stressful conditions I developed a very bad fever and viral infection that had me bedbound for a full 15 days. In fact, no one knew I was ill in bed, without being able to get up and walk, for three days until friends who were constantly calling, broke down the door to my apartment.

There was absolutely no way I could move from my bed – I had a constant fever of 40 degrees and was having cold sweats; was dehydrated and pretty much having delusions with such a heavy feeling in my head that the only thing I wanted to do was sleep. The pains in my body also prevented me from moving. The fever remained at 40 degrees or more for the full 15 days and no amount of antibiotics of other drugs seemed to help. After 15 days of taking a combination of antibiotics, anti-inflammatories and antipyretics, I eventually recovered but did not feel my "usual" self after this. My energy levels never seemed to return to normal and there was certainly something that was triggering my sinuses, which were getting inflamed constantly.

A couple of months after recovering from this ordeal I developed intractable headaches and migraines that again had me holding my head and taking pain killers as if they were going out of fashion – every day. I needed to work as I was a busy clinical psychologist and clinical sexologist at the time and felt an obligation towards my patients, as well as my students; I was teaching biology at a local private school in Larnaca as well as teaching undergraduate courses in psychology at Intercollege, a local private college in Nicosia.

After many months of these persistent headaches, accompanied by an unexplainable fatigue, I eventually went to the local G.P. who took some X-rays and found that my frontal sinuses were loaded with fluid – he immediately prescribed antibiotics. Less than two months later I was back there again for more antibiotics as my sinuses were again blocked and causing headaches and pain, not to mention the tiredness, apathy – and on occasions depression. I was quite incapacitated and this was certainly enough to cause an active person to fall into a depression – otherwise I loved my work. There is nothing more frustrating than waking every morning with band-type headaches that prevented me from concentrating on my work.

Erratic Performance and Behaviour

It was around the same time that I was also invited to teach part-time at a local flight school – they wanted me to teach the human-factor elements of their local Private Pilots course. These topics combine both psychology and biology, so I was duly suited, having degrees in both. I had no qualms about accepting this job offer as one of my deepest passions while still at school was to become an RAF jet pilot but as fate would have it, there were other plans for me. It was not long before the school invited me to take my own private pilots license (PPL). They felt that this would facilitate my teaching, as it would give me the experience of being in the cockpit.

I needed no further persuading – I began ground school immediately and within a short while I was sitting in the left-hand seat flying a Cessna 152 or a Piper Cherokee. But the problem that my instructors could never understand was why my flying was so erratic. On my "good" days when I would get up feeling generally clear-headed and alert I would fly the plane to perfection with perfect takeoffs and landings as we practiced our touch-and-goes. On the "bad" days when I would get up with a headache, sore muscles, lack of sleep and generally feeling like a truck had run over me, I would sit in the cockpit ready for takeoff and upon applying full power, I could hardly steer straight on the runway – much to my instructors horror! Eventually I got my license but it was a tough uphill climb (literally!), with the instructor's blood pressure seeing better times!

To cut a long story short, in the 7 years of frequenting various medics, allergy specialists and an ENT surgeon (who eventually persuaded me to have a septum operation for a supposedly defective septum in my nose), I was in a much worse state than when I first began getting symptoms. In these 7 years I had taken 18 courses of antibiotics and was in a real mess.

My symptoms had now worsened and became more frequent including headaches and migraines, fibromyalgia (pains and aches in all my body), chronic fatigue (or Myalgic Encephalitis as it was diagnosed by one homeopathic doctor), bowel distension, more or less constant stomach pains with dreadful distension, Leaky Gut Syndrome, Systemic Candidiasis with skin itching, rashes, chronic tiredness and more. I sought diagnosis and treatment abroad in the US and the UK. I was getting weaker and weaker and was now becoming ill with whatever I ate. I was getting desperate as my workload and obligations grew – I now had a family with two young children and was building a house, as well as conducting many additional professional duties. Despite ill health, I was invited to do a radio programme and I accepted; I was also asked to write a column in a national tabloid with a large circulation, and I accepted that too. I could barely manage to keep going.

Seeking Help from Natural Medicine

In desperation, I began reading Natural Medicine books. I was fumbling in the dark as even though my initial degree was in biology and psychology, I had not really delved into the fascinating science of Natural Medicine. One of the first books that I read was written by Dr. Richard Mackarness entitled "Not All In the Mind"[1] – that alerted me to the idea that food allergies can have a detrimental impact on both mental health and physical health. He suggests that in evolutionary terms our bodies are not adjusted to high cereal diets and dairy products, which have only been around for the last few hundred years (it takes thousands of years for our bodies to adjust to evolutionary changes).

He also suggests that up to 80% of the population are probably experiencing some type of food or chemical allergy due to eating highly processed food that our bodies are not yet adjusted to. After reading this book I attempted a detoxification and elimination diet by basically cutting out everything apart from fruit and vegetables.

The first couple of days I felt like my head was going to blow off like a grenade – the pain was unbearable and I spent the weekend in bed sleeping, going to the toilet and more sleeping. I had mostly vegetable soups, light salads, plenty of fruit and lots of water. On the third day I woke feeling so refreshed and alert that I could not believe it! I was hopping around like a little child in a candy store after being imprisoned for so long. The feeling of being alive, pain free and with plenty of energy was amazing!

This renewed energy lasted until the end of the detoxification and elimination diet when I then relapsed back into my old state in a matter of days. What was happening? Why did I feel so good on the detoxification diet only to find myself back in the prison of pain and misery again after it? Was it related to the food I was eating? Maybe - I was left with more questions than answers.

Unfortunately, I was not as knowledgeable then as I am now. In hindsight, I knew instinctively that something miraculous had happened in my body during the detox, but ignorance could not explain the mechanisms. One of the main reasons I felt so well was because I had simply cut out the foods

---

1 Mackarness, R. Not All in The Mind. London: Pan Books, 1976.

that I was intolerant to – wheat and dairy – I used to eat cheese sandwiches washed down with coffee most days, as I was too busy to prepare anything else. "Were these food allergies making me feel so bad?" I wondered.

Were those unpleasant symptoms I'd experienced in the first couple of days of the detox related to the fact that the stored toxins were being released from my organs and tissues in a big gush? Again, in retrospect, it is clear that this is exactly what was happening – during any detoxification regime toxins are released by the bucketful in the first few days, then things slow down somewhat and the symptoms abate. You begin feeling really well as the body clears itself of accumulated toxins – some of these can be deeply buried in tissues and joints and can cause pain in these areas.

After reading many books on detoxification and experimenting over time, I eventually flew over to England where I saw one of the authors of a nutrition book, from the Institute of Optimum Nutrition, Patrick Holford, where I became his student. During the three years of intensive study I managed to learn a lot that helped my healing process, but not enough to completely heal myself.

My pursuit for learning was intrinsically motivated by my burning desire to completely heal myself, so spanning a 23 year period I studied and obtained degrees and diplomas in Clinical Psychology, Clinical Sexology, Clinical Nutrition, Naturopathy, Herbal Medicine, Homeopathy, Iridology and Su Jok Acupuncture. I have also studied and trained in numerous diagnostic and therapuetic techniques such as VEGA testing, Bioresonance Therapy, Rife technology, Bach Flower remedies, Thermography, Darkfield Microscopy and Live Blood Analysis, Low Intensity Laser Therapy, Autonomic Response Testing, Field Control Therapy, Biological Terrain Analysis, heavy metal analysis using atomic fluorescence and inductively coupled plasma optical emission spectrometers as well as many varied detoxification techniques.

Regaining My Health!

After these long, interesting years of study I eventually managed to regain my health and optimise it. This year, 2009, I am 52 years old and have plenty of energy and the well-being to do all the things that I like doing including flying a small private plane, horse riding, maintaining antique cars and motorbikes, water skiing, writing books, researching and running the busy DaVinci Natural Health Centre,[2] of which I am the Founder Director, based in Larnaca, Cyprus. I am also the Academic Director of the DaVinci College of Holistic Medicine,[3] as well as being involved with many other projects and activities too numerous to mention.

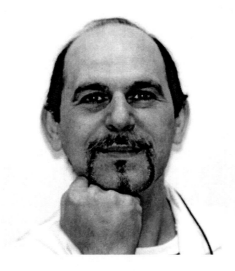

Dr. George J Georgiou, 2009

My Diverse and Evolving Clinical Practice

My psychology and sexology practice has expanded and diversified and over the years I have been offering a wide range of health services to my patients. While my passion for maintaining my own health has not abated, I have developed a new passion: to help my patients recover their health, just like I did. I felt disappointed when a patient did not respond well to my treatments.

When some of my patients failed to see any health benefits, I asked myself, "what could I have done better or different." I kept researching and reflecting on the why and the how - I strove to improve and optimise the therapeutic programmes I was offering that could resolve the multitude of problems facing my patients. I began analysing old and new cases. I researched the literature, tested many new and different therapeutic protocols, refined them or discarded them on the basis of clinical

---

2 www.docgeorge.com
3 www.collegenaturalmedicine.com

outcomes. When I could not find suitable therapeutic protocols available, I formulated new ones. Those that tested positive were retained; the failed ones were discarded.

My continuous training and research, combined with the feedback from my patients, enabled me to optimise and customise the treatment methodology to the needs of individual patients: bespoke medicine. I began observing many of my patients recovering from serious ill-health and eventually experiencing the health transformation that I did. At the beginning I was not so sure: perhaps it was a fluke? Perhaps it was coincidental? Perhaps it was luck?

I was getting some amazing results but I thought to myself: "Let us not get carried away. This could be based on some patients coincidentally recovering and not based on my methodology." But the results were replicable with more and more patients, and with different and varied conditions, even though the treatments differed for each patient having the same disease.

The word spread and I began getting referrals for more serious cases: chronic degenerative diseases such as arthritis, multiple sclerosis, heart disease, diabetes and cancer – even from abroad. These cases were tough and needed special attention – cancer in particular was a real challenge. How do you approach patients that were literally given a few months to live? I had to stretch my knowledge and experience to new limits. I had to change the whole framework in which I worked. Serious cases required private attention for nearly a whole day. I had to get appropriate equipment, invest in a bigger library. I had no space to put it all so I built a larger Centre, fully equipped, with in-house laboratory facilities.

While I was active in clinical practice, I also engaged in academic and empirical research – especially, on heavy metal toxicity. After three years of arduous research in laboratories and in the field, I developed a unique product called HMD®[4] of which I am now the worldwide patent-pending holder of. I have published a number of articles in peer-reviewed journals and I am regularly invited to conferences to talk about my research, clinical methodology, as well as my unique therapeutic protocols.

---

4 www.detoxmetals.com

I have had a rewarding and successful career, blessed with the satisfaction of helping people regain their health and their lives back. There is nothing more spiritually rewarding than having a patient who has been given a zero prognosis from the medical fraternity, regain complete health – this in itself is enough to motivate me to work until the day that I die.

Success Breeds Success and ….. Jealousy

Success breeds success – it also breeds jealousy. My clinical work caused discomfort among the local medical establishment. The "miraculous" natural cures of patients did not resonate well with conventional medicine. I was hounded by the Cyprus Medical Association, constantly being reported to the police and General Attorney for "practising medicine without being a qualified medical practitioner." I was arrested and handcuffed on one occasion (I spent one evening giving health advice to police jail guards)! All this was harassment by the "powers that be" – all motivated by jealousy, greed, ego and self-interest – not by patients' interests. After all, none of my patients complained to me or reported me for negligence or unprofessionalism – it was always the medical association who would undergo the "witch hunt" using every influence that they could to exterminate those that were getting in their way.

I began getting banned from appearing on TV after talks with the allopathic medical doctors – when I presented patients on TV that had been cured of Crohn's, Irritable Bowel Syndrome, Multiple Sclerosis, cardiovascular problems and more the powerful lobby of the medical profession made certain I did not appear again. I also began getting banned from discussing issues of holistic vs allopathic medicine – it appears that the media here in Cyprus is no more democratic or objective with freedom of speech than most of the Illuminati-owned channels abroad. Continuing with this education in Holistic Medicine would certainly have been beneficial to the viewers and their families, but this was not the issue.

Even though I was hounded on a number of occasions, I was never convicted even once as the charges were thrown out by the Attorney General even before reaching a court of law - there simply was "no case." Even the police got criticised by the medical fraternity for "not doing their job properly and not being strict enough with charlatans." The harassments still continue, and so do attempts to lock me away and silence me. As much as I do not like the reaction and the actions of conventional medics and their associations – I understand them fully: there is a lot at stake, ranging from bruised egos to big cash. My treatment methodology is not only effective – it costs a fraction of the money spent on their conventional, ineffective, as well as risky treatments.

The more patients who are treated using Holistic Medicine, the more resistance there is from the medical profession – it's an irony as one would think that they would pay attention, but it is not the motive to heal that is the prime factor, but the gargantuan ego and self interests. In Cyprus where I have been working for over 25 years, I have been attacked by the Cyprus Medical Association more times than I care to remember – usually this takes place about every 5 years where I get a call from the police saying that the Cyprus Medical Association is bringing charges against me for "practising medicine without being a qualified medical practitioner."

The police come round to the Centre with search warrants, take what they want, bully me around and ask a myriad of questions in order to "catch me out" and take photos of anything that they wish. There is no arguing with them as they normally appear in force and move around stirring in my personal desk, taking personal diaries that have no relevance to their case and generally bullying me in order to frighten and weaken the "enemy." It's an inconvenience and an invasion of privacy, but one has to stand firm and be chivalrous in these matters, as truth and innocence triumph in the end – the Higher Powers make certain of this.

Hassled and Arrested!

On one occasion about 15 years ago, two police officers knocked on the door of my old Centre in downtown Larnaca. They had warrants to search the premises – so I let them in to do their search. A very belligerent, haughty sergeant began asking questions in an abrupt manner as if I were a criminal who had already been tried and found guilty. I reminded him that the Cyprus Law states that I am innocent till proven guilty by a court of law.

It was obvious from the beginning that we were not going to resonate together on any meaningful level. He walked around the Centre asking me questions about the various therapeutic devices that I was using, such as "What is this?" – pointing to the VEGA machine and "What is this?" pointing to the BICOM bioresonance machine, and so forth. Initially, I was courteous and began furnishing him with the information he wanted, but it soon became clear that he was not duly gifted with too much gray matter, so at some point in time I offered to give him the reading material to study so that he could answer his own questions.

At that point, having politely refused to answer his questions, he shouted to the young constable who was accompanying him, to go down to the police car and bring up the handcuffs so that I could be taken away handcuffed. I said nothing but stood there looking at him rather surprised. The constable did not move and stood there sombrely staring at me. The sergeant again shouted even louder, "go bring the damn cuffs and let's take him away." At that point the poor constable asked whether this was really necessary and said to the sergeant: "Dr. Georgiou does not appear to be overly violent, so are the handcuffs absolutely necessary?" The sergeant would have none of it, and with a few more outbursts the distressed constable was back with the handcuffs and I was being led away to the police car – it was an odd feeling being led away from a healing Centre where your only motive is to heal people, to a detention centre for hardened criminals.

On the way out of the Centre, the door was sealed with police tape and later that afternoon we were back, but this time with about 10 officers from the Narcotics division. They wanted to see what narcotics I was storing in the various jars of natural herbs that I had in my herbal pharmacy back then. There was more cross-examination by many of these, who could not have been more than 25-30 years old, but with an arrogance that was overpowering.

One of them picked up a kilo jar of a white powdered herb that was actually slippery elm (useful for gut problems as it coats the gut with a mucilaginous coat). I foresaw what he was going to ask so I facetiously said: "If this kilo bottle were truly cocaine or another narcotic then why would I need to be working?" He obviously did not like my answer as they frenetically began systematically testing some of the other herbs. Needless to say, after a couple of hours of finding nothing that even looked like a narcotic, they got tired and decided to call it a day. So it was back in the squad car and away to the police station again.

On arrival at the station I was placed in a small cell where there were two policemen – one was behaving like the "good cop" and the other the "bad cop." It was so obvious that I could not help but snigger at the set up. I am certain that they missed the fact that I was also a clinical psychologist and was aware of such tactics from my medico-legal studies back at university.

I felt frivolous so decided to play a little game. Within a half hour I was behaving towards the "good cop" as if he was the "bad cop," basically ignoring him as much as possible, and befriending the "bad cop" as if he were the good cop. After the initial confusion and "try-harder phenomenon" on their behalf they figured out what I was doing and decided to relax a little. We all smiled and sat down and talked about my escapade – they were curious to understand why I had been arrested!

Then began the questions regarding what I was in for – at that point I asked to see the warrant for my arrest to see what the charge was and who had made it against me. It was not surprising to find the signature of the ex-President of the Cyprus Medical Association on the warrant, as I had seen this numerous times – he was a true "witch-hunter."

The present debacle was based on an allegation from a patient who had reported to the police that he had come to see me in my capacity as a professional Clinical Sexologist for a sexual problem – impotence – only to "discover" that I was not a "qualified medical practitioner." It seemed strange that a patient would report me in this way, particularly one who had come to me with a sexual problem – one would think that he would not want this to become public knowledge. There was something strange in the allegation but I could not remember all the details of this particular patient as I needed to see his history file to get a better picture of what was going on.

I asked the police officers how long I would be held for and discovered that there were rumours of being held for 8 days – I immediately called my wife and asked her to send over some pyjamas, toothbrush, some books and change of clothes. As I was preparing to settle in and psychologically prepare myself for this unanticipated experience, very soon after - within a couple of hours - one of the chief policemen for the Larnaca area came into the cell and began talked to me in a civilized way, apologizing for the "confusion" and the harassment, and said that it was OK to go home immediately.

I had spent a complete day "inside," counselling the policemen on optimal nutrition, who by that point had befriended me and understood the politics involved – that this was yet another frame up by the Cyprus Medical Association (CMA), who really wanted to eradicate successful practitioners of natural medicine as they were "eating part of their pie." These are the exact words used by a past-president of the CMA and actually quoted to a journalist, which was published in one of the leading newspapers on the island!

Consequently I am the current Larnaca Branch President of the Cyprus Natural Therapeutics Association (CNTA) and as a professional body we are aghast at this quote that we have saved in our archives – "eating part of their pie" – it is a repulsive, dishonourable and disgraceful thing to say that goes against the Hippocratic Oath, as well as all the patients on the island who are under the care of the CMA. It is clear that the CMA need to revise their ethical guidelines and adhere more to the Hippocratic Oath.

When I was eventually released from the cell that night and got back to my Centre, I was curious to find out who this patient was. I quickly found his file and noted that he had seen me four times with his fiancée for an erectile dysfunction and was cured on the third visit with one final follow-up visit to make certain that everything was working well. I remembered the couple well and recollected that we had a good, professional rapport – I remember really liking the couple and treating them with a healthy respect, motivated to help them regain their sexual functioning as soon as possible.

I also remember them being very grateful to me when they were discharged and actually invited me for a coffee, which I politely declined. My curiosity really began to grow now as this was sounding more and more bizarre. Why would a satisfied patient who had been cured of a sensitive sexual problem and was appreciative go to the police and report me? How could such a "satisfied" client be so malevolent as to actually turn up at a police station and file a complaint against me? I decided to call the client and get to the bottom of what happened.

Needless to say, when he heard my voice he froze, but I persisted and pointed out that this allegation of "practicing medicine without being a medical doctor" was not only pertinent to myself but included all the other natural medicine practitioners on the island. This was not an isolated incident that involved me alone, but it had far reaching implications. So why did he report me ….. I asked the question many times but he was elusive, brazen and vague.

I then asked him if he had any complaints about my behaviour as a professional towards him. Had I been negligent or said anything that he disliked? At this point he was so apologetic that he was close to tears. He not only said that he was very grateful for the help that I had given him and his fiancée, but had recommended me to others! Well, at that point I was really exasperated and told him straight that he was not making sense.

There was a brief silence before he began his confession - one of his "best male friends" was a medical doctor in the Larnaca area, and whilst discussing manly things over a cup of coffee, he had mentioned my name and how pleased he was to have overcome an embarrassing problem. As soon as the doctor heard my name, which he recognized and did not like the fact that I was working as a Clinical Sexologist, he got irate and began coercing the client to report me to the police for "practising medicine without being a qualified medical practitioner."

The client initially resisted, but he felt obligated towards his medical practitioner and friend who was persuasive in his arguments so after much coercion he did just this, and based upon one single testimonial from a "satisfied" patient the bureaucratic wheels were set in motion that led to my arrest. Something is obviously wrong when the Law or the Cyprus Medical Association can abuse these powers to benefit their members at the injustice of others.

I chastised the client for his actions, asked him if he had any other complaints against me, and got a promise from him to go back to the police and tell them that he had made a mistake – I later heard that this actually took place. Within a couple of months I received a call from the police station informing me that the General Attorney had thrown my case out, yet again. There was no apologize for the false arrest, the handcuffs, the harassment, the inconvenience and most painful – the intrusion into ones own privacy for no apparent reason.

There have been other similar incidences in my 25-year career here in Cyprus, but interestingly when my papers and qualifications turn up at the District Attorney's office in Nicosia, the case is always thrown out and never goes to court. I have never been convicted of any offence of this nature. Ostracised by the medical fraternity I am, but really I have no interest in developing relationships with people that do not have a healthy respect for me based on what they see, as opposed to what they hear. Self-interest is also rampant here in Cyprus but this mindset also does not interest me. My pursuit of science and the truth are far more important to me, with the ultimate goal of helping as many sick people as I can, as this is what gives me the spiritual satisfaction and courage to continue my work in the midst of this persecution and discrimination. I hope this book will seal the truth of this harassment that I have not shared with others to date as the opportunity was not present.

Recently, however, at the beginning of 2009 there have been high-level talks at the Cyprus Ministry of Health regarding passing legislation to regulate natural or CAM medicine here in Cyprus. Very recently on January 19th I took part in a TV debate on Cyprus national TV (PIK 1) with three other medical doctors, one who had reported me to the police last year after providing false witness to the police that the patient later attested and nothing came of it – a real 'witch-hunter' of holistic medicine practitioners, another medical homeopath who believes that only medical doctors can practice homeopathy and a representative of the Ministry of Health. They began the conversation gently about how this legislation of natural medicine is for the protection of the patients, but this was obviously a smoke screen, as really this is for the protection of their own kind, the 2,000 or so medical practitioners that work on the island.

As the show unfolded, their agenda became crystal clear – the medics wanted to have all natural medicine regulatory bodies under their own auspices – they would set the criteria, what practitioners could practice and how, placing incredible restrictions upon them. Only medical homeopaths would be able to practice homeopathy as they see it as being a 'medical' field and non-medical homeopaths could take a homeopathic history, but would then need to call their medical 'mentor' with the case history details and they would diagnose and prescribe the correct homeopathic remedy over the phone.

This is exactly how the medical homeopath presented his scenario to me over the phone the day after the show. I simply mentioned that in most parts of the world, including many European countries, most homeopaths are non-medical and legally allowed to practice given that they are qualified professionals. The issue is not this, however, it is ultimately the aim of the Cyprus Medical Association and the corresponding Ministry to have all patients seeing natural medicine practitioners referred ONLY through a medical doctor.

It does not take a lot of astuteness to understand what the outcome of this will be – it would basically wipe natural medicine, and this Holistic Medicine Model, right off the map here in Cyprus. This agenda certainly does not support the patient as they will be the ones who are at a loss as they will not be able to visit a natural medicine practitioner unless they get a referral from a medical doctor. The chances of this happening are slim, if non-existent. The political agenda of the Cyprus Medical Association is to clearly support their clan so that no one else "eats from their pie," as natural medicine has began to threaten them given that they know that many Cypriots are now turning to natural medicine to treat their chronic diseases that they have so little to offer.

We are currently still in discussions with the CMA and the Ministry as I write this book now – nothing has been finalised or resolved as yet. As the Larnaca Branch President of the Cyprus Natural Medicine Association I intend to protect the benefits of the Cypriot people to choose whatever type of healing modality they wish for themselves and their family, whether it be the medicine model or the holistic medicine model. It is their constitutional and democratic right to do just this and should not be hindered by the self-interests of one group of professionals.

Seeing Repeatable Results

I apologize for the tirade regarding politics but when you are in the midst of it, it touches you deeply. Let's go back to a more positive note! Now that I am maturing as a practitioner of Holistic Medicine, and seeing repeatable results in many facets of health, I am really encouraged to continue and write this book and others like it to get the word out about the holistic approach. I am also optimistic that there will be a paradigm shift in thinking from a model of symptom-suppression using drugs with many side-effects, to one of identifying causes and eliminating these, while gently helping the body to rebuild and repair using natural healing modalities that do the "least harm" – something that Hippocrates said 2,500 years ago and which ironically is still part of the Hippocratic Oath the doctors have to swear to when they complete medical school.

Personally I believe that Hippocrates is, and should remain, the Father of Traditional Medicine and not the Father of Allopathic, modern medicine. I really think that they have chosen the wrong scientist to represent what they practise today as when one reads Hippocrates' work one understands just how natural and gentle his healing approaches and protocols were. His teachings could not have been further from what modern medicine practices today – as we would say in holistic medicine, there is "no resonance."

At the end of this book I have chosen to illustrate 15 "incurable" cases that I have personally seen in clinical practice – I use the word 'incurable' to denote that the medical fraternity refers to these disease processes as "incurable" – but when approached through a different paradigm, that of holistic medicine, they can be cured completely.

There are hundreds of other similar cases that I have seen over the years, but space restrictions do not allow me to illustrate them all in one book. I think that the average reader will get an understanding that these are real people with real health issues, having consulted many medical doctors who failed to cure them. I do not believe that they were not cured because the medical doctors seeing them could not care about their healing – to the contrary, I believe that most medical doctors are honest, conscientious practitioners who care for their patient's welfare and wellbeing. However, based on their medical training that looks at only one aspect of the whole person, mostly the physical and chemical structure only, they will obviously miss all the causative factors that are playing a role on all the other levels of health.

This will become a lot clearer when we begin discussing the premises of "Holistic Medicine" and what they comprise – this is the essence of the next chapter entitled "The Holistic Model of Health."

Chapter 2

The Holistic Model of Health

What is Holistic Medicine

I am certain that everybody reading this book will have come across the term "Holistic Medicine" at some point in time. There is considerable confusion about the meaning of "holistic." If you have ever entered into a discussion about Holistic Medicine you will see that everybody has their own opinion. This is not surprising, since there are no accepted standard definitions for "Holistic Medicine." Most people use the term as a synonym for alternative therapies, basically meaning that they are turning away from any conventional medical options and using alternative treatment exclusively. This is not exactly correct.

Holistic Medicine can be thought of as an approach to how treatment should be applied as opposed to any specific treatment modality itself. Let's consider a working definition that I put together a little while ago:

"Holistic Medicine is a system of health care that combines many modalities and models of healthcare such as naturopathy, nutrition, homeopathy, herbal medicine, energy medicine, psychoemotional modalities of healing as well as spiritual "soul healing" work such as Hellinger's Family Constellations. The goal of these combined therapies is to help the patient or clients achieve optimal physical, mental, emotional, social and spiritual health."

Holistic Medicine needs to look at the whole person and how they interact with their environment and the people around them. It needs diagnostic and therapeutic tools to examine and balance the physical, nutritional, environmental, psychological, emotional, social and spiritual levels of health. It therefore encompasses all modalities of diagnosis and treatment as stated above, including allopathic medicine using drugs and surgery if there are no other safer alternatives.

The ultimate goal of Holistic Medicine is to use all diagnostic and treatment modalities available to optimize the health of the person on all levels of well-being, without doing harm to the person. It is the optimization of all resources to bring about a cure in the person, no matter what school or modality they belong to.

There are a number of diagrams that have tried to explain the multimodal approach of Holistic Medicine – perhaps one of the oldest that was developed in the 1980's by Dr. Dietrich Klinghardt,[1] one of the leading proponents of holistic medicine that has provided many tools for practitioners in this field.

The physical body is at the lowest level and it is the foundation upon which everything else rests. This is the level that most interests medical doctors as well as single-healing modality natural medicine practitioners such as herbal medicine, nutritionists and chiropractors. On the second level is the electromagnetic body – it is the summation of all electric and magnetic events caused by the neuronal activity of the nervous system. This level is generally not examined by medical practitioners as it requires different tools to access this electromagnetic body. Acupuncturists tap into the meridians and chakras that are part of this second level. The third-level body is called the "mental body" and consists of our conscious and subconscious thoughts, attitudes and beliefs. This is where the average psychotherapist will work, but there are also other natural medicine healing modalities such as homeopathy, applied psychoneuro-biology and meditation that can access this level.

On the fourth level, the "Intuitive Body" is the level beyond our level of consciousness – the level of the unconscious, the meditative state and trance state. This is where hypnotherapy, regression therapy and Hellinger's Family Constellation therapy can access this level.

The fifth level, the "Soul" is perhaps the most profound and the one that is least accessed by therapists of all kinds – it is the level where we at one with a Higher Consciousness, a Higher Power, God. Prayer and the Spiritual aspects of religion can access this level.

It is generally believed that the first three levels belong to the personal realm, meaning the individual detached from others. The fourth and fifth levels belong to the transpersonal realm, meaning that these are levels that relate to our relationships with others. The lower levels generally supply

---

1 http://www.klinghardtacademy.com

energy to the higher levels, but the higher levels has an organizing influence on the lower levels.

The premise of Holistic Medicine is to attempt to treat the whole patient on all levels, as opposed to the symptoms. Often a complaint such as migraines may have a myriad of different causes in each patient – so there is no standard therapy for migraines as the causes would be different in each person with migraine. This is why it is important to take into account all the causative factors for each person, and ultimately you will be treating the patient and not the disease per se.

This takes us back to Hippocrates about 2,500 years ago who said:

> **It is more important to know what sort of PERSON has a disease than to know what sort of DISEASE a person has**

It appears that this wise statement made by Hippocrates, the Father of Medicine has been forgotten by modern medicine! Instead of looking at the person and trying to understand WHY they have the bunch of symptoms that make up their diagnosis, we consume ourselves with LABELLING the disease and suppressing its symptoms, when we should clearly be looking for its root causes.

We can extrapolate from this that Holistic Medicine is based on a "health-care system" and not a "disease-care system" – it encompasses Preventative Medicine by attempting to catch developing health issues early on, instead of waiting until they reach pathological parameters. Optimizing health should be the ultimate goal of all Holistic Medicine practitioners.

Often Holistic Medicine is not interested in labelling the disease itself as this does not often give information regarding the causes of the symptoms and signs suffered by the person. Holistic Medicine should first identify the causes of the symptoms, which are the body's way of "talking" to the practitioner, without necessarily being overly concerned with the "diagnosis."

The 5 Levels of Healing – A Guide to Diagnosis and Treatment

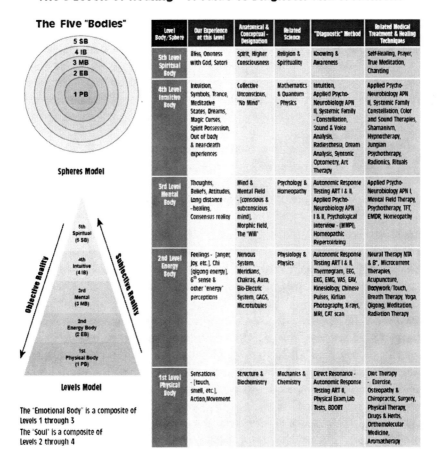

The Five "Bodies"

Spheres Model
(5 SB, 4 IB, 3 MB, 2 EB, 1 PB)

Levels Model
- 5th Spiritual (5 SB)
- 4th Intuitive (4 IB)
- 3rd Mental (3 MB)
- 2nd Energy Body (2 EB)
- 1st Physical Body (1 PB)

Objective Reality / Subjective Reality

Levels Model

The "Emotional Body" is a composite of Levels 1 through 3
The "Soul" is a composite of Levels 2 through 4

Level Body/Sphere	Our Experience at this Level	Anatomical & Conceptual - Designation	Related Science	"Diagnostic" Method	Related Medical Treatment & Healing Techniques
5th Level Spiritual Body	Bliss, Oneness with God, Satori	Spirit, Higher Consciousness	Religion & Spirituality	Knowing & Awareness	Self-Healing, Prayer, True Meditation, Chanting
4th Level Intuitive Body	Intuition, Symbols, Trance, Meditative States, Dreams, Magic Curses, Spirit Possession, Out of body & near-death experiences	Collective Unconscious, "No Mind"	Mathematics & Quantum - Physics	Intuition, Applied Psycho-Neurobiology APN II, Systemic Family - Constellation, Sound & Voice Analysis, Radiesthesia, Dream Analysis, Syntonic Optometry, Art Therapy	Applied Psycho-Neurobiology APN II, Systemic Family Constellation, Color and Sound Therapies, Shamanism, Hypnotherapy, Jungian Psychotherapy, Radionics, Rituals
3rd Level Mental Body	Thoughts, Beliefs, Attitudes, Long distance -healing, Consensus reality	Mind & Mental Field - [conscious & subconscious mind], Morphic Field, The "Will"	Psychology & Homeopathy	Autonomic Response Testing ART I & II, Applied Psycho-Neurobiology APN I & II, Psychological Interview - (MMPI), Homeopathic Repertoirizing	Applied Psycho-Neurobiology APN I, Mental Field Therapy, Psychotherapy, TFT, EMDR, Homeopathy
2nd Level Energy Body	Feelings - [anger, joy, etc.], Chi [qigong energy], 6th sense & other 'energy' perceptions	Nervous System, Meridians, Chakras, Aura, Bio-Electric System, GAGS, Microtubules	Physiology & Physics	Autonomic Response Testing ART I & II, Thermogram, EEG, EKG, EMG, VAS, EAV, Kinesiology, Chinese Pulses, Kirlian Photography, X-rays, MRI, CAT scan	Neural Therapy NTA & B*, Microcurrent Therapies, Acupuncture, Bodywork/Touch, Breath Therapy, Yoga, Qigong, Meditation, Radiation Therapy
1st Level Physical Body	Sensations - [touch, smell, etc.], Action, Movement	Structure & Biochemistry	Mechanics & Chemistry	Direct Resonance - Autonomic Response Testing ART I, Physical Exam, Lab Tests, BDORT	Diet Therapy - Exercise, Osteopathy & Chiropractic, Surgery, Physical Therapy, Drugs & Herbs, Orthomolecular Medicine, Aromatherapy

The 5-levels of healing as postulated by Dr. Klinghardt[2]

This can be clearly illustrated when a person goes to their medical doctor with bowel distension and pain after eating, as well as bouts of intermittent diarrhoea and constipation. The doctor diagnoses Irritable Bowel Syndrome or IBS and usually gives antispasmodic medication to alleviate the symptoms.

A Holistic Medicine practitioner, however, would begin to investigate the causes of these symptoms such as:

---

2 Klinghardt, D. Explore! Volume 14, November 4, 2005

❖ Lack of hydrochloric acid production in the stomach and deficiency in pancreatic enzymes, leading to poor digestion of food with resulting fermentation and bloating.

❖ Food intolerances to wheat, lactose, caffeine and eggs, causing the production of inflammatory chemicals such as cytokinines and COX-2's.

❖ Dehydration - the person only drinks 2-3 glasses of water daily, so is severely dehydrated and his digestive processes suffer as a result.

❖ Eating a lot of junk food which is nutritionally deficient, resulting in a downward spiral of nutritional deficiencies.

❖ The patient is constantly stressed at home due to marital discord, poor communication with his wife and an autistic child.

Once all these causes are rectified, then the IBS disappears forever – the IBS was the result of these causative factors provoking the symptoms and discomfort, and not that the person was lacking in anti-spasmodic medication, or any other medication.

Based on the abovementioned example, it is clear to see that there are no limits to the range of diseases and disorders that can be treated in a holistic way – simply find all the potential causative factors, remove them, then help the body to repair, rebuild and rebalance – but this needs to be done on all levels – physical body, energetic body, etheric body, mind, emotions, and spirit. This is why when an individual seeks holistic treatment for a particular illness or condition, other health problems automatically improve without direct intervention, as the same causative factors could also be responsible for a myriad of other symptoms.

Holistic Health teaches the person to reach and maintain higher levels of wellness, optimizing health as well as preventing illness. People generally enjoy the vitality and well-being that results from their positive lifestyle changes, and this provides the motivation to continue this process throughout their lives.

In Holistic Medicine the healthcare professional and the patient work as partners – this is really the only way of succeeding as healing is not really related to the practitioner's skill but the willingness of the patient to work with the practitioner and implement their bespoke healing programme. Rather than just eliminating or masking symptoms, the symptom is used as a guide to look below the surface for the *root cause*. Whenever possible, treatments are selected that support the body's natural healing system.

The Medical Model of Disease

Recently I have been discussing issues of Holistic Medicine on national TV in Cyprus, where I work and live, in the presence of medical doctors. This has opened up some interesting observations into how allopathic or medical doctors perceive and tackle diseases in their patients. Generally, with few exceptions, allopathic doctors perceive the body as a physical and chemical entity, much like a mechanic would view a machine. Using this "mechanistic" approach, their concern is to examine these structures using a variety of technologies such as X-rays, MRI's, CT scans, gastroscopes, colonoscopes, biochemical lab tests and the like.

These technologies and testing techniques are all measuring the physical and chemical structure of different body parts – the "physical body" which is on the first level of the five levels of healing. They will examine the body organs (their size, shape and whether there are any structural abnormalities) – to the various tissues, down to the cellular level, to determine pathology (disease) of their structure (number of erythrocytes, white blood cells, platelets, histopathological structure of different cells etc) and the biochemical constituents of the blood, plasma and other body fluids.

Allopathic doctors are extremely well trained in looking at the physical and chemical composition of the body, and they spend many years in medical school doing just this. However, this "mechanistic" perception of the body has many limitations as this only allows us to view one perspective of the human body, when in fact there are many different levels that are important in diagnosing and fully understanding the aetiology of disease.

When observing the allopathic profession examining a patient based on this mechanistic approach, it becomes obvious why they sometimes behave in rather irrational ways. Generally, the "Medical Model of Disease" or "Biomedical Model" is based on collating the symptoms, placing them into a diagnostic category with a specific label, and then using some form of drug, surgery or radiation to eliminate the symptoms. The assumption is made that all patients are homogenous. The Biomedical model is a "wait for illness" approach.

This is a "symptom suppression" approach to dealing with disease as it rarely identifies the real causes of disease, let alone removing the causes. The fact that a diagnosis has been placed on a diseased organ does not justify the rationale that the diseased organ is the CAUSE of the diagnosis. Tonsillitis, for example, is not the cause of inflamed tonsils; Irritable Bowel Syndrome (IBS) is not the cause of an irritable bowel, and so forth. The diagnostic labels themselves may be important for the medical doctors themselves, but they do little to help understand the true causes of disease.

The label given to the symptoms of an illness is not the illness itself – it may surprise you to hear that a cancerous tumour is not the disease per se, it is merely a symptom – the disease itself are all the aetiological factors that caused the body to produce the tumour in the first place – there is more on viewing cancer holistically in chapter 11.

If one puts oneself in the position of a medical doctor with this perception, then it is easy to understand why they behave as they do. For example, if there is a part of the gut that is ulcerated and the symptoms cannot be eliminated using medicinal drugs, then the next "logical" step is to remove the organ itself. This may sound rather surprising to the objective onlooker, but personally I have heard from many patients who have been victims of this narrow-minded approach.

Let's Whip Out the Gut!

Late last year I was at the local general hospital seeing a young woman in her 20's who had ulcerative colitis. She was admitted to the hospital as she had slight haemorrhage with diarrhoea, probably related to something that was irritating the gut. During her month's stay in the hospital she had been taking IV cortisone with strong antibiotics (which will destroy all the protective bacteria in the gut and aggravate the inflammation), she had even had chemotherapy (what they give to cancer patients) – God knows what the logic is here – as well as a visit from the psychiatrist, who readily prescribed anti-depressants as he felt that her gut problems were related to her depression (who would not be depressed in these circumstances)?

Recently, her parents were invited to a round-table discussion by the head doctor who, with a solemn expression suggested that the gut should be removed immediately to stop the bleeding and irritation, as nothing else seems to be working!

The doctor added, in a final, desperate attempt, that they may instead decide to give Cyclosporine, a powerful immune-suppressing drug that is given to organ transplant patients to prevent rejection – this literally puts the immune system to sleep. Apart from the chances of catching a nasty bug in hospital which would be near impossible to combat without an immune system - the other side effects of this powerful drug are gum hyperplasia, convulsions, peptic ulcers, pancreatitis, fever, vomiting, diarrhoea, confusion, breathing difficulties, numbness and tingling, pruritis, high blood pressure, potassium retention and possibly hyperkalemia, as well as kidney and liver dysfunction.[3]

I very recently saw another unfortunate tragedy – this time with a 12-year old Swedish girl diagnosed with Crohn's Disease who came to me about one month after the surgeons had removed her complete colon or large intestine and she had a colostomy bag on the side of her abdomen. If you had seen the psychological, emotional and spiritual devastation in this young teenage girl after the surgery it was a sight never to forget.

Yes, I know you are stunned, just as I was – it sounds unbelievable for a relatively simple case that is easy to bring under control simply by altering the diet (by identifying and removing food intolerances and using some healing herbs and homeopathics). There is a case, Mrs. A, in Chapter 12 that was healed of exactly this condition after suffering for 7 years with many symptoms. However, nutrition does not seem to be an issue that is of much concern to gastroenterologists, even though food is the primary material that travels through the entire gut many times per day. The first patient in the hospital was told after querying the food she was eating, that it was a "controlled diet" that had been carefully planned by the hospital dietician – white bread, margarine, marmalade, hamburgers with spices, white macaroni and toxic chicken, as well as various dairy products and sweet foods – obviously the hospital dietician needs to go back to school if she considers this to be a healthy diet!

I made some quick suggestions to her so that she could change her diet immediately – to eat mostly steamed vegetables, vegetable juices and fruit, while taking Omega 3 and 6 fatty acids (which help the body produce natural anti-inflammatory prostaglandins), as well as a mixture of herbs known for their anti-inflammatory effects such as curcumin (tumeric) and boswelia, as well as aloe vera juice. Three days after implementing this simple regime she began feeling a lot better, and there is a lot more that

---

3 www.sideeffects.com

can be done such as identifying and removing her food intolerances, as well as optimizing her diet based on her metabolic type – which will need to wait until she is discharged from the controlled hospital environment and her dietician.

Why the Blinkers?

So, why do all these intelligent doctors who were "A" grade students at school think in this narrow-minded, blinkered and insular way? In order to understand why they are so doctrinaire in their approach to disease, let's take a step back and look at an analogy of man as a whole entity – I will use the analogy of an iceberg to demonstrate the point. When we look at an iceberg we normally see about 10% of the iceberg above the waterline, the remaining 90% is below it.

This is important to note, as most medical doctors are trained to observe only what is above the waterline – the 10% of causative factors that involve the physical and chemical structure of disease. This is the main part of the curriculum in most medical schools as most of the funding for research comes from the pharmaceutical companies who want the budding doctors to prescribe their drugs. They therefore have a big say in what is to be included in the curriculum and nutrition, environmental medicine, energy medicine and the psychoemotional and spiritual aspects of the person make up very little.

If we return to the iceberg analogy, we see that just like the iceberg in its entirety is composed of the 10% above the waterline, PLUS the 90% below the waterline, so is man composed of many different levels, some we can see and measure and some we cannot. However, they all interact to determine whether we are healthy or not – all these levels make up the HOLISTIC MODEL OF HEALTH that this book is all about. The tip of the iceberg where doctors spend most of their time looking is based on the Biomedical Model of Disease as doctors tend to examine the physical body for pathology or disease and are not really trained in looking at the whole health spectrum from perfect health all the way through to pathology. This is why there is very little advice that you will obtain from your average medical doctor about Preventative Medicine.

The tip of the iceberg represents the physical and chemical composition of the body – we have already mentioned that medical doctors are extremely well trained at examining these parts in detail and using this knowledge to diagnose pathology. This knowledge about the physical body, and all the medical technology that has emerged over the last 30-40 years has certainly played an important role in saving many lives, particularly in emergency medicine – this needs to be respected and honoured as it is a big contribution to the health of mankind.

It is when the medical profession have to deal with complex, chronic diseases that have taken years to develop and are multi-causal, that they freely admit defeat – there is really not much that they can do to cure these diseases, they can treat and manage them and provide palliative care only. Why is this?

Its simply that they are only looking at one level of the body, the physical level – they can identify and label most disease known to man, but they will not be able to eradicate those that are related to a multitude of factors on the many different levels of health. For example, many chronic diseases are now related to the accumulating toxicity from heavy metals and xenobiotics that are ubiquitous in today's world. It is rare that you will find a medical doctor looking for these – it is not really a part of their curriculum. It is also rare that the doctor examines the diet of the person and fully understands its implications – the field of clinical nutrition or orthomolecular nutrition is again not part of their curriculum. Nor is helping patients overcome psychoemotional issues that may remain unresolved and be a major cause to the illness.

When the focus of the person is on the tip of the iceberg, ignoring the other 90% below the waterline, then this is akin to having one's nose firmly pressed against a tree, knowing everything about the tree in exacting detail, but missing the real culprit, which is in the forest! You obviously need to move back from the tree in order to see the forest!

Now let's examine the parts of the iceberg below the waterline, the BIG part making up 90% that modern medicine does not regularly look at. It is only in seeing this part too that we can really begin to understand the causative factors of degenerative diseases – once these causative factors are identified then they must be offloaded to facilitate the body's natural healing process. This is a brief overview as we will expand on all these factors and more in Part B of the book.

Nutrition and Health

We all know that nutrition plays an imperative role in health – you have all probably heard the saying "We are what we eat" – well, you had better believe it!

Why do we eat?
We eat to nourish all our cells with vital nutrients such as vitamins, minerals, trace elements, amino acids, fats and phytonutrients.

Therefore, the foods that we choose to eat should be nutrient-dense, rich in nutrients, not ones that are empty and deficient.

How many of us consciously choose foods on this basis? You will find that many people around you eat because they like the taste of food, not because they are thinking about nourishing their cells. The general attitude of most people seems to be let's eat anything as long as it has a nice taste and we like it. It's amazing how many people treat their bodies as if they were 'walking dustbins' with no respect to what the body really requires to function optimally.

Over two thousand years ago Hippocrates[4] wrote about the negative effects that food could have on different people:

"For cheese does not prove equally injurious to all men, for there are some who can take it to satiety, without being hurt by it in the least, but, on the contrary, it is wonderful what strength it imparts to those it agrees with; but there are some who do not bear it well, their constitutions are different, they differ in this respect, that what in their body is incompatible with cheese, is roused and put in commotion by such a thing; and those in whose bodies such a humor happens to prevail in greater quantity and intensity, are likely to suffer the more from it. But if the thing had been pernicious to the whole nature of man, it would have hurt all."

There is an emerging science of orthomolecular nutrition (not dietetics). "Orthomolecular" is a Greek word coined by Professor Linus Pauling,[5]

---

4 Adams, Francis. The Genuine Works of Hippocrates. Baltimore: Williams, 1939.

two times Nobel prize winner, which means "correct molecules" – choosing the correct or necessary molecules that the body requires to function correctly. This is a science that is already helping many people with chronic, degenerative diseases to regain function – most probably because it was the nutritional deficiencies over time that led to the degeneration in the first place, so correcting these reverses the main cause.

If any part of your body is deficient in the numerous nutrients that it requires daily to function, then it is only a matter of time before symptoms appear. The body cannot build enzymes, hormones, blood, muscles, immune responses, let alone detoxify itself without many of the vitamins, minerals, trace elements and more that it requires. It is akin to a builder trying to build a house without bricks, or without cement – the end result would be defective and most likely dangerous.

There is also another emerging science which explores the effects of certain foods on health – it is now well known that certain individuals react adversely to particular foods. This is the embryonic science of Food Intolerance or Allergies[6] – "embryonic" even though it was identified and studied by certain scientists more than 50 years ago (Dr. Von Pirquet, Dr. A. Rowe,[7] Dr. H. Rinkel,[8] Dr. R. Mackarness[9]). Virtually everyone is intolerant to certain food substances – often they do not realise this as they are "masked food allergies" meaning that the symptoms can appear many hours, or even days after eating the suspect food.

These masked food allergies cause the body to produce inflammatory chemicals such as cytokinines and COX-2[10] – which will no doubt create further symptoms and imbalances. There are many recent studies (too numerous to mention here) that have been published in peer-reviewed journals, yet still allopathic doctors and dieticians (who know very little about orthomolecular nutrition and the effects of food on the body), still

---

5 http://osulibrary.oregonstate.edu/specialcollections/coll/pauling/index.html

6 Brostoff, J. and Gamlin, L. Food Allergies and Food Intolerances. Rochester: Inner Traditionals International, p.119, 2000.

7 Rowe, AH. Food Allergy: Its Manifestation, Diagnosis, and Treatment. Philadelphia; Lea & Febiger, 1931.

8 Rinkel, HJ., Lee, CH, Brown, D Jr., Willoughby JW, and Williams JM. The Diagnosis of food allergy. Arch Otolaryng 79:71, 1964.

9 Mackarness, R. Not All in The Mind. London: Pan Books, 1976.

10 Kitts, D., Yuan, Y., Joneja, J., Scott, F., Szilagyi, A., Amiot, J., Zarkadas, M. Adverse reactions to food constituents: allergy, intolerance and autoimmunity. Can J Physiol Pharmacol 75:241-254, 1997.

ignore statements made by the World Health Organization and other organizations, which say that over 80% of all chronic diseases are preventable by changing dietary habits and lifestyle.

Instead, doctors believe that patients with "incurable" symptoms, like the patient that I mentioned above with ulcerative colitis, are neurotic and "imagining" their symptoms. If the patient disagrees and resists drug treatments they will inevitably get a visit from the locum psychiatrist. Medical doctors believe that patients get better because "someone is taking an interest" in their case and "giving them attention" (don't laugh, as a distinguished gastro-enterologist said just this to a patient of mine who appeared on national TV in Cyprus recently, talking about how her Irritable Bowel Syndrome had been cured by "my giving her attention." She aptly responded that her gut "did not need a psychologist" but someone to identify the food intolerances that were inflaming her gut!) This intransigent and obdurate attitude is very frustrating to the patient and their families!

Man and the Environment

Man interacts with the environment daily, and it is getting tougher and tougher to avoid toxins, radioactive fallout, electromagnetic radiation, microwaves from mobile phones, geopathic stress (which I explain below), and much more. All these factors, if we are exposed to them for long enough, can be very detrimental to our health.

I have heard the argument that these factors cannot really play a role in chronic diseases as we are now seeing an increase in childhood cancers, leukaemia's and diabetes, so how can young children be affected by the environment from a very young age?

Well, there are numerous studies that have shown that infants are actually born with an array of toxins, all directly transported from the mother. An interesting study that was done by the Environmental Working Group[11] a few years ago in the USA took neonate cord blood and analyzed it for numerous toxins.

---

[11] Environmental Working Group. A Present for Life: Hazardous Chemicals in Umbilical Cord Blood. Greenpeace International and WWF-UK. Sept 2005.

> **They found an average of 287 toxic chemicals in these newborns, of which 180 of these were carcinogenic!**

A similar study found toxins and heavy metals in newborns in the North Pole born to Inuit Eskimos,[12] so it is clear that we cannot escape these toxins in today's world – this is why we all need to learn how to detoxify and clean our bodies on a regular basis. What would your bedroom look like if you had not cleaned it for 20, 30, 40 or more years? – it would be nothing short of a stable full of rats, mice, cockroaches, parasites, bacteria and viruses – the body is no different!

Other studies have shown that these toxic chemicals can be directly transferred across the placenta from the mother to her baby[13,14] – another reason why detoxification is important before deciding to become pregnant. Large amounts of mercury have also been found in young babies due to the preservative Thimerosal that contains 50% mercury, which is placed in vaccinations – there is a lot of evidence to suggest that this is one of the main reasons why the rate of autism and ADHD has greatly increased.

We also need to be aware of the effect of various energies such as microwave ovens, mobile phones, electromagnetic and geopathic stress on the body. If a pregnant mother were sleeping on a geopathic stress line then inevitably the baby would be affected, as well as herself – there have been many experiments to show that if a person is sleeping on two crossing geopathic stress lines then they will inevitably develop cancer in a matter of a few years. These stress lines upset the natural electromagnetic waves of the body, causing a variety of diseases.

---

[12] Bjerregaard, P., Hansen, JC. Organochlorines and heavy metals in pregnant women from the Disko Bay area in Greenland. *The Science of the Total Environment* 245, 2000.

[13] Houlihan, J., Kropp, T., Wiles, R., Gray, S., Campbell, C. BodyBurden: The Pollution in Newborns. *Environmental Working Group.* July 14, 2005.

[14] Iyengar, GV., Rapp, Human placenta as a 'dual' biomarker for monitoring fetal and maternal environment with special reference to potentially toxic trace elements. Part 3: Toxic trace elements in placenta and placenta as a biomarker for these elements *The Science of the Total Environment*, March 2001.

Energetic Man

Man is also made up of electromagnetic waves and other particles that all resonate at set frequencies. Even as far back as 1923, Georges Lakhovsky, a Russian engineer working in France, built a simple apparatus[15] capable of registering microvoltage measurements from human cells, plants and microbes. In his studies of normal and diseased cells, Lakhovsky found that there were marked differences in their oscillation patterns.[16]

Each group of cells emitted frequencies specific to its organ or tissue of origin. Cancerous cells emitted a different, abnormal pattern.[17] Lakhovsky also discovered that harmful factors such as faulty nutrition, environmental pollutants containing toxic chemicals or heavy metals, bacteria or viruses, weaken and distort cellular electro-magnetic fields prior to the onset of illness and death. After years of research he concluded that health is nothing but a state of electro-magnetic equilibrium of body cells, while diseases and death represent just the opposite – a broken energetic balance.

Around the same time, Professor Harold Saxton Burr[18] of Yale Medical School confirmed Lakhovsky's findings in his own series of experiments – he called these electro-magnetic fields emitted by different body tissues "L-fields," with "L" representing Life. Regrettably, this line of research was never continued after the death of Burr and others. Modern medicine, dominated and essentially controlled by the pharmaceutical industry, offered no inducements to spur research into Energy Medicine. Even today there is no profit to be made from Energy Medicine, hence there is no particular interest to "Big Pharma."

Professor Robert Becker, MD,[19] a pioneer of Electromedicine in the U.S. and Chief of Orthopaedic Surgery at the VA Hospital of SUNY in Syracuse, was able to induce tissue and bone healing in many hopeless cases by applying small currents through the tissues' electrical pathways.[20] Mainstream medicine, he said, was based upon a scientifically outdated model that relied exclusively on the chemical-pharmaceutical approach, to

---

[15] Lakhovsky, G. Neoplastic Formation and Cellular Oscillatory Imbalance. Treatment of Cancer by the Multiple-Wavelength Oscillator. USA: Gaston Doin and Co, 1932.
[16] Lakhovsky, G. The Waves Which Cure. Gauthier-Villars and Co, 1929.
[17] Lakhovsky, G. Contribution to the Etiology of Cancer. Gauthier-Villars and Co, 1927.
[18] Burr, H.S. Bluprint for Immortality, Neville Spearman Publishers, 1972.
[19] Becker, RO, Selden, G. The Body Electric. New York, Morrow, 1985.
[20] Becker, RO et al., Clinical Exp. With Low Intensity Direct Current Stimulation of Bone Growth, *Clin. Orthop. & Rel. Res*, vol. 124, pp. 75-83, 1977.

the exclusion of the more fundamental dimension of body energetics. As a result, he concluded that the tremendous healing potential of energy-based modalities such as homeopathy, acupuncture, visualization and electromedicine were neglected, to the great detriment of mankind.

In 1994, two biophysicists from the Max-Plank Institute of Physics in Gottingen, Germany, Drs. Erwin Neher and Bert Sackmann,[21] were awarded a Nobel Prize for their discovery of the essential role that the flow of charged atoms (the ions of body fluids and tissues) plays in physiological processes in living cells. Professor Fritz-Albert Popp[22] and Professor Herbert Frohlich[23] established that cells in the body interact through coherent oscillations: they have demonstrated that electromagnetic communication between cells constitutes the primary process governing chemical reactions.

This vast body of scientific evidence makes it apparent that the physiology of all living systems is being controlled via computer-like electromagnetic communications. Homeopathy is indeed unique among all therapies in its ability to influence cellular memory.

So why does the medical profession not know this? Simply because it is not taught in the medical schools they attend, as the curriculum is controlled by the pharmaceutical industries – who are interested in discovering and patenting medicinal drugs for huge profits. The truth is that there is no profit to be made in homeopathics – which they cannot patent – as you cannot patent something that is natural, so they are not interested. It is a sad fact of the greed that prevails in the health industry: "Let's keep looking at the body as a physical and chemical factory because we can keep giving drugs to change the chemistry, as this is where the profits are!"

The Psycho-Emotional Person

We all know that chronic stress can cause heart disease, including hypertension and strokes; a compromised immune system which can lead

21 Betz, WJ & Sakmann, B. Effects of proteolytic enzymes on synaptic structure and function. *J. Physiol.* 230: 673–688, 1973.
22 Popp, FA and an, Y. Delayed luminescence of biological systems in terms of coherent states, Physics Letters 293:93-97, 2002.
23 Fröhlich, H. and Kremer, F. Coherent Excitations in Biological Systems, Springer-Verlag, 1983.

to infections, allergies or even cancer; and gastrointestinal conditions such as ulcers and irritable bowel syndrome. In fact many of the "sudden deaths" that we hear about even in young people, are probably caused mainly by either acute shock or chronic stress.

There is a new branch of medicine called psychoneuroimmunology (PNI), which looks at the connection between the mind and stress, and diseases of the body, with many research studies that have demonstrated the clear relationship between stress and disease.

Perhaps one of the most interesting researchers in this field that has published much is Dr. Ryke Hamer, M.D.[24] After twenty years of research and therapy with over 31,000 patients, Dr. Hamer finally established firmly, logically and empirically how biological conflict-shock results in a cold cancerous or necrotic phase and how, if the conflict is resolved, the cancerous or necrotic process is reversed to repair the damage and return the individual to health.

Twenty years ago, Dr. Ryke Geerd Hamer, a German doctor with his own practice in Rome, Italy, received a call in the middle of the night. His 17-year old son Dirk had been shot while on holiday in the Mediterranean. Three months later, Dirk died and shortly after, Dr. Hamer, who had been healthy all his life, but who was utterly devastated by this catastrophe, found he had testicular cancer. Rather suspicious about this coincidence, he set about doing research on the personal histories of cancer patients to see whether they had suffered some shock, distress or trauma before their illness.

In time, after extensive research of thousands of patients, Dr. Hamer was finally able to conclude that disease is only brought about by a shock for which we are totally unprepared. This last point is very important. If we can in any way be prepared for the shocking event, we will not become ill. In fact, Dr. Hamer does not like to say 'cancer'. Rather, it is a special biological response to an unusual situation, and when the 'shock' situation is resolved, the body sets about returning to normality. This is a very simplified account, of course. The books explain in detail the complete process.

---

24 Hamer, RG. Summary of the New Medicine. Avici di Dirk Publishers, Germany, 2000.

He presented his work to the university in Germany with which he was affiliated. Without testing or proving his hypothesis, they asked him to deny his findings. Since he could not possibly contemplate denying what he had scientifically proven beyond a shadow of a doubt, he refused. As a result, his licence to practise medicine was withdrawn and the situation remains unchanged to this day. Even though the University of Tubingen was ordered by a court of law to hold tests to prove the theories, they have never done so.

Holistic Medicine – The Whole Iceberg

This completes the analogy of the iceberg – it should be clear that modern medicine practitioners who have their perception fixed on the tip of the iceberg, are not going to be able to identify and eliminate ALL the causative factors of chronic diseases. Instead, they will identify ONLY the structural and biochemical pathologies in the body and try to alleviate the symptoms using drugs, surgery or radiation.

This is one of the main reasons why modern medicine has such abysmal results in treating chronic diseases such as hypertension, diabetes, arthritis, cancer and asthma – diseases that normally have multiple causative factors. They never even look for poor nutrition which leads to gross deficiencies in nutrients, poor digestion and absorption; high levels of toxic metals and organic xenobiotics such as organochlorine pesticides, PCB's from plastics, Bisphenol-A, lead, mercury, arsenic, cadmium, as well as electromagnetic and geopathic stresses, not to mention psychological and emotional stresses from family, society and work.

If you were a patient with a chronic disease, would you not want to know what the causes of your disease processes were? Certainly you would, but often we hear from medical doctors that the cause is "idiopathic" – another word for "unknown!" We also hear "psychosomatic" a lot, meaning that the causes are psychological and emotional. This is not a deep analysis of this particular aetiological category, but a "dustbin" of modern medicine where all the "unknowns" are dumped – this would include all the patients who do not get better with drugs or surgery, mainly because the true causes of their problems have not been properly diagnosed.

Modern medicine rarely asks the patient what they eat or drink, let alone look at food intolerances and allergies. I was shocked to see a 33 year old man who was referred to me by his mother – he had a heart attack two months previously, with a serious diagnosis of "deep vein thrombosis" hanging over his head; with gross oedema (swelling) of the leg. He was being treated by the medical profession with Warfarin, a blood- thinning drug, for the last month, but generally was not getting better. What I found shocking was that no medical doctor, of the numerous that he had seen, had asked him about his lifestyle habits. He was smoking 2 packs of cigarettes per day, drinking large quantities of alcohol daily, eating lots of junk food and drinking only 2-3 glasses of water daily!

Within 4 days of drinking more water, cutting out the junk food, stopping smoking and drinking and beginning a detoxification diet of fruit and vegetables, his swelling had greatly reduced and he was feeling so much better. This man could easily have died of his deep vein thrombosis: a very dangerous condition.

It's important to work in a holistic fashion with these chronic patients – the therapist must begin working through the levels of the potential causative factors – this is what we do at the DaVinci Natural Health Centre in Larnaca, often identifying more than 15-20 possible causative factors. When these are eliminated we see all sorts of degenerative diseases cured in amazingly short periods of time.

This book will take you through most of the potential causative factors of the majority of chronic diseases in the world today. These factors are really not very difficult to identify and eliminate. If one works within a holistic medicine framework with most chronic health problems – the success rate is high in most cases – some of which are illustrated in this book.

The next chapter will look at what the specific causative factors are and how they can be resolved.

Chapter 3

Finding the Causes of your Disease

Introduction

At the heart of medicine lies the individual and their own unique story - that story typically includes the chief complaint, the history of any present illness, the past medical history, family history, dietary history, supplement and medication history, lifestyle, social, and exercise history, physical exam findings and laboratory evaluation.

In conventional medicine, the aim is to arrive quickly at the diagnosis - this is particularly critical in the acute care setting where rapid diagnosis leads to rapid treatment. Treatment in this setting must be prompt, as it is often designed to "lock down" and control physiology. The chief complaint and history of the present illness become the critical aspects of the story; the rest of the patient's story is truncated when other information is seen as superfluous to reaching the diagnosis.

In acute care, the patient's history is condensed to the main complaint and the history of the present illness, while the most important criteria is finding the correct diagnosis. Let's take an example of a patient who suffers from wheezing attacks – the history of the present illness may indicate a previous history of asthma with tightness in the chest and shortness of breath. The diagnosis now becomes "asthma attack" and the treatment will be with corticosteroids and bronchodilators.

These typical medical models are fine with acute disease, but when the same model is applied to chronic disease problems arise. When the physician wants to proceed directly to the diagnosis and name the disease quickly, they are missing a lot of other pertinent information as the patient's whole story is not understood and each complaint becomes a discrete issue that is treated in isolation to the complete picture.

The result is a focus on treating each symptom complex as a separate and distinct "disease" with a separate treatment for each; so depression is treated with antidepressants, hypertension with antihypertensive drugs, high cholesterol with Statin drugs, gastroeosophogeal reflux disease (GERD) with hydrogen-proton inhibitor drugs that block hydrochloric acid production and so on. Each of these symptoms becomes a distinct diagnostic entity in itself and the patient ends up being treated with a cocktail of drugs based on each of these individual symptoms or syndromes.

The patient's individual story never has a chance to be heard and understood in context. It is apparent that in the rush to diagnose and treat, modern medicine concentrates on the branches and leaves of the tree and not the trunk and the roots. Holistic or functional medicine should not be viewed as an alternative but as a bridge to a more effective CHRONIC CARE model.

In the Holistic or Functional health model, the patient's full story is of central importance. Questions that are asked and need answers include: where does the symptom come from? That is, what are the antecedents and triggers? What maintains the symptoms? That is, what are the mediators? And what can be done to change that dis-eased homeostatic balance point the patient is locked into? That is, what are the underlying points of leverage where intervention can be most effective?

In order to answer these important questions, it is not enough to just look at the present symptoms and history of the present illness. It is important to investigate further and take the entire patient's history in order to understand the sources or causes of these symptoms.

Can the symptoms be due to tooth and scar foci, toxic metals, mineral and vitamin deficiencies, fatty acid deficiencies, hormone and enzyme deficiencies, hypochlorhydria or hydrochloric acid deficiency, with pancreatic enzyme deficiencies, internal biochemistry based on the pH, resistivity and redox potential of urine, saliva and blood, Indican's test of gut toxicity, food intolerances, Metabolic Typing to determine the 'octane' of fuel or food that our particular constitution requires, environmental allergens, immune status, parasites, viruses, bacteria, fungi, moulds, candida, electromagnetic and geopathic stress, tissue integrity, hereditary weaknesses, organ functioning, psychoemotional and spiritual states, as well as systemic entanglements that go back many generations and can cause a myriad of health issues.

These fundamental clinical imbalances are the key to the underlying mechanisms of disease – the diagnosis remains useful but is less important. This expanded model allows the clinician to choose from a wider array of therapies such as minerals and supplements, herbs, homeopathics, exercise, counselling, diet, manipulative therapies, acupuncture and more.

Let's apply this model to a simple case of chronic headaches – the medical model would generally place a diagnosis based on the present history – migraines – and treat using Triptan or a similar drug. However, this case may not be as simple as it seems.

The headaches could be a result of structural integrity problems – a subluxation of the cervical spine or whiplash after an accident, or exposure to toxins such as mercury from amalgams or aspartame taken as a sweetener, digestive issues such as hypochlorhydria and pancreatic insufficiency leading to food putrefaction in the gut, mineral and vitamin deficiencies, dehydration, hypoglycaemia, drug side effects, chronic antibiotic use leading to dysbiosis and systemic Candidiasis, lack of exercise, spiritual and psychoemotional reasons such as loneliness, overwork, marital discord, sexual identity issues and many more causative factors.

You can see how easy it is for the medical model to miss most of these potential causative factors – the result using drugs will not be a complete cure but simply treatment of the symptoms by simply suppressing them. You can see how the Holistic model encompasses the full and unique story of the patient. It integrates underlying mechanisms of disease into the differential diagnosis paradigm as well as increasing the range of potential treatment options.

This Holistic or Functional Model is the only way I know of getting to the bottom of chronic diseases and helping the body to heal - the beauty of this intensive approach is that even international patients can come in for the full assessment, collate all the information, design a bespoke treatment programme, all in a few days. Then they can return to their homeland and implement the treatment while staying in touch by e-mail and phone. It has been working successfully this way for many years now.

The IDEL Diagnostic Programme

Over the years I have devised the IDEL Diagnostic Programme1 for doing all this and more – IDEL is the acronym that stands for 'IDentify' and 'ELiminate.' Without removing the root causes it is literally impossible to cure chronic diseases – the best that one can hope for is a temporary alleviation of symptoms using drugs or natural remedies. To be absolutely honest, this simple enlightenment took me about 20 years to put together, as it requires a large database of knowledge and clinical experience to collect and make sense of this data.

This testing method may sound rather extravagant and long-winded but it is really the only way that I know of collecting enough information about the patient to determine the causative factors of their disease. I am often faced with patients who come in with thick files after having seen five, six or more health practitioners who have all run their own tests and determined a treatment plan. The problem with this approach is that the naturopath will look at their patients only from the naturopathic perspective; the homoeopath will examine the patient only from the homoeopathic perspective and treat accordingly; the herbal medicine practitioner will also do the same according to their level of training in that one modality. Sometimes you may get lucky and find practitioners with two modalities who obviously have a wider vision. It is indeed rare, however, to find practitioners who understand and offer a wide range of the various healing modalities in a coherent and synergistic way.

The DaVinci Natural Health Center aims to cover this gap. The IDEL diagnostic program is perhaps a unique composite of methodology where many levels of health are assessed using different diagnostic and therapeutic modalities concomitantly, to get to the bottom of someone's health problems quickly and efficiently.

Using the IDEL diagnostic programme, misdiagnosis and treatment failure is reduced to the minimum as it takes the guesswork out of the 'diagnosis.' I place the word diagnosis in inverted commas as I am not merely looking to label the disease, but am more concerned with identifying the causative factors. Having a label for a disease does not magically render it curable. Look again at most of the 'incurable' chronic diseases mentioned in this book' testimonials section (Chapter 12) – heart disease, diabetes, cancer,

---

1 www.docgeorge.com/IDEL-Diagnostic-Programme.html

arthroses, neurological disorders, etc. Why these are considered invincible by the medical profession?

The main reason for their failure to cure such patients is that they have not really examined the myriad of reasons that have caused the health problem in the first place – in chronic degenerative diseases this is rarely one cause but many causes that have been accumulative over the years and are responsible for the 'pathogenesis'[2] of the disease. Instead, they have spent time using expensive biochemical tests and looking at the structure of the body parts using sophisticated scans, only to place a label on the disease (the diagnosis) which usually leads to giving drugs to suppress the symptoms without even looking at the causes.

It is no wonder that most of these chronic, degenerative diseases are considered 'idiopathic' - meaning there is "no known cause." Also, "psychosomatic" is another category that chronic diseases are thrown into, as well as 'hereditary' – in other words: blame the genes, which could occur rarely, but it is not always the case. All this is misguided conjecture and has no relevance to the true causes of chronic diseases. Maybe you should challenge your medical practitioner next time they mention any one of these potential causes and ask them to prove their hypothesis as Medicine is supposed to be evidence-based. I bet that in most cases they will be dumb-founded that a patient has had the nerve to challenge such a "medical diagnosis!"

So coming back to the IDEL Diagnostic Programme - the real beauty of the programme is that it guides the practitioner and the patient to the potential causative factors underlying the disease, and to finding a way of safely eliminating them, while concomitantly helping the person to repair and rebuild their body. I use the word 'safely' as I use no drugs, dangerous diagnostics, or surgeries. The tools I use are the diverse protocols based on the varying facets of Natural Medicine. These will become clearer as we examine the results and look at the treatments offered.

Here is a summary of the potential causative factors that are commonly picked up by the IDEL Diagnostic Programme – these issues are rarely addressed by the medics even though they can all be extremely detrimental to health.

---

2 This is a Greek word meaning the birth of the disease.

Potential causative factors

These causative factors include poor diet, nutritional deficiencies, bacteria, viruses, fungi, moulds, parasites, Candida, enzyme and hormone deficiencies, hypochlorhydria (low hydrochloric acid production in the stomach), food intolerances and other allergens, hidden inflammatory processes in the body, toxaemia, toxic metals and other xenobiotics, electromagnetic and geopathic stress, mobile phone stress, X-ray stress, vaccination stress, unhealed scars and teeth infections (foci), imbalanced pH, redox potential and resistivity and many more. We carefully examine and identify all of these factors and others using functional testing methods and complex equipment.

Regardless, it is certainly worth anyone's while to look in greater depth at the IDEL Diagnostic Program. The following is an overview as to its various components and how it works in practice.

Complete health history

It is inconceivable to undergo any medical treatment without the practitioner recording a patient's personal and family health history, that is, the background to symptoms, past medications and treatments, biochemical tests and reports of various scans – including dental X-rays. The practitioner should also have other related information such as the patient's stress, exercise, nutrition, and occupational profiles.

Personally, as I am not a medical practitioner, I do not undergo the normal scans that medical doctors ask for, nor the majority of blood tests, even though I have been trained to interpret them. I don't really need to do these tests as the patient usually brings a huge file full of scans, blood and urine results as well as other more esoteric tests. I carefully scrutinize these and look for pathology and other clues to add to the puzzle of the pathogenesis of the disease. These clues I will then add to the myriad of data that I collect from many of the functional tests that I conduct, as we will see in more detail below.

When I mention functional tests I mean tests that are really looking at the function of the body as opposed to its structure – when a doctor scans the liver, for example using ultrasound, he is looking at the structure of it – which may be quite normal, but this really does not tell us much about its function. Certain urine and saliva tests, including blood tests, as well as thermography, for example, will give me a much better idea of the functioning of the liver which is more important information than merely looking at the structure. Even iridology and thermology will give me information on the function of organs but not about their structure. Both are important to know, but the functioning of the body is far more important.

Iridology

In the Orient, the eyes are often described as being 'The window to the soul.' 'The eyes never lie' is also a common adage. So it is with iridology. Here, a special microscope is used to study the iris of each eye. The two are then compared and analysed against specific topographical maps, in terms of morphology, colours, shapes, and so on. Iridology can also help the practitioner identify the body's genetic strengths and weaknesses, and the levels of inflammation and toxaemia in the organs and tissues; as well as the efficiency of the eliminative systems and organs. In this way, the practitioner is able to determine several problems in a patient's constitution in addition to any developing health issues.

Iridology is what many have called the combination of "science and art" of microscopic analysis of the iris and the dynamics of the pupil. Many consider iridology a "fringe" practice, but it has enormous potential when practiced correctly. The iris and inner papillary border[3] are the visible aspects of the autonomic and central nervous systems that we have.

In Iridology structural markings in the iris and eye colours (pigments) carry both personal and genetic significance. The colour of the iris illustrates certain genetic and constitutional traits. Some signs are important for what they look like, some markers are important for where they are – the iris can be a projection of a map of the body and its various systems, as in Reflexology or Auricolotherapy.

The beauty of Iridology is that it provides us with analytical or diagnostic clarity on many levels. It helps the practitioner to pinpoint the foundation or cause to a problem or identify the contributing pathways to a particular symptom or collection of symptoms. For example, migraines can be triggered via many different causes, such as erratic blood sugar levels,[4] low progesterone levels, liver congestion, chronic sinusitis, certain food

---

3 Andrews, J. Iris & Pupillary Signs, 3rd Edition, 2008
4 Andrews, J. Endocrinology & Iridology, 2006

allergies initiated via the intestinal immune system[5] or even neuromuscular tension connected to the cervical vertebrae – this could prove to be an overwhelming list of symptoms for the patient and the practitioner! Yet a professionally trained iridologist will be able to differentiate between all these causes and focus on the root cause of the problem, through microscopic analysis of the iris, pupil and inner pupillary border as well as the sclera.[6]

I find iridology very fascinating and rewarding as it gives a lot of information at the blink of an eye (literally!) – it's always interesting when I see a spinal subluxation[7] in the iris and ask the patient whether they have neck or lower back discomfort – they are always amazed at how I can determine this from just looking into their eyes!

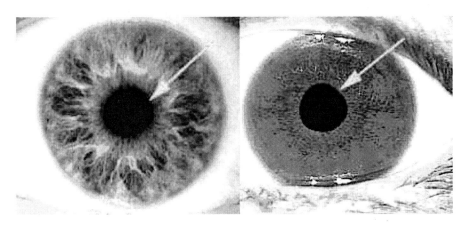

Pupiltonia – flattening of the pupil edge showing spinal subluxations

The iris in the picture above shows such a subluxation – if you look carefully around the pupil area where the green arrow is pointing, you will see that there is a flattening at the 2 o'clock position – this is an indication of a cervical or neck subluxation in the C2-3 region.

I can also tell if a person has a predisposition to high cholesterol levels – you don't really have to be a rocket scientist to determine that one as you can see in the picture below, a large white circle surrounding the iris which is often referred to by iridologists as a 'cholesterol ring.'

---

5 Andrews, J. Immunology & Iridology. 2003.
6 Sclerology is the science of identifying markings on the sclera (white part) of the eye
7 For more details on this condition please see the following section

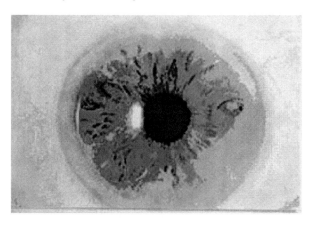

Cholesterol ring

When I was last in Lebanon, hiring a car for the day, the manager came up to greet me and I took one look at his eyes, and there was this characteristic cholesterol ring glaring at me. I smiled and asked him how high his cholesterol levels had been at his last blood test – he curiously looked at me and blurted – 'How do you know that I suffer from high cholesterol levels?' I continued to explain how and by the time I returned the car he had also examined several members of his family and indeed confirmed that many other members also had a similar marking – he actually upgraded the car for me at no extra charge as he was so amazed at what the iris can reveal.

Iridology is so quick and easy that it is disappointing why more practitioners do not use it in their clinical practice. Agreed, to become a master at it takes many years of practice and study, but certainly within a year or so the average practitioner who applies themselves would be able to spot at least 20-25 different health issues within 5 minutes of examining a person's iris. It's really the only medical test that can actually determine constitutional weaknesses and strengths as well as predict how strong or fragile a person really is. The iris below, which is known as a daisy iris with various largish lacunas or holes scattered about, indicates that the integrity of the connective tissues of this person are weak. Such people are likely to be fragile, and will not be able to push themselves too far without getting ill.

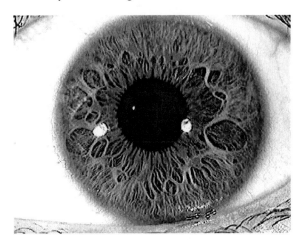

Weak connective tissue constitution

My intention here is not to teach you iridology but to help you see just what wonderful visual medicine iridology really is. Medical doctors that usually pooh-pooh iridology are doing so from a position of ignorance as they probably have not even opened one single text book about iridology – and this is really a shame given that the Father of Iridology was a medical doctor – his name was Dr. Ignatz von Peczely. Subsequently there have been many medical doctors practicing this art and science mainly in Germany, Russia and Asia as well as other parts of the world.

There is presently a lot of scientific research[8] being conducted on iridology around the world, here are some examples:

Intestinal tumours – embryological topography research examining the possibility of a more reliable method of screening for identification of various types of intestinal carcinoma. This research is a combined effort between John Andrews and Dr. Lo Rito in Italy and associated international colleagues.

Pituitary – ongoing research looking at the iris, embryology and IPB (inner pupillary border – posterior epithelial cells) signs in relation to pituitary and hypothalamic outpatients from endocrinology departments in UK hospitals.

---

8 Advanced Iridology Research Journal

IPB signs – documentation and correlation on 'new phenomena' located on the inner pupillary border and only recently observed due to advancements in technology through Iris Supplies of Australia.

Longitudinal Iris Development Study – twenty-five years duration mapping the development of the iris, pupil and IPB from birth through to the age 25 to categorize the stages of development exerting change on the iris and identifying, if possible, what has influenced this? This project could be instrumental in helping to demystify many of the points of controversy maintained in iridology in the English speaking world. The dubious points that leave Iridology open to denigration and ridicule.

Structural Problems – Spine and Feet

The spinal column extends from the skull to the pelvis and is made up of 33 individual bones called vertebrae. Running along the centre of the spine is the spinal cord, which is made up of billions of neural cells. Between each vertebra are spinal nerves connected with all internal organs, glands, muscles, and other tissues of our body. There is a direct relationship between the health and alignment of our spine, the health of our nervous system and of all our tissues and organs.

I am often picking up spinal subluxations from the iridology exam – subluxations are when vertebrae in the spine have moved out of place and are impinging on spinal nerves, that adversely affect the neural impulses running down them to feed the organ systems. I give the analogy of the electricity company delivering 150 volts to your house instead of 220 volts because of a pinched main feed – inevitably certain electrical equipment will begin malfunctioning and this is the case with organ systems of the body – in fact they can atrophy (shrivel) and malfunction over time.

This is why I work closely with an osteopath, who has also been trained in muscle testing – this way he can draw correlations between the nerve impingement and dysfunctions, and symptoms in other parts of the body. Chiropractors also can adjust spinal subluxations, but I have never met one in Cyprus who uses muscle testing too.

Some time ago, I was forever seeing a local chiropractor for spinal adjustments – this puzzled me as a short time after he would adjust my spine I was back again for another adjustment – 5-6 visits per year was quite common in my case, but I was also seeing the same phenomenon in many other patients whom I was also referring. I began searching for an answer as to why the spine was being misaligned continuously, even after a professional adjustment.

This led me to Professor Rothbart's work. The spine was being misaligned by a problem in the foot that is called 'Primus Metatarsus Supinatus' (PMS) or 'Rothbart's foot'[9] after Prof. Rothbart, who discovered it. It's a long story, but simply put if you are born with a defect of the feet, as many people are, which causes hyperpronation[10] (a leaning of the body), then this will affect the spine and one's posture. This will result in many of the symptoms that you go to a chiropractor for – low back pain, knee pain, neck pain, muscle pains and an increased propensity for musculoskeletal injuries. You can read the full story and therapy in Prof. Rothbart's newly-released book entitled: Forever Free From Chronic Pain: The Pain Sufferer's Guide to Getting Your Life Back, available on amazon.com – I had the honour of writing the forward for this book.

---

9 Rothbart BA, Liley P, Hansen, el al. Resolving Chronic Low Back Pain. The Foot Connection. The Pain Practitioner (formerly American Journal of Pain Management) 5(3): 84-89, 1995.
Rothbart BA. Medial Column Foot Systems: An Innovative Tool for Improving Posture. Journal of Bodywork and Movement Therapies (6)1:37-46, 2002.
Rothbart BA, Yerratt M. An Innovative Mechanical Approach to Treating Chronic Knee Pain: A BioImplosion Model. The Pain Practitioner (formerly American Journal of Pain Management) 4(3): 13-18, 1994.
Rothbart BA Proprioceptive Insoles. From a Podiatric Point of View. Health and Healing Wisdom. Price-Pottinger Nutrition Foundation Journal, Vol 29(3):11, 2005.
10 Rothbart BA. Medial Column Foot Systems: An Innovative Tool for Improving Posture. Journal of Bodywork and Movement Therapies (6)1:37-46, 2002.
Rothbart BA, Liley P, Hansen, el al. Resolving Chronic Low Back Pain. The Foot Connection. The Pain Practitioner (formerly American Journal of Pain Management) 5(3): 84-89, 1995.

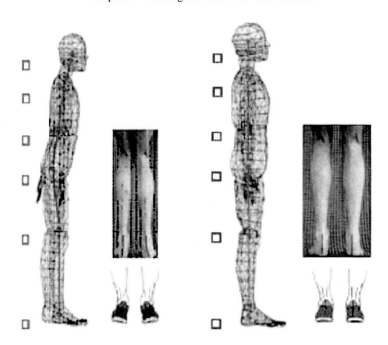

Hyperpronation (left) and after adjustment (right)

Headaches, plantar fasciitis, shin splints, blisters and calluses are all common problems of hyperpronation: a condition in which as we age and become more sedentary, our muscles become weaker and it becomes harder to maintain the body as upright as possible. Over time the body moves toward a collapsing posture – bio-implosion:[11] a forward leaning posture: head forward of the spine, rounded shoulders, forward-rotated pelvis, knees travelling inward, collapsing ankles and an unstable gait. All of these changes are visible. Some are less pronounced than others, but to the experienced observer it is obvious.

Prof. Rothbart was able to adjust the problem by designing and patenting proprioreceptor insoles,[12] which are easy to fit into the patient's shoes. These will rectify the hyperpronation, the body posture will return to

11 Rothbart BA, Yerratt M. An Innovative Mechanical Approach to Treating Chronic Knee Pain: A BioImplosion Model. *The Pain Practitioner* (formerly *American Journal of Pain Management*) 4(3): 13-18, 1994.
12 Rothbart BA Proprioceptive Insoles. From a Podiatric Point of View. Health and Healing Wisdom. *Price-Pottinger Nutrition Foundation Journal*, Vol 29(3):11, 2005.

normal and the symptoms related to the bad body posture will basically disappear[13].

At the DaVinci Natural Health Centre we can examine the patient for Rothbart's Foot and find the solution to these chronic problems by fitting Posture Control Insoles (PCI). We have worked with athletes, achieving amazing success regarding their performance and efficiency, as well as helping alleviate many other chronically painful conditions.

Vega Testing and Autonomic Response Testing (ART)

I have always said to my friends that if I were ever stranded on a remote island somewhere in the Pacific and had to work as a therapist, the only piece of equipment I would take with me would be my VEGA machine and the testing ampoules. The VEGA machine is a bio resonance testing device that has its roots in the work of Dr Reinhold Voll, MD, who ingeniously merged and transformed traditional Chinese acupuncture into a modern form of electromedicine called EAV (Volls' so-called ElectroAcupuncture).

In the early 1950s, Reinhold Voll,[14] a German medical doctor, developed an electronic testing device for finding acupuncture points electrically. He was successful in finding acupuncture points and demonstrating that these points, known to Chinese acupuncturists for millennia, had a different resistance to a tiny electrical current passed through the body, than did the adjacent tissues.[15] Many other researchers have also verified that electrical conductance at the acupuncture points is significantly greater than the surrounding tissue.

Voll then began a lifelong search to identify correlations between disease states and changes in the electrical resistance of the various acupuncture points. He thought that if he could identify electrical changes in certain acupuncture points associated with certain diseases, then he might be able to identify those diseases more easily, or earlier, when treatment intervention was likely to be more effective. Voll was successful in identifying many acupuncture points related to specific conditions and

---

13 For information see www.rothbart.org.
14 Voll, R. 1980. The phenomenon of medicine testing in electro-acupuncture according to Voll. American Journal of Acupuncture 8:97-104.
15 Voll R.: Topographic Positions of the Measurement Points in Electroacupuncture. (Illustrated Vol. I). Med. Liter. Verlagsgesellschaft, Uelzen, 1977.

published a great deal of information about using acupuncture points diagnostically.[16] He found, for example, that patients with lung cancer had abnormal readings on the acupuncture points referred to as lung points. Changes also occurred in the electrical conductance of the acupuncture points supplying musculoskeletal structures that are inflamed.

Voll discovered that certain acupuncture points showed abnormal readings when subjects were reacting allergically.[17] He made several serendipitous discoveries related to "allergy" testing. He noted some unusual readings on certain acupuncture points when a patient had a bottle of medicine in his pocket. He could remove the bottle and consistently get different readings when the bottle was in his pocket compared to when it was not. At first he was baffled as to how a closed bottle of medicine outside the body could affect the acupuncture readings. It was even more baffling when he discovered that the glass bottle of medicine could change the readings when it was in contact anywhere along the closed electric circuit involved with the testing procedure.[18]

Personally, I have spent more than 15 years working with the VEGA[19] machine and I can say that I truly resonate with it. The analogy that I give to illustrate this is that the VEGA is akin to a musical instrument. We often see a maestro playing a guitar so beautifully that we are in awe - how beautiful those notes seem to flow and with what ease the maestro plays. Of course, if we take the same instrument that the maestro is playing in our own hands, without devoting a lot of time and arduous effort in really learning to play it, then our attempts to perform like the maestro will be in vain.

This is really what happens with the VEGA machine – in the wrong hands it can make more wrong predictions than pure guesswork – in the maestro's hands it can be as accurate as any medical scanning device at determining anything that you ask of it. It will accurately determine what food intolerances a person has; whether they have viruses or residual particles of viruses in their tissues that may have been left from an old infection or vaccination. It can identify bacteria, parasites, fungi and

16 Voll, R: Twenty Years of Electroacupuncture Therapy Using Low Frequency Current Pulses. *Amer. J. Acupuncture*, 3(4): 291-314, 1975.
17 http://www.youtube.com/watch?v=Jltzy072hxY
18 Kenyon JN. 21st century medicine: a layman's guide to the medicine of the future. Wellingborough, Northants: Thorsons, 1986.
19 Fehrenbach J, Noll H, Nolte HG, et al. Short manual of the Vegatest-method. Schiltach: BER, 1986.

moulds and tell what drugs or remedies a person is adversely reacting to. It can also identify organ weaknesses and prioritise them; it can identify whether the person has electromagnetic stress, X-ray stress, mobile phone stress, geopathic stress and the like; as well as being able to identify the specific potency of any remedy that a person needs to take.

All these tests can be done quickly and in less than an hour as it is not difficult to scan all the organs of the body, test for food intolerances,[20] identify the weak organs, identify the specific potency required to make a homeopathic sarcode in order to strengthen a weak organ; as well as scan for vaccination stress, viruses, bacteria, fungi, Candida and parasites.

The VEGA helps the practitioner to take the guesswork out of working out the pathogenesis of disease, as well as guessing which dosage or homeopathic potency the patient is resonating with. It is my belief that when there is a paradigm shift in thinking from mechanistic to holistic, then most health practitioners of all disciplines will be proud owners of a VEGA machine.

In the early days when I began using the VEGA, I was astounded by its accuracy as I was testing the organ systems of an athlete who wanted to optimize his health and sports performance. I really did not find much as this athlete was fairly healthy and was on an optimal diet and supplement programme. But one thing that came up on the VEGA was the reproductive system – it was showing weaknesses in the testes, epididymis and prostate.

It turned out that he was indeed sterile but did not mention this in his history as he was ashamed and embarrassed, as this was a real blow to his vision of having a family with his wife. Further testing showed that he was afflicted with systemic Candidiasis and certain protozoa, along with vaccination stress. When these issues had been addressed with a 90-day protocol, his wife became pregnant a couple of months later. This is a professional athlete who had consulted at least 5 doctors about his sterility problem, but no amount of medical testing could determine what the VEGA had helped me to diagnose in less that 30 minutes.

---

20 Krop J, Swiertzek J, Wood A. Comparison of ecological testing with the Vega test method in identifying sensitivities to chemicals, foods and inhalants. *Am J Acupuncture* 13 253-259, 1985.

I also use ART testing (Autonomic Response Testing) which is an intriguing biofeedback system of evaluation and treatment and, as mentioned above, a means of tapping into the autonomic nervous system to elicit health information. The technique was co-developed by Dietrich Klinghardt, M.D., Ph.D and Lousia Williams, D.C., N.D.[21] ART uses a combination of bioresonance and biofeedback techniques such as Applied Kinesiology, EAV, Nogier pulse, Chinese pulse, heart rate variability and other techniques to assess the health or dysfunction of the autonomic nervous system.

Effectively, through VEGA and ART the body is stimulated with the energetic signature of a particular food, drug, supplement or even medical treatment and its response measured. In this way, items that trigger negative responses from the body can be avoided because they are, for example, allergenic, toxic or just unnecessary. Conversely, whatever invokes a strong positive physical response can be identified and used – or continue to be used - in treatment, instead of blindly relying on statistical average clinical studies that may have no bearing at the individual level. This is bespoke medicine, specifically designed for each patient, the ultimate form of Medicine. It is also an inexpensive healing approach, which is an additional benefit for the patient.

I have had fun with ART testing! I remember not long ago a hugely built taxi driver was brought, hobbling into my office, with his aunt holding one arm and his sister the other. They sat him down in front of me and he began explaining how frustrated he was, as he could no longer drive his taxi because he was suffering from acute vertigo, with balance and coordination problems. I could not help but notice the mobile phone that he threw onto my desk as soon as he sat down. It was certainly a new model that I remember reading about, but it looked liked it had been dragged through the fields – all scratched and well worn, with the colour literally fading into a dull grey. I immediately asked him how long he spent talking on his mobile daily. He said that it depended on the day, but was certainly between one and two hours. I was intrigued as I was aware from previous patients, including members of my family, who seem to have their mobiles strapped to their heads with sellotape, that excessive use of microwave radiation from mobiles could cause labyrinthitis (inflammation of the inner ear), a condition characterised by the previously mentioned symptoms faced by our taxi driver.

---

21 www.klinghardtneurobiology.com

I asked the big man to stand up and got his auntie to call his mobile. Meanwhile I asked him to stretch out his arm so that I could perform a muscle test – I could happily have swung on his arm like a chimp on a branch he was so strong! He smiled while I heaved with all my strength, trying to budge his arm – but to no avail. When the mobile phone began ringing I asked him to answer it and place it up to his ear so that he could talk to his auntie, while I continued the muscle testing. I told him that I would only be using a couple of fingers to see what happened. As he happily chatted on the phone I used just one finger to push his arm down – in fact the arm dropped like a brick with the use of such minimal force from my feeble finger. He was amazed and stunned, and immediately asked me to repeat the experiment. I did so with only one finger as before, and again his huge arm, with biceps like a bodybuilder's, dropped like a ton weight. He was now staring at me in amazement, looking very puzzled indeed and was trying to understand what was happening. We repeated this once again at his request and he blurted out: "What the hell is happening here? Why have I lost all my strength?"

I began to explain to him that this muscle test was an indirect way of testing the autonomic nervous system (ANS). When something stresses the ANS, such as the mobile phone in this particular case, it sends a stress signal to a part of the brain called the thalamus which then sends another stress signal down the sensory and motor nerves to the muscle being tested, hence making it weak. The muscle is merely an indicator, which tells the practitioner that the microwave radiation – from the phone in this particular case – was making the muscle weak.

Further testing on the VEGA – where I had a mobile phone stress ampoule already made up – revealed that indeed there was a conductivity drop and the mobile phone stress was stressing his ANS. It took a further couple of minutes to find a potency that resonated with this ampoule and him, and a homeopathic potency of this ampoule was then made using a potentizer – the VEGA also worked out what dosage he should be taking – 5 drops daily. After only a week he called me and said that the vertigo and coordination problems had disappeared and he was now back to driving his taxi. Hip-Hip for the VEGA and ART!

Sorry for rambling on about all these experiences, but I feel that it would be interesting to share these precious moments of discovery, as it is a revelation when you use lateral thinking to piece things together. There was another difficult case of a 66 year old sweet and polite lady who had a stroke, along with many other chronic problems stretching back over many years. She suffered from hemiparesis of one hand – she literally had no sensation of hot and cold or pressure on this hand. During the initial IDEL Diagnostic testing, one of the things that we discovered on using ART testing was a scar focus on her knee – an old cut from many years back from when she fell over on rough ground. I was again muscle testing her arm while she was lying down and as soon as I touched the scar in question the arm went very weak. She was amazed and wondered what was happening (see more details on scar and tooth foci below).

I again explained that when one cuts the skin one is also cutting the autonomic nervous system (ANS). Sometimes that cut does not heal correctly and the ANS does not connect its fibres correctly, causing the membranes of the skin to lose their polarity. In effect, the scar will act as an impulse generator causing interference with the normal electromagnetic fields of the body. This can cause a myriad of symptoms which are really very difficult to relate to the scar itself. Its akin to disconnecting the correct wire in the basement of the house that switches off the lights on the first floor.

After identifying the scar focus[22], I treated her with a soft laser. This helps to repolarise the membranes, therefore eliminating the focus itself, which stops interfering with the electromagnetic fields of the body. One day, a while after the last of the three laser treatments, she phoned me and said, 'You know what? Last night I was in the cinema with my husband and half way through the film I scratched the back of my hand!' She was ecstatic with excitement as this was the hand that had been literally paralysed and not registering any sensation, let alone the feeling of scratching – within a few more days she had also regained the sensation of hot and cold – it was truly amazing how eliminating a scar focus could help the body recuperate in this way. Praise is for ART testing for allowing us to do this type of cutting-edge work.

The currently most widely known definition of disturbance fields was coined by Pischinger[23] who wrote that disturbance fields consist of nondegradable material in the soft connective tissue.

By the age of 30, approximately 80% of patients in many Western countries have a focus, of which over 80% of these are head foci (teeth,

---

22 For a fuller explanation please see the section on tooth and scar foci later in this chapter
23 Pischinger, A. The Extracellular Matrix and Ground Regulation: Basis for a Holistic Biological Medicine. North Atlantic Books, USA, 2007.

paranasal sinuses, middle ear, tonsils). The remainder are found in the abdomen and scars on the skin, e.g chronic adnexitis, chronic cholecystitis, chronic prostatitis, abnormal bacteria flora, etc.

Hunecke verified the significance of scars as disturbance fields when he noticed that symptoms would disappear when the scars where injected with procaine, a topical anaesthetic used in medicine and dentistry – this created the birth of neural therapy.[24]

Dietrich Klinghardt was the medical neurologist that reawakened the significance of tooth and scar foci with his work in neural kinesiology, also called Autonomic Response Testing (ART). As Dr. Klinghardt says: "A scar injection (or injection to a tooth, ganglion or other dysfunctional structure) can stop abnormal neurological signals (from scar, tooth or other dysfunctional group of cells).

Abnormal signals stemming from a often remote untreated focal area are often the cause of ANS dysfunction in the brain, leading to areas of vasoconstriction, impaired transport in the ground system and inhibition of trans-membrane transport and impaired transit of nutrients across the ground system or matrix. This in turn creates a focus-specific vulnerable area within the brain with decreased immune function, decreased oxygen and nutrient uptake, and decreased detoxification abilities. The outcome is a region with increased toxic metal (and other toxin) deposition and uninhibited growth of fungi, bacteria and viruses."[25]

With the correct treatment, either using neural therapy, low light lazer therapy and other techniques it is possible to eradicate all these ANS blockers in the body and allow the body the freedom to repair itself.[26]

Heart Rate Variability (HRV) testing

I have placed this Heart Rate Variability (HRV) test immediately below the VEGA and ART testing as it is another test which taps into the autonomic nervous system. In fact, where most of the tests that I conduct

---

24 Dosch, P. Manual of Neural Therapy According to Huneke. Georg Thiem Verlag, USA, 2007.

25 http://www.klinghardtacademy.com

26 Stittmatter, B. Identifying and Treating Blockages to Healing: New Approaches to Therapy: New Approaches to Therapy-Resistant Patients. Georg Thieme Verlag, USA, 2004.

measure very specific aspects of health, the HRV is a test of the overall performance of all of the body's physiological systems. It is therefore an excellent method of monitoring body changes over time.

HRV refers to the beat-to-beat alterations in heart rate. The Autonomic Nervous System (ANS) is the portion of the nervous system that controls the body's visceral functions, including the functioning of the heart, movement of the gastrointestinal tract and secretion by different glands, among many other vital activities. It is well known that mental and emotional states directly affect the ANS.

While the rhythmic beating of the heart at rest was once believed to be monotonously regular, we now know the rhythm of a healthy heart under resting conditions is actually surprisingly irregular. These moment-to-moment variations in heart rate are easily overlooked when average heart rate is calculated. HRV derived from an electrocardiogram (ECG), is a measurement of these naturally occurring, beat-to-beat changes in heart rate.

It is believed that HRV will become as common as pulse, blood pressure or temperature in patient charts in the near future. In the last ten years more than two thousand published articles have been written about this test. HRV has been used as a screening tool in many disease processes. Various medical disciplines are looking at HRV. In diabetes and heart disease it has been proven to be predictive of the likelihood of future events.

It is found that lowered HRV is associated with aging,[27] decreased autonomic activity, hormonal tonus, specific types of autonomic

---

[27] Effects of age and physical activity on the autonomic control of heart rate in healthy men. Melo RC, Santos MD, Silva E, Quiterio RJ, Moreno MA, Reis MS, Verzola IA, Oliveira L, Martins LE, Gallo-Junior L, Catai AM. *Braz J Med Biol Res.* Sep;38(9):1331-8, 2005.

neuropathies (e.g. diabetic neuropathy)[28,29] and increased risk of sudden cardiac death after acute MI.[30]

Other research indicated that depression, panic disorders and anxiety have negative impact on autonomic function, typically causing depletion of parasympathetic tonus. On the other hand an increased sympathetic tonus is associated with lowered threshold of ventricular fibrillation. These two factors could explain why such autonomic imbalance caused by significant mental and emotional stress increases risk of acute MI followed by sudden cardiac death.

Aside from that, there are multiple studies indicating that HRV is quite useful as a way to quantitatively measure physiological changes caused by various interventions both pharmacological and non-pharmacological during treatment of many pathological conditions having significant manifestation of lowered HRV. This is one of the main reasons why I use the HRV – it is always interesting to monitor improvements in HRV as treatment progresses – as the causative factors unload from the body, the ANS becomes less stressed and the HRV improves.

Digital Infrared Thermal Imaging (DITI)

This is yet another way of eliciting information from the autonomic nervous system (ANS). As the ANS controls most of the organs and bodily functions, anything we can find out about its imbalances will greatly help us to determine which direction we need to move in to correct these imbalances.

Digital Infrared Thermal Imaging (DITI), or more simply Thermography, is another form of convenient and inexpensive analysis of the human body by tapping into the thermal energetic activity of the organs and tissues. Thermography can detect disease, inflammation and injury by revealing the thermal abnormalities present in the body. A special camera that measures bodily temperature differences is used to determine

---

28 Kudat H, Akkaya V, Sozen AB, Salman S, Demirel S, Ozcan M, Atilgan D, Yilmaz MT, Guven O. Heart rate variability in diabetes patients. *J Int Med Res.* 34(3):291-6, May-Jun 2006.
29 Kardelen F, Akcurin G, Ertug H, Akcurin S, Bircan I. Heart rate variability and circadian variations in type 1 diabetes mellitus. *Pediatr Diabetes.* 7(1):45-50, Feb 2006.
30 Evrengul H, Tanriverdi H, Kose S, Amasyali B, Kilic A, Celik T, Turhan H. The relationship between heart rate recovery and heart rate variability in coronary artery disease.. *Ann Noninvasive Electrocardiol.* 11(2):154-62, Apr 2006.

dysfunctional organs and tissues. It can also assess pain and pathology anywhere in the body.

Throughout the test there is zero radiation exposure, so it is 100% safe for everyone; 100% non-invasive, and without any injections. It offers privacy and there is no physical contact. Thermography is also cost effective, and yields instant images through digital technology. An even more significant advantage is that it can provide important clinical information much earlier than other forms of imaging, such as mammography with X-Rays, which are, in fact, carcinogenic.

X-rays, CT-scans, Ultrasound and MRI scans are all tests of anatomy that are assessing the structure of the body - thermography on the other hand measures physiological changes and functioning of the body, not only structural issues.

Thermography detects hidden inflammation

Inflammation is the precursor to many cancers and other degenerative diseases such as arthritis, heart disease, stroke, diabetes and high blood pressure. Early detection of inflammation using Thermography may help prevent many negative health conditions from developing.

Thermography specializes in:

- ❖ Breast imaging
- ❖ Pain diagnostics
- ❖ Early-Stage Disease Detection

Thermography can also:

- ❖ Visualize pain and pathology.
- ❖ Assess pain and pathology anywhere in the body.
- ❖ Is a very useful adjunctive procedure to other diagnostic tools, such as X-ray, Magnetic Resonance Imaging (MRI) scans and ultrasound.
- ❖ Is very cost-effective, risk free and provides you with instant images.
- ❖ Thermography is used in early detection of cardiovascular disease.
- ❖ Thermography also plays an important role in cardiovascular disease prevention as it can assess heart function and detect

inflammation in the carotid arteries, which may be a precursor to a stroke and blood clots.

There are also many other uses of thermography such as:

- ❖ Arthritis - can help in its early detection and can differentiate between osteoarthritis and rheumatoid arthritis.
- ❖ Neck and Back Problems - pain and joint degeneration appear very clearly on thermography scans and help to identify the source of the pain in the body.
- ❖ Dental Issues - thermography can also detect TMJ, gum disease, infected teeth, NICOs and other dental issues that are precursors to many other serious diseases.
- ❖ Sinusitis and Headaches - there is often a relationship between headaches and sinusitis - the thermography scan will show this very clearly.
- ❖ Immune Dysfunction, Chronic Fatigue Syndrome and fibromyalgia - when there is inflammation detected by thermography in the thoracic spine areas of T1 and T2 this correlates well with immune system dysfunction.
- ❖ Carpal Tunnel Syndrome - this is an often misdiagnosed condition - the thermography can help to identify the source of the pain which may be from the cervical spine.
- ❖ Digestive Disorders - thermography can often detect Irritable Bowel Syndrome, diverticulitis and Crohns Disease and correlate these with other inflammatory issues in the body.
- ❖ Other Health Issues - these would include bursitis, herniated discs, ligament and muscle tear, lupus, nerve problems, whiplash, cancer and many others.

More broadly, thermography is a safe and effective means to help in the diagnosis of: breast cancer, diabetes, nervous system disorders, metabolic disorders, repetitive strain injuries, headaches, neck and back problems, temporomandibular joint (TMJ) disorders, pain syndromes, arthritis, vascular disorders, soft tissue injuries, and strokes. At the Da Vinci Natural Health Center, once the images are recorded and inspected locally, they are subsequently sent to the US where qualified and specialist MD thermologists analyse and write a comprehensive report on them, which is then sent to the patient. The images shown below of the left and right breast would normally be in colour and the darker shades that are seen would be bright red indicating a hyperthermia or high temperature compared to the rest of the surrounding area.

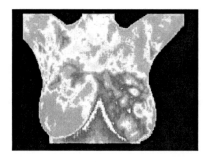 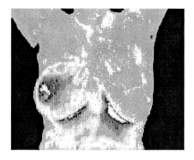

Thermogram showing left breast pathology (left) and right breast pathology (right)

Tooth and Scar Foci

Another one of the tests included in the IDEL Diagnostic Programme is the identification of tooth and scar foci, mainly by using the variety of ANS-sensitive tools which we have mentioned above such as VEGA, ART, FCT, Thermography and others. When I first came across this protocol I was sceptical, but since seeing the results with my own eyes I strongly believe in it, and all my patients now get checked for tooth and scar foci thoroughly.

Tooth foci

So what are tooth foci? 'A Focus of infection has been defined as 'A circumscribed area infected with micro-organisms which may or may not give rise to clinical manifestations.' A Focal Infection has been defined as 'Sepsis arising from a focus of infection that initiates a secondary infection in a nearby or distant tissue, or organs.' In other words, it could be an infected tooth, or a scar somewhere on the body that is causing an "interference field" in another remote part of the body.

In recent years there has been a reawakening of the dangers of oral infections and their potential disastrous effects on systemic health. The substances that are spread from such a focus include the bacterial, viral and fungal organisms that survive in such foci. It will also include the endotoxins produced by anaerobic organisms in the foci such as Siphonospora31 that excrete lethal toxins known as Thioethers.

---

31 George, M., Ivančaková, R. Root Canal Microflora, Acta Medica, Hradec Králové, 50(1):7–15, 2007.

Current research indicates that other toxins produced by anaerobic organisms are also released into the body – these include hydrogen sulphide products and methyl mercaptans, both of which are highly poisonous products – these paralyse the acupuncture meridians which run through that particular tooth. This meridian will subsequently adversely affect a whole bunch of organs and tissues in the body. You can read more about this in Chapter 9.

There are now maps of the teeth connected to their various meridians with lists of symptoms and organs that can be affected. Dr. Rau of the Paracelsus Clinic in Switzerland systematically tested a group of about 150 women all with breast cancer and found in nearly every case that there was a tooth focus on the Stomach Meridian – this has also been validated by myself in numerous cases that I have tested.

Published case reports include the following disease states as being directly related to Oral infections:

Disease States related to Oral Infections			
Mediastinitis	Maxillary sinusitis	Blindness	Endopthalmitis
Cavernous sinus thrombosis	Necrotising mediastinitis	Light reflex interference	Lung abscess
Pharyngeal cellulitis	Superior Orbital Fissure Syndrome	Brain abscess	Aspiration pneumonia
Cardiac problems	Proptosis	Meningitis	Acute hemiplagia
Necrotising fascititis	Opthalmoplegia	Psychotic episodes	Metastatic paraspinal abscess
Gasarion ganglion	Trigeminal neuralgia	Endocarditis	Septicemia
Myocardial infection	Deuodenal ulcers	Splenic abscess	Leg abscess
Blood disorders	Immune reactions	Inflammatory Bowel Disease	Low birth weight
Infertility	Death	Toxic shock	Kidney damage
Arthritis	Rheumatic changes	Infection of artificial joint prosthesis	Brain tumours

In other words all areas of the body may be affected by the presence of infected foci in the mouth. Dr. Weston Price conducted his own research on tooth foci - he decided to implant an extracted root-filled tooth under the skin of an animal. He felt that if bacteria were present and carrying illness, their presence in a tooth might offer the same kind of proof physicians found when they injected the bacterial culture to produce disease in an animal. That is exactly what took place. He found that by implanting the root-filled tooth, the disease of the patient was transferred to animals. Whatever disease the patient had, the animal with the extracted tooth under its skin developed.

In other words, if the patient had heart disease, the animal developed heart disease. If he had kidney trouble, disease of the kidney was transferred to the animal. If he had a problem in his joints, the animal's joints became similarly involved. The principle held true for the whole spectrum of human ailments. Whatever the disease, the animal would develop that of the patient.

Scar Foci

Scar foci are when a cut to the skin has not healed properly and it leaves the autonomic nerve system, near the surface of the skin, in a state of depolarization. This can create interference fields in the normal, subtle electromagnetic fields of the body. A scar on the foot, for example can cause chronic migraines or a myriad of other health problems. These scars are identified in much the same way by ART testing, and then by using low intensity laser therapy it is possible to repolarise the tissues and heal the scar focus. More about scar foci is discussed in chapter 9.

Digital Homeopathy

Even though I trained as a classical homeopath many years ago I have never been quite comfortable working as one – I always had the feeling that there was a lot of guesswork involved in homeopathy whereby the practitioner had to choose between many different remedies that sort of fitted the symptom picture, and even when the remedy was found they had to then guess the potency. There did not seem to be any hard and fast rules for either choosing the appropriate remedy or the potency and no objective testing to determine this either.

However, having practiced the art and persevered, I became convinced that homeopathy worked because when I did find the correct remedy and the correct potency, the results could be miraculous – literally a cure overnight! I have now witnessed this enough times to know that homeopathy is a powerful healing tool that I should pursue, but I always had my mind open as to how best to use it.

Having studied with Dr. Dietrich Klinghardt, a German medical doctor and neurologist and his associates, I quickly learned that it is possible to find the appropriate remedy, as well as the potency, by using the muscle testing he has called Autonomic Response Testing (ART), which I touched on earlier in this chapter.

My perseverance to find more refined methods led me to another doctor who has a modified version of the muscle testing called Field Control Therapy (FCT) – his name is Dr. Savely Yurkovsky,[32] a Russian-trained medical doctor. What Dr. Yurkovsky taught me was how to factor pernicious agents against the various organ systems and then make homeopathic isodes (see below) of these pernicious agents based on the information that you receive from the patients themselves. This becomes really quite bespoke, as the patients, through muscle testing, are telling you what remedy they need and what potency of that remedy best suits them.

This branch of homeopathy that deals with the administration of causative agents, isodes and autoisodes (remedies prepared from bodily fluids such as blood, saliva, urine, pus and other discharges), can be classified as causative homeopathy. Unlike classical homeopathy, causative homeopathy aims its prescription solely against the offending agents rather than the symptoms produced by these agents.

There is a large body of evidence that has demonstrated the efficacy of causative homeopathy. In 1974, during a meningococcal meningitis epidemic in Brazil, 18,640 children were vaccinated with one low-potency dose of Meningococcinum, a homeopathic remedy prepared from meningococcus bacteria taken in one low potency dose. Only four children developed meningitis, compared to 32 reported cases amongst 6,340 "control" children who did not receive the remedy.[33]

Back in 1932 in France, the homeopathic isode, Diphtherinum, prepared from an infectious agent causing diphtheria, was given as an immunization to 45 children. Every child developed circulating antibodies against diphtheria (confirming that this remedy had appropriately stimulated immune responses). Several years later, as the children's antibody levels

---

32 www.yurkovsky.com
33 Castro, D., Nogueira, C.G. Use of the nosode Meningococcinum as a preventive against meningitis. *Journal of the American Institute of Homeeopathy*. V.68, 211-219, 1975.

declined, Diphtherinum was readministerd and restored the high antibody concentrations.[34]

Homeopathic Sarcodes and Isodes

As I mostly resonate best with my VEGA machine, I have modified both approaches and developed my own methods of diagnosing and testing using the VEGA. What I have found works well in the field of homeopathy is making homeopathic sarcodes – these are homeopathic potencies of healthy organs – to help strengthen organs such as kidneys, liver, bone marrow, pancreas, thyroid and whatever other organ the testing shows is imbalanced or weak. One can also make isodes of pernicious agents such as mercury, phthalates and other xenobiotics, again at the potency that the patient is resonating with. The potencies usually run into the M and LM potencies, which are considered to be high potencies in homeopathy.

The patient takes these sarcodes and isodes for a few days and then they are re-tested – sometimes they will have done their work in a few days, whereas other times it requires higher potencies of the same sarcode or isode to go down a layer and do deeper work, much like peeling the layers of an onion. It is also possible to use this testing method to go very deep into the body to see what is resonating with the DNA of certain tissues and organs and making a sarcode of that tissue and DNA to repair it. This is really very bespoke testing and the avenues one can investigate are only restricted by the creativity of the practitioner. I believe that this art of practicing "Resonant Homeopathy" will one day be taught to all homeopaths so that they can widen their horizons beyond Hahnemann's traditional teachings.

Orthomolecular Nutrition

Perhaps the largest portion of my time studying has been in trying to get my head around the topic of nutrition. Even though I spent three years studying nutrition, my learning about this complex topic really began after I had completed my studies. What a complex and confusing topic it is with so many differing opinions from so many different schools of nutrition. No wonder many of my patients say to me, 'Hey doc, how do we know that what you are going to advise us about nutrition is the truth, given that so

---

34 Chavanon, P., La Diphterie (1932), 4e edl, Imprimerrie St-Denis, Niort.

many others have told us different things?' They are right, as this is how I felt for years while experimenting on myself.

After completing Nutrition College I began experimenting religiously on myself, and my poor patients. Wow! I was getting some dramatic failures back in those days with patients calling me up who were vomiting, feeling dizzy, losing muscle mass, not being able to function properly, as well as developing many other symptoms. I knew the power of nutrition as I was seeing the results on my patients as well as on myself, the problem was that the same diet did not fit all people. Where one person would really take off and be bounding with energy on an alkaline detoxification diet using fruits and vegetables, another would feel suicidal and could hardly get up in the morning to go to work. I was confused about what was happening and read voraciously everything that I could get my hands on regarding nutrition and the optimal approach.

I became quite ill myself when I decided to follow Dr. Peter D' Adamo's blood type diet – most people know it these days – where certain blood groups should avoid certain food families based on their Lectin content.

Lectins are found in ALL foods, certain foods more than others, and the same food may contain varying amounts of lectins depending on processing, when and where the plant was grown and species. The most common potentially toxic lectin containing food groups are:

- ❖ Grains, especially wheat and wheat germ but also quinoa, rice, buckwheat, oats, rye, barley, millet and corn.
- ❖ Legumes (all dried beans, including soy and peanuts).
- ❖ Dairy (perhaps more so when cows are fed grains instead of grass – a speculation based on research showing transference of lectins into breast milk and dairy and potentially more harmful in pasteurized, processed milk because of the reduction of SIgA, an immunoglobulin that binds dangerous lectins[35] NOTE: Only breast milk is good for babies.
- ❖ Nightshade family of vegetables (includes potato, tomato, eggplant and pepper).

Each of these groups has a history of being implicated as allergenic. These include all foods made from the following substances: milled grains,

---

35 Davin JC et al. The high lectin-binding capacity of human secretory IgA protects nonspecifically mucosae against environmental antigens. *Biol Neonate* 59(3):121-5, 1991.

flours, oils, vinegars, peanut butter, cereal or legume oils (soy, canola, corn), additives, thickeners, grain vinegar and products containing grain vinegar, grain alcohol including grain based vodka and all beers and ales.

There has been some information that lectins may be inactivated by soaking, sprouting, cooking or fermenting. Soaking legumes over night, draining the water, rinsing and draining again does seem to remove or inactivate many of the lectins. Heating seems to remove others in some foods but not all. There is little data to prove that any of these methods remove lectins completely as few foods have been tested, and of those that have lectins many seem to remain after processing.

So, back to Dr. D' Adamo's work – apart from talking about these lectins, which can be avoided to a certain degree even though the liver happily processes most of these anyway, he also talks about people with certain blood groups such as mine – A rhesus negative – eating a more vegetarian diet. So for 7 months I followed pretty much a vegetarian diet eating very little meat, some fish and pulses, nuts, seeds and avocados but large servings of fresh fruit, vegetables, salads and vegetable juices. Literally from the beginning, the following are common symptoms that I developed while being on this diet:

- ❖ Constant bowel distension with flatulence.
- ❖ Muscle wasting that was particularly visible on the face, with hollows around my cheek bones and eyes.
- ❖ Elevated cholesterol level from 170 to 240 – checked on blood tests twice over the 7 month vegetarian diet.
- ❖ Band-type headaches most mornings that would last many hours and were incapacitating – I subsequently discovered that these would occur whenever I ate large bowls of fruit at night as a main meal.
- ❖ Difficulty concentrating, remembering details, focusing and generally my cognitive functioning had lost its focus.
- ❖ Tiredness – most of the day and even when waking at night with pronounced muscle pains

It was not until a doctor friend came over from Greece to spend a few days and saw me and said, 'What are your doing? You are not looking too well' I immediately responded, 'Well I am eating all this healthy food as I am experimenting with a new diet that is mostly vegetarian.' He smiled and simply said, 'Ah yes, but what is your Metabolic Type?' I said that I did not know even though I had skimmed Bill Wolcotts' book "The Metabolic Typing Diet"[36] some two years back. I therefore went back to the book and read it properly this time, became very interested and trained as a Metabolic Typing Consultant by following courses and taking exams.

Nutritional Testing for Metabolic Typing®

The Metabolic Typing® diet is primarily a way of optimizing the percentage of proteins, fats, and carbohydrates required in an individual's metabolism. The method combines various nutritional and biochemical theories into a unique way of broader nutritional and health advice.[37]

Certain researchers such as George Watson, Roger Williams, William Kelley and others believed that people's metabolisms functioned differently when it came to two factors, which are largely determined by heredity:

1. Autonomic nervous system dominance. There are two branches of this system. One of these branches, the sympathetic nervous system, is often referred to as the 'fight or flight' branch. It helps you burn energy. The other branch is the parasympathetic nervous system. This branch helps you conserve energy. It also helps you digest food. Advocates of this diet believe that one branch tends to be stronger or more dominant than the other.

2. Rate of cellular oxidation. This refers to the rate at which cells convert food into energy. Some people are fast oxidizers, because they rapidly convert food into energy. In order to balance their systems, fast oxidizers need to eat heavier proteins and fats that burn slowly. In contrast, slow oxidizers convert food into energy at a slow rate. In order to balance their systems, it is recommended that they eat mainly carbohydrates rather than protein and fat.

For an accurate assessment of your Metabolic Typing®, a trained health practitioner can provide a thorough assessment that may include urine and blood tests, but taking the intermediate questionnaire will also provide an

---

36 Wolcott, B., Fahey, T. The Metabolic Typing Diet. Doubleday, New York, 2000.
37 For more details see http://www.metabolictyping.com.

accurate assessment[38] –Wolcott in his book and website[39] talks about three general Metabolic Types:

1. The Protein Type - if you are a protein type it means one of two things - either your cells tend to burn carbohydrates too quickly (meaning you're a fast oxidizer), or the parasympathetic branch of your autonomic nervous system is stronger and more dominant than the sympathetic branch. This means you need a high-protein intake in order to strengthen your sympathetic system, and in turn acidify your too-alkaline metabolism. Or you need protein to slow down your overly rapid cellular oxidation rate, thereby alkalinizing your too-acid metabolism.

2. One of the best foods for a Protein type is high-density, high-fat proteins known as "high-purine" proteins. These include foods like red meat, dark meat chicken and turkey, and various kinds of seafood such as salmon, tuna, herring, sardines, mussels, caviar and anchovies. Most protein types can also eat freely of whole fat foods in the form of cheese, eggs, cream and milk. It's especially important for protein types to include a significant amount of protein at every meal, and to moderate their intake of carbohydrates (grains, vegetables and fruits), especially the carbohydrates that are high in sugar and starch.

3. The Carbo Type - carbo types generally need a higher percentage of carbohydrates in their diet in order to strengthen the parasympathetic branch of their nervous system, which is weaker than the sympathetic system. This helps to alkalinize their too-acid metabolism. Alternatively, they require more carbohydrates to speed up their naturally slow cellular oxidation rate, thereby bringing it into balance by acidifying their too-alkaline metabolism.

The best foods for Carbo types are typically low-fat, relatively low-protein diets - ones that include liberal amounts of carbohydrates in the form of vegetables, fruits and whole grains. However, carbo types need to remember that a "low-protein" diet does not mean a "no-protein" diet. In fact, most carbo types will find that they need to include protein at most meals, but they need

---

38 See www.docgeorge.com and click on Metabolic Typing Test.
39 http://www.metabolictypingdiet.com

to focus on leaner, lighter meats, seafood and poultry than protein types. They should restrict their consumption of red meat in favour of light meat chicken and turkey and lighter seafood such as haddock, cod, perch, sole, catfish and flounder.

If you're a carbo type you should stick to low-fat dairy products, but you can eat a very wide selection of vegetables, fruits, and grains. However, many carbo types, like protein types, do best by focusing on vegetables that contain low or moderate levels of sugar and starch.

The Mixed Type - the mixed types are somewhere in the middle of the other two types, which have more pronounced or clear-cut metabolic imbalances. This type needs to eat a mixture of protein type foods and carbo type foods. This will accomplish two things: 1) it will support both the sympathetic and the parasympathetic branches of the autonomic nervous system; and 2) it will keep their cellular oxidation rate, which is neither too fast or too slow, in balance.

Mixed types need to consume relatively equal ratios of proteins, fats and carbohydrates. They also need to eat a mixture of high-fat, high-purine proteins and low-fat, low-purine proteins. The same applies to all of the other foods contained on the protein type and carbo type diets - including grains, legumes, vegetables and fruits.

A quick overview of my own personal Metabolic Typing test results appear below:

- ❖ My Metabolic Type: Autonomic
- ❖ Sympathetic Oxidative: Fast
- ❖ Endocrine: Thyroid
- ❖ Dominance: Fast
- ❖ My Macro-nutrient Ratios: Carbohydrate 30%, Protein 40%, Fat 30%.

So now I knew why I was ill when I tried following the vegetarian diet that was recommended for my blood type – I was a protein type requiring 40% protein with each meal or snack, along with only 30% carbohydrates and 30% fat. This was the octane of fuel that my body required to functional optimally and this ratio of foods was controlling nine parameters of my biochemistry, which my vegetarian diet had turned upside down!

Within one month of being on this diet I had regained my muscle mass, energy, concentration, my cholesterol levels dropped from 240 to 180 even though I was again eating meat and fat and the bloating and headaches completely disappeared. It was amazing how quickly my body found its balance as soon as it was receiving the 40:30:30 ratio of food mentioned above that fitted my genetic makeup.

The Metabolic Typing® Diet is something that I use frequently with my patients now and it works well. It is bespoke and addresses the genetic and biochemical individuality of the person and does not guess this – there is no diet that fits all and the adage 'One man's meat is another man's poison,' is fitting here.

In my long, arduous journey reading through hundreds of nutrition books, there was another striking piece of research that really caught my attention and made a lot of sense. This was the work of the late Dr. Weston Price, DDS, a dentist by profession, but also an astute researcher with a congenial spirit of enquiry. Alongside him there is also Dr. Francis Pottenger, MD who is probably best known for his cat studies were he compared how cats fared when he fed them a nutritious raw diet versus a deficient cooked diet.[40]

Price travelled the world over in order to study isolated human groups, including sequestered villages in Switzerland, Gaelic communities in the Outer Hebrides, Eskimos and Indians of North America, Melanesian and Polynesian South Sea Islanders, African tribes, Australian Aborigines, New Zealand Maori and the Indians of South America. Wherever he went, Dr. Price found that beautiful straight teeth, freedom from decay, stalwart bodies, resistance to disease and fine characters were typical of primitives following their traditional diets, rich in essential food factors.

The striking thing is that all these human groups were eating very different diets – some like the Eskimos were eating large amounts of fat, blubber, and fish with little or no vegetables and fruit. The Swiss villagers were eating plenty of dairy produce with fruit and vegetables, and very little meat and so on. What Dr. Price found, however, which is crucially

---

40 I will not mention much about Dr. Weston Prices' research here as I will be expounding on its significance in Chapter 3. All I wish to say here is that he published a classic text book that is worthwhile reading entitled *Nutrition and Physical Degeneration* and is available from the Price-Pottenger Nutrition Foundation (PPNF) – *www.price-pottenger.org*

important for us today too, is that regardless of what food these people were eating it was all organic, home-grown in fertile soils rich in minerals, not sprayed with pesticides and herbicides; and the animals eaten were all wild and free-grazing, eating off the land. These people were also eating local produce and would not import food over thousands of miles as we tend to do today.

Live Blood Analysis (LBA)

Following on from what we have said above about nutrition, there is another test that I use, from a single drop of blood, that is sometimes known as nutritional microscopy –so called because there is a lot of information that can be elicited from this analysis regarding the nutritional status of the patient, the status of their digestion and other nutritionally-related factors.

This test is rarely seen in allopathic medicine as nutrition is not really part of their main curriculum unfortunately, so inevitably tests related to nutrition will also not be of interest. The practitioner takes one drop of blood from the patient's finger and places it on a slide with a cover slip. This is then placed under a compound microscope with a special condenser called a carotid condenser, which allows light to be scattered at right angles to the slide. What this does in effect is to create a darkened background on the slide that allows the various components of the blood to light up and phosphoresce.

Perhaps the most striking thing is that the blood is still living and moving. This is why it is often referred to as 'Live Blood Analysis,' or 'Darkfield Microscopy.' Live blood under the microscope provides an incredible sight that can be also viewed by the patient, either directly through the microscope, or via a monitor.

Normally, most microbiologists would kill the blood with various chemical stains in order to see the various structures in Technicolor. This, however, loses a lot of the qualitative aspects as well as the behavioural aspects as dead blood really has no behaviour – it is dead! Looking at blood in its living form is fascinating for both the patient and the therapist – even though I have now been doing this for years it is still as fascinating as the first time I saw a live blood sample.

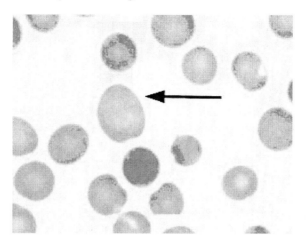

Macrocyte

The image above shows a macrocyte, an abnormally large erythrocyte or red blood cell - 10 to 12 microns in diameter. This is normally a sign of Vitamin B12 deficiency which causes maturation failure in the process of erythropoeisis. Most often megaloblastic anaemia is the consequence of deficiency of Vitamin B12 or folate or both.[41]

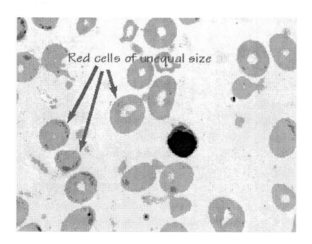

Red cells of unequal size

Anisocytosis

---

41 Leavell, BS and Thorup, OA. Fundamentals of Clinical Haematology, 4th ed. W.B. Saunders Co. Philadelphia. pp 22-23, 1976.

The image above shows red blood cells of differing sizes – some small and some large – this is known as Anisocytosis – this is another early sign of iron deficiency, as well as vitamin B12, folic acid. The more severe the anisocytosis, the more severe the anaemia.[42]

There are many other parameters of health that can be seen in live blood analysis that can be directly correlated to nutrition.[43]

As soon as you see the blood sample on the screen, you cannot help but comprehend how alive it really is – lots of tiny particles moving around by Brownian motion – these are really particles of colloidal protein that Professor Enderlein, a German microbiologist and researcher, referred to as 'protits.' They are present in all human fluids, as well as plants and no one really knows their function as they do not contain genetic material such as RNA or DNA.

However, when the body's pH changes, then there is a physical phenomenon that occurs which is well-known in physics, and is called 'Zeta Potentials.' The zeta potential is a measure of the magnitude of the repulsion or attraction between particles. As the blood becomes more and more acidic then these little particles begin sticking together or flocculating to form long strings of strange-looking structures, all of which were named by Prof. Enderlein.

Basically the more toxic the person is, the more their pH will have shifted from normal, so the more morphologies can be seen in their blood. This is a clear indication that the person is really off-balance, toxic and requiring immediate intervention: to bring the internal milieu[44] (or biological environment) back to some sort of balance with the correct pH – this is best achieved by getting the patient to detoxify with fruits, vegetables and juices for 15 days.

In addition to this aspect of live blood analysis, there are many other things that can be determined such as whether the person is anaemic, is deficient in folic acid and vitamin B12, has leukaemia or sickle cell anaemia, has a predisposition to a heart attack or stroke, is getting enough oxygen

---

42 Miaele, JB. Laboratory Medicine: haematology, 6th ed. Ladeg, DE ed., CJ Mosby Co. St. Louis. p.476, 1977.
43 Practitioners that are interested in studying live blood analysis in depth can go to www.collegenaturalmedicine.com
44 I explain this more fully in the next section: Biological Terrain Analysis (BTA)

delivered to the cells and tissues of the body, has a lot of free radical damage or has a good, active immune system given that you can actually see the white blood cells such as the neutrophils literally walking across the screen – this is really mind-blowing to the majority of patients who witness this!

While it does not amount to a diagnosis for any specific organ or disease, LBA grants a unique way to analyse the health of blood and its constituent cells. It can also offer insights and indications as to the pH of the blood, the quality and vitality of red and white blood cells (the tendency to degenerate, anisocytocis, cell atrophy, autolysis due to toxins, cellular contamination), as well as revealing signs of liver stress/damage, cholesterol, undigested fat and protein, hormonal imbalances, sugar imbalances, yeast and bacterial infections; as well as parasites and other aspects of the internal ecology of humans and other animals.

I often photograph interesting findings and record live blood on video, so that a visual record of the quality and behaviour of the blood being tested at various stages of treatment can be held and compared with other samples, taken from the same patient, to help monitor the patient's progress. I call this "visual medicine" for both doctor and patient as it is a visual representation of the internal workings of this fluid, which is life-giving and the body could not survive without.

In the 18th and 19th centuries, live blood analysis was the main tool of medical practitioners and researchers. Many medics at the time were glued to their microscopes, observing a world unseen to the naked eye. The constituent cells of blood and all kinds of microbes and germs were common objects of observation.

Louis Pasteur was the most prominent and famous supporter of the theory – and now mainstream dogma – that all microbes and bacteria have only one form (monomorphism) and the primary way to fight them is in an outright war waged with antibiotics. This view was opposed by the alternative scientific perspective of Antoine Bechamps. He demonstrated that microbes could alter their form, literally evolving as different germs (pleomorphism, that is, having many forms), depending on their biological environment (their internal 'milieu).

What Bechamps observed was that a deteriorating internal biological environment caused or allowed microbes to evolve into more virulent forms. This theory implies that the optimal way to fight these microbes is to reverse the internal milieu using proper nutrition, proper detoxification and a natural lifestyle. Not, in other words, by attacking them with antibiotics. Using drugs may win a few battles, but the war is sure to be lost as the drugs harm the milieu even further than the original invaders.

Bechamps' scientific analysis was further developed by Professor Doctor Gunther Enderlein, who formulated a comprehensive model of the pathological processes observed in live blood. He wrote hundreds of articles and published a book in 1925 entitled 'Bacterial Cyclogeny.'[45] Thereafter, many scientists have confirmed the basics of pleomorphism, as well as documented specific cases of the phenomenon in several different species of bacteria. For example, two French biologists, Sonea and Panisset, published a book in 1983 called, 'A New Bacteriology,'[46] which noted that bacterial pleomorphism was a proven scientific fact by the 1980's. In 2001, Dr Peter Schneider in his article, 'Prof. Enderlein's research in today's view: can his research results be confirmed with modern techniques?'[47] provided updated scientific evidence about the validity of Enderlein's live blood analysis work using modern scientific techniques.[48]

Biological Terrain Analysis (BTA)

Biological Terrain Analysis (BTA) is an American term for what has been known as the 'Internal Milieu,' something that Bechamps mentioned last century when he said that the internal milieu is the factor that is most important in keeping various bacteria alive and spreading.

The one hundred trillion cells in the human body are bathed in a nutrient-filled fluid matrix called the Biological Terrain. Other names for this fluid include the interstitial matrix and the internal milieu. This environment, like the soil, feeds and nourishes all of the cells in the body. The outermost wall of every cell is called the cell membrane. This membrane is permeable, which means that certain elements can flow in and out of this

---

45 Enderlein, G. Bacteria Cyclogeny, Enderlein Enterprises Inc., Gemany, 1999.
46 Sonea, Panisset A New Bacteriology. Jones & Bartlett Publishers, 1983.
47 Ullmann, R. A Modern Scientific Perspective On Prof. Dr. Enderlein's Concept Of Microbial Life Cycles, Biochemist; BioResource : Articles: A Modern Scientific Perspective, 2001.
48 I have written a course for people who wish to study this fascinating topic to Diploma level which is available at my website www.collegenaturalmedicine.com. There is also an interesting section on Live Blood Analysis on my other website www.docgeorge.com.

membrane. The cells absorb electrolytes, vitamins, minerals, enzymes and fluid in very specific amounts. The cell, to maintain cellular health and create substances called energy-rich intermediates, then utilizes these nutrients.

The body, to produce energy in the form of ATP (the energy that fuels many critical actions and reactions in the human body), then uses these substances. The waste products from these cellular reactions within the cells are then released back into the Biological Terrain for proper filtering and disposal by the body. The integrity of the cell, its cell membrane and the vitality of the Biological Terrain increase the probability that the cell will grow and thrive.

This procedure entails the clinical monitoring of the body's internal biochemical environment to gain an understanding of cellular pathology and biochemical imbalances. Measurements include pH, oxidative stress, and mineral concentrations from urine, blood, and saliva. BTA is a powerful health screening analysis that provides valuable biochemical information about cellular function and metabolism in the body's tissues, organs, and systems.

The information in question includes data on oxygen transport, nutrient delivery, waste removal, mineral retention, cellular absorption, and multiple metabolic chemical interactions. The information is complex and it is often difficult to understand what is happening biochemically in the body – here are some examples of the types of problems that can be found from the BTA analysis that would be difficult to affirm using any other test:

- ❖ Low hydrochloric acid production in the stomach – hypochlorhydria.
- ❖ Low enzyme production due to weak pancreatic function.
- ❖ Mineral depletion – pointing to the presence of heavy metals as well as malabsorption problems.
- ❖ Electron transport system deficiency – low adenosine triphosphate (ATP) production, implicating heavy metals and mineral deficiencies, as well as a lack of coenzyme Q10 which is required for ATP production.
- ❖ Lymphatic congestion.
- ❖ Kidney and liver congestion.

The nine values measured are analyzed and plotted by the BTA instrument's computer software onto a report that contains graphs and charts. The data are then assessed by the practitioner and used as a teaching guide to share with the patient. Although the testing procedure does not diagnose any specific pathology or disease states, it does serve as an analytical guide post that tremendously aids in the overall evaluation of the patient.

What is exciting about this particular test is its ability to pick up pre-pathological changes in the body that predispose one to bacterial and viral infections, as well as many chronic diseases.

Hair Tissue Mineral Analysis (HTMA)

In clinical work I have found one test that I use often, and find to be invaluable, is the Hair Tissue Mineral Analysis (HTMA).49 This involves taking a small sample of hair by cutting the first inch-and-a-half of growth closest to the scalp at the nape of the neck, or even pubic hair if someone is completely bald. It is then sent to a licensed clinical laboratory where the hair is prepared through a series of chemical and high temperature digestive procedures and is finally analysed for levels of minerals and toxic metals, by using sophisticated measuring devices called spectrometers.

Hair is considered an ideal tissue for sampling and testing.50 Firstly, it can be cut easily and painlessly and can be sent to the lab without special handling requirements. Secondly, clinical results have shown that a correctly obtained sample can give an indication of mineral status and toxic metal accumulation following long-term or even acute exposure. Hair is used as one of the tissues of choice by the US Environmental Protection Agency in determining toxic metal exposure. Indeed, a number of studies have concluded that human hair may be a more appropriate tissue than blood or urine for studying a community's exposure to harmful trace elements.

Although our aim is to rid the body of harmful toxic metals, conversely trace minerals are essential in countless metabolic functions in all phases

---

49 Bland, J. Hair tissue mineral analysis. an emergent diagnostic technique. Thorsons Publishers, USA, 1983.
50 Watts, DL. Trace Elements and Other Essential Nutrients: Clinical Application of Tissue Mineral Analysis.

of the life process.[51] For example, zinc is involved in the production, storage, and secretion of insulin and is necessary for growth hormones. Magnesium is required for normal muscular function, especially the heart. A deficiency in magnesium has been associated with an increased incidence of heart attacks; anxiety and nervousness. Potassium is critical for normal nutrient transport into the cell – deficiency can result in muscular weakness, depression and lethargy. Excess sodium is associated with hypertension, but adequate amounts are required for normal health. Even vitamin status can be indirectly assessed from HTMA[52].

HTMA can detect recent exposure (from the last couple of months) of toxic metals in your blood that ultimately end up in the hair tissues as well. The way I use the test is to take an initial baseline sample to see the levels of minerals and toxic metals that are actively circulating in the blood during the last couple of months – this is basically the time it takes to grow the inch-and-a-half of hair that is taken. I then put my patients on a natural chelator which I researched and discovered and have the worldwide patent-pending for – it is a natural chelator that has undergone double-blind, placebo controlled trials with 350 people and is called HMD®. A further HTMA is taken after 2 months to see how many metals have been mobilized from storage sites in the body – usually we find a percentage increase of metals in the second test.

51 Wilson, LD. Nutritional Balancing and Hair Mineral Analysis: A Comprehensive Guide. LD Wilson Consultants, Inc., 1993.
52 More information can be found at http://www.detoxmetals.com

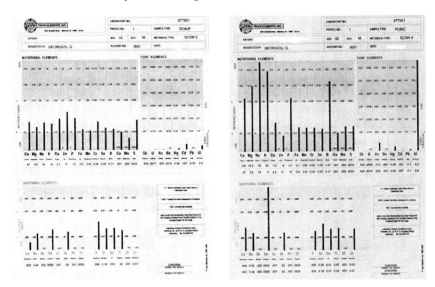

HTMA results two months apart after using HMD®

The two reports above are from the same patient, taken two months apart. On the left is the baseline sample before any natural chelator or minerals were given. Generally there is a low level of minerals with a little Cadmium and Aluminium burden. This is what has been circulating in the blood over the last couple of months, but is not a reflection of what is stored in the body tissues and organs. On the right are the results of the second hair test, taken two months after the first, while on the HMD® protocol. Notice that there is a huge increase in the levels of aluminium with some arsenic also appearing – these are the heavy metals that were in the storage organs that were mobilized by the HMD.®[53]

On a number of occasions I have heard practitioners say to a patient, based on the initial HTMA showing no detectable metals, that they are squeaky-clean. This is simply not true! The initial hair test does not tell us about the metals that are stored in the body tissues and organs, only those that have been running around the blood in the last couple of months. Seeing no metals in the initial test, therefore, has no bearing on how squeaky-clean we may be. This is why it is important for the practitioner to discuss the HMD® protocol with the patient and get them to repeat the test in a further two months, having taken the HMD®. Using this protocol and testing hair

---

53 This protocol using a pre-post hair sample can be found at
www.detoxmetals.com/THMA.html

every couple of months gives the patient and the clinician the data to decide whether the patient should continue chelating or not.

So, where do all these toxic metals come from? Well, exposure to heavy metals is ubiquitous these days. The classic example of exposure is mercury amalgams in the mouth. If you are a dentist working with dental amalgams, or a dental assistant; or if you just work at a dentist's office – even as a cleaner – you are seriously at risk. If you work with industrial metallurgy or use heavy metals, or even if you simply consume fish – especially tuna, swordfish, shellfish, shrimp or other scavenger fish like catfish; lobsters or oysters – you are also at risk.

Urine Indican Test (Obermeyer Test)

The digestive system is one of the most important systems in the body – when it does not function correctly then it is possible to produce many different toxins in the gastrointestinal tract that will adversely affect the liver and bowel, often causing inflammatory diseases. There is a urine test that I use called the Indican Test or Obermeyer Test to determine the degree of indole (3-hydroxy indole) in the urine, which reflects the level of toxicity in the gut. It is a simple test that used to be conducted in most doctors' offices[54] and was quick and accurate in giving a general assessment of gut toxicity.

For those who are interested in the biochemistry, here is a brief version of the logic behind the test. The essential amino acid tryptophan is converted to indole, as intestinal bacteria cleave to the tryptophan side chain. Following absorption, indole is converted to 3-hydroxy indole (indolyz or indicans) in the liver, where it is then conjugated with potassium sulphate or glucoronic acid, and then transported via the blood to the kidneys for excretion. The production of high levels of indicans reflects bacterial activity in the small and large intestines.

These elevated levels are considered an indicator of intestinal toxemia and overgrowth of anaerobic bacteria. Conditions behind elevated levels of urinary indicans can include[55] inflammatory bowel disease, celiac disease, hypochlorhydria, achlorhydria, gastric ulcers, biliary and intestinal obstruction, jejunal diverticulosis, scleroderma, postgastrectomy, Hartnups

---

54 Todd J: Clinical Diagnosis and Management by Laboratory Methods. WB Saunders, Phil, pp 592-3, 1979.
55 Curzon G and Walsh J: Value of measuring urinary indicant excretion. *Gut* 7:711, 1966.

disease,[56] pancreatic insufficiency, diminished peristalsis and blue diaper syndrome or hypermotility of the small intestine.

Detection of indicans depends on its decomposition to indoxyl and subsequent oxidation to indigo blue. It is then concentrated into a layer of chloroform for easier measurement. Results are typically presented on a five-level scale, the first level being normal, and the fifth level being the worst.

A positive test may indicate one of the diseases listed above: hypochlorhydria bacterial overgrowth in the small intestine, and/or malabsorption of protein.[57] A colon hydrotherapy is usually recommended when the level of indoles is high, as well as optimization of the diet based on the person's Metabolic Type; also the use of probiotics such as acidophilus and digestive enzymes to improve digestion.

Breath-Testing for Digestive Problems

When bacteria metabolize or ferment carbohydrates, they produce acids, water and gases. The major gases which are produced from the bacterial metabolism of disaccharides (including lactose, commonly known as milk sugar) include carbon dioxide (CO_2) and hydrogen (H_2).[58] Methane (CH_4) production has been identified in those who fail to produce H2 following ingestion of non-digestible sugars.[59]

The feasibility of using the appearance of such gases to study intestinal absorption and intermediary metabolism has been recognized for many years[60] and its use has grown markedly.

Recent studies have recommended that all patients suspected of having Irritable Bowel Syndrome (IBS) should be tested for disaccharide

56 Asatoor A, London D, Craske J, and Milne M: Indole production in Hartnup's disease. *Lancet* i:126-8, 1963.

57 Greenberger N, Saegh S, and Ruppert R: Urine indican excretion in malabsorption disorders. *Gastroenterol* 55:204-11, 1968.

58 Bond, JH, Levit, MD. Quantitative measurement of lactose absorption. Gastroenterol. 70(6):1058-62, 1976.

59 Bjrneklett, A, Jenssen, E. Relationship between hydrogen (H2) and methane (CH4) production in man. Scand J Gastroenterol. 17:985-92, 1982.

60 Solomons, NW, Schnieder, RE, Garcia-Ibanez, R, Pineda, D, Viteri, FE, Lizarralde, E, Schoeller, D, Klein, P, Rosenberg, IH, Calloway, D. Use of tests based on the analysis of expired air in nutritional studies. Arch Latinoam. Nutr. 28:301-17, 1978.

malabsorption. Indeed, Vernier and co-workers in Italy found **68%** of 230 patients with a suggested diagnosis of IBS had lactose malabsorption which was relieved in most cases by dietary control.

Bond and Levitt, in 1978,[61,62] used breath-H_2 to indicate that some disaccharides (complex sugars) were not broken down (hydrolyzed) and absorbed in the small intestine during the digestion of foods. It was based on evidence that the disaccharides reached the colon intact, resulting in a change in the H_2 in expired air after the sugar was ingested. The most prominent clinical application of the test was for the diagnosis of lactose malabsorption or lactose intolerance.

At the DaVinci Natural Health Centre we use the MicroH2 breath hydrogen test (BHT) by Micromedical[63] to measure changes in the hydrogen concentration of the breath formed by bacterial metabolism of unabsorbed lactose in the colon. It is a simple, accurate, and sensitive indirect test for lactase deficiency in adults.

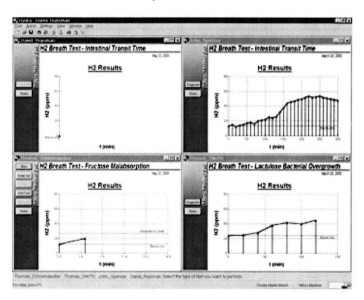

Results from H2 Monitor

61 Bond JH, Jr, Levitt MD. Use of pulmonary hydrogen (H_2) measurements to quantitate carbohydrate absorption. Study of partially gastrectomized patients. *J Clin Invest.* 51(5):1219–1225, May 1972..
62 Bond JH, Levitt MD. Quantitative measurement of lactose absorption. *Gastroenterology.* 70(6):1058–1062, June 1976.
63 http://www.micromedical.co.uk/update/download.asp

Final comments on the IDEL diagnostic methodology

I utilise the above diagnostic methodology with all my seriously ill patients. It takes me around 5 hours to complete all the tests so I normally spend a whole morning with just one patient. It is a different modus operandi compared to the 10-15 minutes the average medic spends with a patient these days, but there is no way of getting to the root causes of patient's problems without thorough investigation.

This testing methodology provides me with crucial information on the state of vitality of my patients, their inherent strengths and weaknesses, their degree of systemic as well as specific degeneration of organ systems and tissues as well as their capacity to undergo potential treatment programmes. Also understanding the person's psychosynthesis and their Spiritual path in life and what traumas they have experienced are important factors that can cause or maintain disease processes.

Once the information is collated within a few days, I proceed with designing a bespoke treatment plan for the patient. This way, treatment protocols are always designed to the needs of individual patients and are dynamically adjusted according to progress made and follow up testing.

I proceed now to explain in more detail the main therapeutic pillars I utilise in clinical practice in order to reverse diseases that are generally considered as incurable. The next Chapter is devoted to Nutrition and Nutritional Therapy. I elected to begin with Nutrition as I consider it as the axis of our health.

Chapter 4

Detoxification: The Essence of Life

We are all toxic

In Chapter one I talked about the importance of detoxification with regard to regaining my health. As a consequence of my healing journey and new-found health, I have developed a number of detoxification protocols which I am now implementing with hundreds of my patients every year at the DaVinci Natural Health Centre in Cyprus.

I am absolutely certain that the topic of detoxification will one day become a true science, with all the biochemical pathways mapped out of how the body cleanses itself when the detox protocols mentioned here are used. Do not underestimate the power of these simple protocols – as a clinician I have seen miraculous changes in many chronically ill patients after detoxifying. In fact, there is an academically oriented clinical course entitled "Toxicology and Detoxification" that has been written for the Bachelor and Doctor of Science in Holistic Medicine.[1]

So how do you know that you are toxic? Do you suffer from tiredness, lethargy, a 'heavy' feeling, digestive problems, bowel distension, headaches, muscle aches, poor concentration and memory, insomnia and many other symptoms too numerous to list? Well all these symptoms can be related to toxins in your body that have accumulated over time. But what are toxins exactly?

A toxin is defined as any compound that has a detrimental effect on cell function or structure. Strictly speaking, scientists differentiate between a "toxin" and a "toxicant" – a toxin is anything that the body produces that is harmful, whereas a toxicant is any chemical that enters the body from the outside.

The topic of toxicology is a very large and complicated one – this is only a very brief introduction for purposes of familiarity – there will be more said on the specific toxins and their effect on health in Chapter 7 entitled: Killing Ourselves With Toxic Chemicals.

---

[1] www.collegenaturalmedicine.com

For the sake of avoiding confusion, this differentiation will not be used here, and toxicants as well as toxins will be grouped into "toxins" which is a more familiar expression to all. Whether a toxin actually causes harm in a particular situation is based on a multiplicity of factors such as: potency (acute toxicity being the strongest), rate of exposure, dose and individual sensitivity. Toxins can cause a variety of harmful effects ranging from cancer (carcinogen) to upset stomachs, to learning and developmental disorders. The table below shows some common signs and symptoms of toxicity:

Headaches	Backache	Runny nose	Fatigue
Joint pains	Itchy nose	Nervousness	Skin rashes
Cough	Frequent colds	Sleepiness	Hives
Wheezing	Irritated eyes	Insomnia	Nausea
Sore throat	Immune weakness	Dizziness	Indigestion
Tight or stiff neck	Environmental sensitivity	Mood changes	Anorexia
Angina Pectoris	Sinus congestion	Anxiety	Bad breath
Circulatory deficits	Fever	Depression	Constipation
High blood fats	Unexplained irritability	Chronic fatigue	Muscle twitching

Signs and Symptoms of Toxicity

Life is toxic! There are toxins in the food you eat, the water you drink and the air you breathe. Even your own body produces toxins as a result of its many metabolic processes that keep you alive.

Signs that detoxification is needed if you have:

- ❖ Unexplained headaches or back pain
- ❖ Joint pain or arthritis
- ❖ Memory failure
- ❖ Depression or lack of energy
- ❖ Brittle nails and hair
- ❖ Abnormal body odour, coated tongue or bad breath
- ❖ Unexplained weight gain
- ❖ Psoriasis

❖ Frequent allergies
❖ A history of heavy alcohol use
❖ A history of natural and synthetic steroid hormone use
❖ An exposure to cleaning solvents, pesticides, diuretics and certain drugs.

Benefits of detoxification

There are a number of benefits of detoxification such as:

❖ The digestive tract is cleansed of accumulated waste and fermenting bacteria.
❖ Liver, kidney and blood purification can take place, which is not possible during regular eating patterns.
❖ Mental clarity is enhanced as chemical and food additive overload is reduced.
❖ Reduced dependency on habit forming substances such as sugar, caffeine, nicotine, alcohol and drugs.
❖ The stomach size is returned to normal as bad eating habits can be stopped.
❖ The hormonal system is enhanced which is especially true for growth hormones.
❖ The immune system is stimulated.

It never ceases to amaze me that most of these symptoms, if not all, can disappear in less than 15 days! After detoxifying on an alkaline diet for 15 days, patients report high energy levels, clear and glowing skin with a brilliance that is obvious (I have said on many occasions that I should take before-detox and after-detox photos of patients as the change is striking), weight loss of several pounds, which is an excellent motivating factor to continue with a detox programme, clear-headedness, higher thresholds for stress and tension, reduced cellulite, good body tone and a great feeling of being relaxed.

'How can you achieve this?' you may ask. Well, the secret is in using a variety of detoxification protocols, which I will share with you below. Detoxification has become a household word and a colloquialism that could mean anything from drinking a glass of carrot juice to entering a detoxification centre if you are an alcoholic or drug addict. The term has now become a misnomer for many things that it is not. In the context that we are using the term, detoxification is the process of removing the toxins that have been accumulating in the body tissues and organs throughout a person's life. These toxins will have been acting as metabolism blockers by literally poisoning the cells and not allowing them to function correctly.

Sources of toxins

So where do toxins come from? There are many sources, some of which I will mention here.

The three main sources are:

a) Exogenous toxins:

Exogenous toxins (Greek: 'from outside') are those that enter our bodies from the outside, i.e. food additives, pesticides, herbicides, fungi from food, industrial pollutants, viruses, bacteria, parasites and electromagnetic pollution such as X-rays, electromagnetic radiation and geopathic stress. These external toxins may also come from other sources such as water, beverages, alcohol, medicines, accidents and injuries. Various industries have polluted our environment with an array of toxic heavy metals such as aluminium, antimony, arsenic, beryllium, bismuth, cadmium, lead, mercury, nickel, thallium and uranium.

b) Endogenous toxins:

Endogenous means (Greek: 'from within') – these are toxins that are found or generated within the human body – this can occur when the body's normal metabolic mechanisms function inefficiently. For example, it typically takes several steps to convert the amino acid methionine into cysteine. If one step is sluggish, an intermediate called homocysteine accumulates in tissues. Accumulation of homocysteine can damage the vascular system and contribute to heart disease.[2] Other toxins can be associated with tuberculosis, syphilis or other diseases due to microbes; excess hormone secretions; constipation: producing toxins in the gut; pathogenic bacteria: causing food to putrefy and produce toxins in the gut;[3] and emotional stress can be a large contributor of toxins in the body.

---

[2] Graham, I, Daly, L, Refsum H, et al. Plasma homocysteine as a risk factor for vascular disease. *JAMA*. 277;1775-1781, 1997.
[3] Donovan P. Bowel toxemia, permeability and disease: new information to support an old

The human intestine also contains at least 50 genera of bacteria comprised of nearly 400 species. There are roughly 10^{12} of gut bacteria for every gram of gut content. The rich diversity of intestinal microbes originates when a newborn is inoculated with the mother's vaginal and faecal flora during birth.

These bacteria in the gut constitute a continuous source of gut-derived metabolites that will reach the systemic circulation. The term *dysbiosis* refers to a state of imbalance in the beneficial organisms in the colon.[4] Among the organisms that may be associated with dysbiosis are:[5] Klebsiella pneumoniae, Citrobacter freundii, Bacteriodes fragilis, Proteus vulgaris, Enterogtoxigenic Escherichia coli, Clostridium dificile, Camplylobacter jejunii, Candida albicans, Candida tropicalis, Geotrichum spp.

The metabolites that may be associated with microbial overgrowth of the bowel may include:[6] Arabinose, Benzoate, Hippurate, p-Hydroxybenzoate, p-Hydroxyphenylacetate, p-Hydroxyphenyllactate, beta-Ketoglutarate, Hydrocaffeate, Tartarate and Citramalate.

c) Autogenous toxins:

Autogenous toxins (Greek: 'Born within') are generated within the body from miasmic influences, which are inherited tendencies that can pass through up to seven generations. Examples of these are psora, sycosis, tuberculosis, syphilinum and others. There is no detection of these pathogens on scientific testing, but their deep presence can affect the body's organs primarily by inhibiting a good immune response and lowering its resistance.

Let's look at some specific sources of toxins that we encounter daily:

---

concept. In: Pizzorno JE, Murray MT. Textbook of Natural Medicine. St. Louis, MO: Elsevier Ltd; 1993.

[4] Hawrelak JA, Myers SP. The causes of intestinal dysbiosis: A review. *Alt Med Rev.* 9(2):180-197, Jun 2004.

[5] Backhed F, Ley RE, Sonnenburg JL, Peterson DA, Gordon JI. Host-bacterial mutualism in the human intestine. *Science* 307(5717):1915-1920, 2005.

[6] Catanzaro JA, Green L. Microbial ecology and dysbiosis in human medicine. Alt Med Rev. 1997;2(3):202-209.

Cigarettes, alcohol, caffeine and drugs are all substances that the body cannot use for building and repair, so will add to the mounting waste. A lot of these toxic wastes are stored in the tissues and organs of the body.

Heavy metals such as mercury from fish and amalgam fillings; aluminium found in cheeses, baking powders, cake mixes, self-raising flour, cosmetics, toothpastes, antiperspirants and some drugs such as antacids. Arsenic is given to chickens as a growth promoter; cadmium is found in tea and coffee, as well as cigarette smokers. Lead is found in paints, fuels, rubber, plastics, inks, dyes, toys, building materials and hair restorers.

Roxarsone - 4-hydroxy-3-nitrobenzenearsonic acid - is by far the most common arsenic-based additive used in chicken feed.[7] It is mixed in the diet of about 70% of the 9 billion broiler chickens produced annually in the U.S. In its original organic form, roxarsone is relatively benign. It is less toxic than the inorganic forms of arsenic-arsenite [As(III)] and arsenate [As(V)]. However, some of the 2.2 million lb of roxarsone mixed in the nation's chicken feed each year converts into inorganic arsenic within the bird, and the rest is transformed into inorganic forms after the bird excretes it. Arsenic has been linked to bladder, lung, skin, kidney and colon cancer, while low-level exposures can lead to partial paralysis and diabetes.

Pesticides from the vegetables that we eat, heavy metals such as mercury from amalgam fillings and fish products, cadmium from smoking, lead and arsenic from pollution and much more.

Plastics containing Bisphenol A, the building block of polycarbonate plastics, which are everywhere – in pesticides as fungicides; antioxidants, flame retardants, rubber chemicals, a coating in metals, cans and food containers; refrigerator shelving, returnable containers for juice, milk and water; nail polish, compact discs, adhesives, microwave ovenware and eating utensils.

A diet that is high in animal fats will add to the waste. There are many different drugs and chemicals that are given to animals these days, ranging from antibiotics, hormones, feed concentrates, etc. All these chemicals will

---

[7] Hileman, B. Arsenic in Chicken Production: A common feed additive adds arsenic to human food and endangers water supplies. *Chemical and Engineering News*. Volume 85, Number 15, pp. 34-35, April 9, 2007.

accumulate in the fat cells of the animals that we then eat – so we slowly build up an accumulation of these chemicals over time.

Sluggish bowels can lead to a great deal of toxicity throughout the body. Try to imagine a 10 metre tube running from mouth to anus packed with meat, sausage, fish, fruit salad, beef burgers, sugars, milk and other goodies – all fermenting and putrefying for days on end. This fermentation produces highly toxic substances such as putrescine, neuracine, cadaverine – these are so poisonous that a small amount injected into a laboratory animal will kill it in minutes. All these toxic substances, apart from causing disease processes in the body, will also act as metabolism blockers, and will therefore have consequences on weight-loss too. This process of 'self-poisoning' by these putrefying foods in the gut is called 'autointoxication.'

Food additives and preservatives, of which there are thousands being used. Not only do these block metabolism, but many are also carcinogens.

Refined foods such as white sugar, white flour, white rice, etc. All these foods are deficient in nutrients, but calorie loaded. Apart from this, they also help to create a lot of sludge and debris in the body. If you remember from your childhood days, you probably used white flour and water to make a glue to make your kite, or to glue your coloured paper in your exercise book at school. White flour and its products when eaten, becomes glue in the intestine and sticks to the internal wall. When mixed with sticky sugar and fat, it becomes a rubber-like substance that blocks absorption of foods through the intestine, as well as being a constant source of toxins. If you don't believe me, read Dr. Jensen's book entitled 'Tissue cleansing through bowel management'[8] – there are also plenty of photos of what actually comes out of the intestine if you do a proper detox – disgusting!

Thousands of new, toxic chemical compounds are produced each year by the chemical industry, most of which are approved by various so-called 'Environmental Protection Agencies' (EPA's) without any serious toxicological studies. The cumulative number of toxic chemicals polluting our planet today exceeds 100,000.

---

[8] Jensen, B. Dr. Jensen's guide to better bowel care: A complete program for tissue cleansing through bowel management. USA: Avery Publishers, 1999.

Many claim that some of these chemicals, such as the flame retardants used in children's clothing, have potentially life-saving applications. But how many of these chemicals do we ingest or are absorbed by our bodies and those of our children? – And at what cost to our health? What is the capacity of the human body to eliminate them? Has anyone conducted a general contracting cost-benefit analysis as to whether the benefits offered, for example, by fire hazard protection, truly outweigh the toxicity generated within us, our children and the environment? The answer is: no. There are no comprehensive, scientific answers, other than to confirm the obvious: toxicity levels in humans and animals across the globe are rising fast. Whether we realize it or not – we are all toxic.

In an article published in the October 2006 *National Geographic* entitled, 'The pollution within,' journalist David Ewing Duncan had himself tested for 320 synthetic chemicals and certain heavy metals at a cost of $16,000, paid for by the magazine. According to the article, Duncan was considered a healthy individual. Nevertheless, he had higher than average amounts of chemical toxins, such as flame-retardants (known as PDBE's), phthalates, Polychlorinated Biphenyls (PCBs), pesticides and dioxins, as well as heavy metals such as mercury.

Duncan's article alludes to some of the possible ways toxic chemicals may have accumulated in his body: some might have originated in childhood, while others may have been picked up in airplanes due to his extensive work-related travel – however, in this, he and his doctors were merely speculating. Duncan also describes his pre and post-mercury toxicity results after a fresh fish dinner and breakfast. Duncan had fresh halibut for dinner and fresh swordfish for breakfast, (cooked in his toxic non-stick pan), both of which were caught in the ocean just outside the Golden Gate Bridge in the San Francisco Bay area.

He tested himself for serum mercury before and after the meals, and found that his blood mercury levels had shot up from five micrograms per litre to over 12. The doctors conducting the tests advised him not to repeat that experiment ever again, yet I'm sure this dangerous diet is adhered to by thousands, unaware of the impact of toxicity on their health – after all, fish is promoted as a health food. Nevertheless, drawing conclusions on the experience of only one healthy adult is not robust, toxicological science. So let us review the research.

It is difficult to fathom how we can live in houses that make us sick, but the term "sick building syndrome" (SBS),[9] first employed in the 1970s, describes a situation in which reported symptoms among a population of building occupants can be temporally associated with their presence in that building. Typically, though not always, the structure is an office building.

Typical complaints may include eye and/or nasopharyngeal irritation, rhinitis or nasal congestion, inability to concentrate, and general malaise-complaints suggestive of a host of common ailments, some ubiquitous and easily communicable. The key factors are commonality of symptoms and absence of symptoms among building occupants when the individuals are not in the building.

There has been extensive speculation about the cause or causes of SBS. Poor design, maintenance, and/or operation of the structure's ventilation system may be at fault. The ventilation system itself can be a source of irritants. Interior redesign, such as the rearrangement of offices or installation of partitions, may also interfere with efficient functioning of such systems. Low levels of specific pollutants found in new furniture, carpeting and other furniture and fittings may also be one of the causes.

A 1984 World Health Organization report suggested that as many as 30 percent of new and remodeled buildings worldwide may generate excessive complaints related to indoor air quality.[10]

In a nationwide, random sampling of U.S. office workers, 24 percent perceived air quality problems in their work environments, and 20 percent believed their work performance was hampered thereby.[11]

Toxic from birth

In September 2005, Greenpeace International, in tandem with the World Wildlife Fund, published a document entitled, 'A Present for Life: Hazardous chemicals in umbilical cord blood.'[12] The research showed

---

9 Burge, S. et al. Sick Building Syndrome: A Study of 4373 Office Workers. *Ann. Occupational Hygiene*. 31: 493-504, 1987.

10 U.S. Environmental Protection Agency, Office of Air and Radiation. Indoor Air Facts No. 4: Sick Building Syndrome. revised, 1991.

11 Kreiss, K. The Sick Building Syndrome: Where Is the Epidemiologic Basis? *American Journal of Public Health* 1990; 80:1172-73.

12 Schuiling, J., van der Naald, W. A Present for Life: Hazardous chemicals in umbilical

convincingly that newborns tested for hundreds of different xenobiotics[13] showed high levels of these toxins. Specifically, the blood tests demonstrated that these infants had an average of 287 toxins in their bodies – 180 of these, known carcinogens. Some of these chemicals included the commonly-used artificial musk HHCB, which was found in almost all blood samples and at higher levels than the other artificial musks. Musk ambrette, a chemical banned from use in cosmetics in the EU since 1995, was still found in 15 maternal and 12 cord blood samples.

Other banned alkylphenol compounds, extensively used in industrial cleaning agents, were also found. Additionally, the study quantified the antibacterial agent triclosan in human blood, and it was found in almost 50% of the samples. DDT, the notorious pesticide banned from agricultural use worldwide, was found in all blood samples. Similarly, the organochlorine by-product and pesticide hexachlorobenzene – also subject to a global ban – was found in the samples. Perfluorinated compounds like PFOS and PFOA, used to make non-stick pans and water-repelling coatings, were present in all but one maternal sample. PFOS was detected in all cord blood samples and PFOA in half of them.

Another US-based study, 'Baby care products: possible sources of infant phthalate exposure,' published in *Paediatrics*, February 2008,[14] concluded that phthalate toxicity is widespread in infants. Babies coming into contact with lotions, powders and shampoos had increased urinary concentrations of phthalates, in direct proportion to the number of products they had been exposed to. This association was strongest in young infants, who are more vulnerable to the developmental and reproductive toxicity of phthalates, given their immature metabolic capability and increased dosage per unit of body surface area. Thus, babies become heavily polluted with toxic and carcinogenic substances by their unsuspecting, well-meaning parents. Essentially, we are unwittingly poisoning our own children.

One could argue that these studies conducted in the United States – where the toxicity levels are perhaps higher than in other countries – exaggerate

---

cord blood. Greenpeace International and WWF-UK, Sept. 2005.

13 A xenobiotic is an artificial or natural substance found in an organism that simply should not be present. The term covers chemicals, medical drugs, naturally occurring heavy metals and all the pollutants released into the environment from human activity.

14 Sathyanarayana, S. Karr, CJ., Lozano, P., Brown, E., Calafat, AM., Liu, F., and Swan, SH. Baby Care Products: Possible Sources of Infant Phthalate Exposure. *Pediatrics*, Vol. 121 No. 2, pp. e260-e268, Feb 2008.

the problem. Perhaps in poorer parts of the world, parents use fewer of the culprit infant lotions and powders, or do without them. Yet, does general environmental toxicity have boundaries?

To address this question, let's examine a similar study conducted on pregnant women living well within the Arctic Circle, which most people feel is a pristine part of the earth. The research was published as an article in *The Science of the Total Environment* entitled, 'Organochlorines and heavy metals in pregnant women from the Disko Bay area in Greenland.'[15] The study showed high concentrations of heavy metals, such as mercury, and organochlorines in the blood and fatty tissue of the Inuit population. This was attributed to their high consumption of the meat and blubber of marine mammals, which are clearly toxic.

In this study, 180 pregnant women and 178 newborn babies were sampled, amounting to 36% of the total number of births in the Disko Bay area during 1994–1996. So, the main food supply of the native population in Greenland, that is, marine mammals, is heavily toxic. It is therefore obvious that pollution has no boundaries. While not within the scope of this book, the fact that the Inuits were unlikely to have been the main polluters of their coastal waters raises serious additional questions of global ethics, politics and economics.

A further study published in the journal *Environmental Research* has shown there is a correlation between the levels of methylmercury in a pregnant or lactating woman's blood and urine and that of her yet-to-be-born or newborn baby, with toxins passing from the mother to the foetus through the placenta. There has since been much research indicating the grave effects on the health of children of high mercury levels, for instance, autism and developmental delays.

The University of Cincinnati published a study in February 2008, entitled: 'Plastic bottles release potentially harmful chemicals (Bisphenol A or BPA) after contact with hot liquids.' BPA is another synthetic chemical classified as an endocrine disruptor, widely used in plastics. The study concluded that the most important factor regarding exposure to BPA from plastic bottles is not whether the container is new or old. Rather, it is the temperature of the liquid contained, that is crucial to the amount of BPA

---

15 Bjerregaard, P., and Hansen, JC. Organochlorines and heavy metals in pregnant women from the Disko Bay area in Greenland. The Science of the Total Environment 245, 2000.

that is released. Hot liquids such as tea, coffee or milk increase the release of BPA up to 55 times! Other similar studies have shown that if you repeatedly scrub, dish-wash, and boil polycarbonate baby bottles, these also release significant amounts of BPA.

BPA is widely used in products such as reusable water bottles, tin linings, water pipes, dental sealants and baby bottles, and has been shown to affect reproduction and brain development. Consider a baby bottle – it is supposed to be scrubbed clean and steam sterilized before a hot liquid, such as formula milk, is poured into it and left to cool ahead of feeding a baby. The whole procedure amounts to unintentional infant poisoning! Will these infants be given the chance to naturally detoxify themselves into adulthood? The evidence indicates that this is not the case.

Today in 2009 as I write, there are moves by manufacturers, retailers and regulatory agencies, who are considering eliminating the chemical bisphenol-A (BPA) from sports bottles and baby bottles. Wal-Mart Canada announced that it would immediately stop selling baby bottles, sippy cups, pacifiers, food containers and water bottles that contain BPA and Canada's Ministry of Health declared that the Canadian government is taking action to reduce BPA exposure, especially in newborns and infants.

Mercury is a well-established, cumulative neurotoxic agent that can have serious adverse effects on the development and functioning of the human central nervous system, especially when exposure occurs prenatally.[16] Given the potential threat that methyl mercury poses to the optimal development of cognitive function, clinicians and regulatory agencies are concerned about the levels of methyl mercury that a pregnant women regularly ingests, and the levels organic mercury in diets, especially from fish containing methylmercury, which is a major source of mercury exposure to the general population. While cases in which treatment with dental amalgam resulting in elevated the blood mercury concentration have been reported, other clinicians have indicated this is not the case.[17] Therefore, this issue remains controversial.

---

16 Methylmercury. Geneva: World Health Organization; Environment Health Criteria 101, 1990.
17 Behrman RE, Kliegman R, Jenson HB. Nelson Textbook of Pediatrics. 17th ed. Elsevier Science Saunders; 2004. Heavy metal intoxification; pp. 702–703.

In one study conducted by a Korean research group[18] they showed that the amount of mercury (from eating fish) in the mother's blood correlated with levels found in cord blood. Blood mercury level in the group who ate fish more than four times per month was significantly higher than that of the group who did not consume fish ($p = 0.02$). In follow-up studies, blood mercury levels were decreased in the study group but slightly increased in the control group ($p = 0.014$). The maternal blood mercury level in late pregnancy was positively correlated with mercury levels of cord blood ($r = 0.58$, $p = 0.047$), which was almost twice the level found in maternal blood. Pregnant women who consume a large amount of fish may have high blood mercury levels. Further, cord blood mercury levels were much higher than that of maternal blood.

North Americans are also toxic

In July 2005, the US Department of Health and Human Services, Centers for Disease Control and Prevention, published a 475-page document entitled, 'Third national report on human exposure to environmental chemicals,'[19] which clearly indicates the growing number of chemical toxins present in all age groups in North America.

A Canada-based study has also compared heavy metal intake in different age groups and their corresponding intake guidelines. The report: 'Metallic lunch: an analysis of heavy metals in the Canadian diet,'[20] shows that Canadians young and old are ingesting unhealthy levels of toxic substances, such as cadmium and lead. In addition, Canadian children are also being exposed to potentially unsafe levels of copper, manganese, molybdenum and nickel.

Another study, 'Human health implications of environmental contaminants in Arctic Canada: A review,'[21] published in *The Science of the Total*

---

18 Kim, EH., Kim, IK., Kwon, JY., Kim, SW., and Park, YW. The Effect of Fish Consumption on Blood Mercury Levels of Pregnant Women. *Yonsei Med J.* 31; 47(5): 626–633, Oct 2006.
19 A full colour report can be downloaded from
http://www.cdc.gov/exposurereport/pdf/thirdreport.pdf
20 Download the full report at
http://www.environmentaldefence.ca/reports/Metallic%20Lunch%20Report_final.pdf
21 Van Oostdam J, Donaldson SG, Feeley M, Arnold D, Ayotte P, Bondy G, Chan L, Dewaily E, Furgal CM, Kuhnlein H, Loring E, Muckle G, Myles E, Receveur O, Tracy B, Gill U, Kalhok S. Human health implications of environmental contaminants in Arctic Canada: A review. Sci Total Environ. 1;351-352:165-246, Dec 2005.

Environment has found extensive toxicity in the Inuits to chemicals such as chlordane and toxaphene pesticides, as well as PCB's. Toxicologists studying the impact of chemicals on health usually have a reference range of values which indicate the 'safe levels' of these chemicals. New research is showing, however, that even low-dose exposure is cumulative over time and can lead to decreased performance in areas of motor function and memory among children. Similarly, disruption of attention, fine motor skills and verbal memory, is also observed in adults exposed to low mercury levels.

Europeans of all age groups are toxic

A study conducted by the World Wildlife Fund set out to explore whether there was any link between the types and levels of contamination found in three generations of families, and to examine possible links between contamination and a family's lifestyle, consumption patterns and use of everyday products. The study entitled, 'Contamination: the next generation - Results of the family chemical contamination survey,'[22] summarizes the findings of an analysis of 104 different chemicals in the blood of 33 volunteers from 7 families living in England, Scotland, and Wales. The volunteers in each family spanned 3 generations, comprising a grandmother, mother, and 2 children. In all, 14 children, 13 adults, and 6 grandmothers took part in the study. The ages of the volunteers ranged from 9 to 88. On analyzing the results, all 3 generations, including the children, were shown to be contaminated by a cocktail of hazardous artificial chemicals, some of them everyday domestic products. Every child carried in his or her body the same range of toxic substances: organochlorine pesticides, PCB's, brominated flame-retardants, phthalates and perfluorinated ('non-stick') chemicals. Five such substances found in each parent and grandparent, were also found in every child.

While it might be expected that the chemical load increases with age, the study demonstrated that this is not always true. Children can be more contaminated by higher numbers and levels of certain newer chemicals than their parents or even their grandparents, despite being exposed to these chemicals for only a fraction of the time.

---

22 WWF-UK. Contamination: the next generation. Results of the family chemical contamination survey. October 2004.

Another interesting report compiled by the World Wildlife Fund – UK (2005): 'Still dirty: a review of action against toxic products in Europe,' highlights the occurrence of hazardous chemicals in everyday products and notes which EU member states have taken measures to help protect their citizens and wildlife. One of the report's observations is that phthalates used in plastics and cosmetics have been linked to reduced sperm counts. The report also documents that lead is still in use in the EU, despite its proven toxicity to children and wildlife.

Other chemicals found, such as alkyl phenols and alkyl phenol ethoxylates – industrial chemicals used in plastics, pesticides, and detergents – are toxic and mimic the female hormone oestrogen, causing feminization of male fish. Brominated flame-retardants, persistent chemicals widely used in electronic equipment, fabrics and plastics, are now found in human breast milk and wildlife, even in remote areas.

Cosmetics beautify but they also poison

Are hair dyes worth perishing for? Is your lipstick making you sick? What about beauty creams and other cosmetics? Over 50% of women of all ages colour their hair. Men increasingly dye their hair, too. Research shows a connection between the use of commercial hair dyes and various diseases, including cancer.[23] Newer studies state that because of the prevalence of hair dye use, further studies are necessary to address the effects of specific colours and types of hair dyes with the possible role of individual susceptibility. So, are you susceptible?

I have seen and tested a number of patients who were suffering from many serious, inexplicable, symptoms whose doctors were mystified as to the reasons for their deteriorating health. One 34 year old lady came up really high on tin toxicity, with all the accompanying symptoms – skin rash, stomach complaints, nausea, vomiting, diarrhoea, abdominal pain, headaches and palpitations. As she was not eating anything from tin cans, she investigated and found it in her lipstick. Stannous fluoride or tin fluoride is also found in some toothpastes.

---

23 Ames, BN, Kammen, HO and Yamasaki, E. Hair dyes are mutagenic: identification of a variety of mutagenic ingredients, 1975. See also Watanabe T, Hirayama T, Fukui S, Mutagenicity of commercial hair dyes and detection of 2,7-diaminophenazine, Kyoto Pharmaceutical University, Japan, 1990.

Independent laboratory testing initiated by the 'Campaign for Safe Cosmetics' in 2007, found that lipsticks from top brands contain lead also. Two-thirds of the 33 cosmetics samples tested contained detectable levels of lead.[24] It was lucky that this lady's lipstick only contained tin, which was eliminated using the heavy metal detox agent HMD[®3].

Almost all cosmetics can cause allergic reactions in certain individuals. Nearly one quarter of the people questioned in the FDA's 1994 cosmetics survey responded 'Yes' to having suffered an allergic reaction to personal care products including moisturizers, foundations, and eye shadows. In book: 'Drop dead gorgeous: protecting yourself from the hidden dangers of cosmetics,'[25] Kim Erickson, with a forward by Dr Samuel Epstein, reveals how manufacturers exploit loopholes in legislation designed to protect the public. So, cosmetic users: beware.[26]

Given that just about everything you put on your skin gets absorbed into your bloodstream, it is interesting that there is such a lack of regulation of carcinogenic ingredients in skin care products. There are over 150 toxic, cancer-causing ingredients currently used in cosmetic products alone. Sunscreens are particularly suspect given that they are recommended, without serious research, as cancer prevention products, whereas in fact they contain many chemicals that actually promote cancer. Another book worth reading that describes the consequences of many of these chemicals on cosmetics is Judi Vance's book entitled: "Beauty to Die For: The Cosmetic Consequnce.[27]

Mercury is everywhere

One of the causative factors that led to my health saga (which I discussed in chapter one), was the extraction of over 10 mercury amalgam fillings, a number of years back. My Holistic dentist and I at the time were not so knowledgeable, and we proceeded to remove all the amalgams as quickly as possible. THIS IS A CRITICAL MISTAKE! Notice that this is

---

24 For more details see: http://www.safecosmetics.org
3 See www.detoxmetals.com
25 Erickson, K. Drop-Dead Gorgeous: Protecting Yourself from the Hidden Dangers of Cosmetics, McGraw Hill, 2002.
26 In response to the toxic onslaught from cosmetics, the Environmental Working Group began an initiative to register the fairly safe cosmetics, which can be accessed at: http://www.cosmeticdatabase.com.
27 Vance, J. Beauty to Die For: The Cosmetic Consequence. USA: iuniverse.com, 1999.

CAPITALIZED! Removing mercury amalgams quickly, particularly when not using a chelation protocol to remove the mercury released is the best way of making you so toxic with mercury that the chances of developing a chronic disorder such as cancer and multiple sclerosis increases exponentially. After poisoning my own self out of ignorance of these phenomenons, I have consequently spent many years studying and developing natural products for detoxification that also work for mercury – one of the products is the above mentioned HMD®, for which I have a world-wide patent-pending, but this will be discussed in more depth in Chapter 7.

Mercury in amalgam fillings

Mercury used in amalgam tooth fillings remains a big issue of dispute. Amalgam was found to be a cheap and long-lasting substance to fill teeth with, but the danger of mercury poisoning was overlooked or ignored. The use of amalgams is now prohibited in many countries. Norway recently announced a ban on the use of mercury, including dental amalgam, that took effect on January 1, 2008. Sweden announced a similar ban and dentists in Denmark will no longer be allowed to use mercury in fillings after April 1, 2008.[28]

The biomedical literature contains numerous articles on the adverse health impact before as well as after amalgam removal. The International Academy of Oral Medicine and Toxicology[29] has even produced video evidence showing mercury vapour released from amalgam fillings, even though they may be over 30 years old.

Chewing gum, drinking hot beverages, brushing teeth and dental polishing increase the methyl mercury released from amalgam fillings.[30] If you doubt how lethal mercury can be, particularly for the nervous system and the brain, a video produced by the University of Calgary Faculty of Medicine, entitled 'How mercury causes brain neuron degeneration'[31] may persuade you. It clearly shows how mercury degrades neural fibres in a petri dish in zero time. Despite all this damning evidence, in the USA

---

28 www.mercurypolicy.org
29 www.iaomt.org
30 Gebel T, Dunkelberg H. Influence of chewing gum consumption and dental contact of amalgam fillings to different metal restorations on urine mercury content. Zentralbl Hyg Umweltmed. 199(1):69-75, Nov 1996.
31 http://commons.ucalgary.ca/mercury

alone, around 180 million mercury amalgams are placed in peoples' mouths every year.

Before we leave the topic of mercury amalgams, I would like to broadcast a loud warning AGAIN to all those reading this – PLEASE DO NOT REMOVE YOUR AMALGAMS UNLESS YOU ARE FOLLOWING AN ADEQUATE CHELATING PROTOCOL!! There is research which clearly shows that once the dentist's drill is on the amalgams, there are huge mercury deposits released into the blood and faeces – up to 100 times the initial level before the dentist starts working on your amalgams.[32]

Mercury in vaccines

Many vaccines and inoculations use Thimerosal as a preservative. Following a 1999 recommendation in the US, this is generally being phased out, though it remains in use in several countries. Thimerosol contains around 50% toxic mercury; often being linked to autism. There is an interesting article published in *Medical Hypotheses*, 'Autism: a novel form of mercury poisoning,'[33] showing how exposure to mercury can cause immune, sensory, neurological, motor and behavioural dysfunctions, similar to traits defining or associated with autism. The authors of this paper conclude: "A review of medical literature and US government data suggests that: (i) many cases of idiopathic autism are induced by early mercury exposure from thimerosal; (ii) this type of autism represents an unrecognized mercurial syndrome; and (iii) genetic and non-genetic factors establish a predisposition whereby thimerosal's adverse effects occur only in some children."

The similarities extend to neuroanatomy, neurotransmitters and biochemistry. By the age of 10, a child may be many hundreds of times over what is considered a 'safe' dose of mercury poisoning from his injections. There is no safe dose of mercury.

There are a variety of chemicals that have been found in vaccinations such as:

---

32 Bjorkman, L, Sandborgh-Englund, G, Ekstrand, J: Mercury in saliva and faeces after removal of amalgam fillings. <u>Toxicol Appl Pharmacol</u> 144(1): 156-162, 1997.
33 Bernard, S., Enayati, A., Redwood, L., Roger, H., Binstock, T. Autism: a novel form of mercury poisoning. *Medical Hypotheses* 56(4), 462–471, 2001.

❖ Mercury - the heavy metal used in the disinfectant and preservative thimerosal, and known to cause brain injury, autism, attention deficit hyperactivity disorder (ADHD) and autoimmune diseases.

❖ Aluminium - a toxic metal additive used to promote antibody response, associated with Alzheimer's disease, brain damage, seizures and cancer.

❖ Formaldehyde - a preservative, as well as a nerve-damaging and cancer-causing agent.

❖ Ethylene glycol - (antifreeze).

❖ Monosodium glutamate (MSG) - a breakdown product of protein, and common flavour enhancer well known for poisoning brain cells.

❖ Sulphites - cause genetic damaging to some animals.

❖ Neomycin - an antibiotic, also previously registered for use in US pesticides, and known to cause reproductive and developmental harm such as birth defects, infertility, sterility and impairment of normal growth and development.

Servicemen and women who are subjected to many different injections during their tours of duty are at risk of toxic poisoning. Most fish are contaminated with mercury and other toxic substances, as the *National Geographic* reporter (mentioned above) easily discovered. Even polar bears living in the Arctic, thousands of miles from any industry, have been found in poor health and dying because of toxic poisoning.[34,35] No animal or human living on this planet earth is free from the risk of contamination.

Toxins accumulate in the body over time. Some people experience toxicity symptoms from birth, while others experience symptoms gradually. Children with autism, Attention Deficit Disorder and similar neurological problems are usually found to have high levels of mercury, which is thought to be a major contributory factor in these conditions. Disruptions of the endocrine system and other metabolic functions develop over time, leading to chronic disease – any known disease, including multiple sclerosis and cancer.

34 Brown, V. Toxic Chemicals: A Threat to Wildlife and Humans. WWF. December 2003.
35 WWF International Arctic Programme. The Tip of the Iceberg: Chemical Contamination in the Arctic. 2006.

Toxicity and the fertility threat

In 1992, a study in the *British Medical Journal* entitled 'Evidence for decreasing quality of semen during the past 50 years,'[36] reported that semen quality is seriously declining. In 1997, Dianne Dumanoski and others published a book entitled, 'Our stolen future: are we threatening our fertility, intelligence and survival?'[37] This groundbreaking book revealed that chemicals in the environment have affected human reproductive patterns in ways that may threaten the survival of the species. Yueliang Guo and others in 2000 published a study in the *Lancet*, 'Semen quality after prenatal exposure to polychlorinated biphenyls and dibenzofurans.'[38] The study reported that boys prenatally exposed to such chemicals have sperm with abnormal morphology, reduced motility and reduced strength. These results are consistent with studies on animals exposed in the womb to such toxic chemicals.

Another study entitled, 'Chlorinated pesticides and heavy metals in human semen,'[39] published in 2000, measured concentrations of chlorinated pesticides and heavy metals (lead and cadmium) respectively, in semen samples collected from men amongst the normal population in India. The study concluded that the presence of these xenobiotics in human semen relates to the use of pesticides, emission of exhaust from motor vehicles and industrial operations.

A 2006 study entitled, 'Persistent pesticides in human breast milk and cryptorchidism'[40] investigated a possible human association between maternal exposure to 27 organochlorine compounds used as pesticides and cryptorchidism among male children. The study concluded that the link between congenital cryptorchidism and certain persistent pesticides in breast milk, as a proxy for maternal exposure, suggests that testicular descent in the male foetus may be adversely affected.

---

36 Carlsen E, Giwercman A, Keiding N, Skakkebaek NE. Evidence for decreasing quality of semen during past 50 years. *BMJ.* 12;305(6854):609-13, Sept 1992.
37 Theo, C., Dumanoski, D., Myers, JP. Our stolen future: are we threatening our fertility, intelligence and survival? Penguin, USA: 1999.
38 Guo YL, Hsu PC, Hsu CC, Lambert GH. Semen quality after prenatal exposure to polychlorinated biphenyls and dibenzofurans. *Lancet.* 7;356(9237):1240-1, Oct 2000.
39 Kumar R; Pant N; Srivastava S P. Chlorinated pesticides and heavy metals in human semen. *International journal of andrology* 23(3):145-9, 2000.
40 Damgaard, IN., Skakkebæk, NE., Toppari, J., Virtanen, HE., Shen, H. Schramm, K., Petersen, JH., Jensen, TK., Main, KM. Persistent Pesticides in Human Breast Milk and Cryptorchidism. *Environmental Health Perspectives* Volume 114, Number 7, July 2006.

A similar study: 'Concentrations of persistent organochlorine compounds in human milk and placenta are higher in Denmark than in Finland' investigated why there was a significantly reduced male reproductive health status, including a higher prevalence of cryptorchidism and hypospadias in Danish men, as compared with Finnish men. Exposure to environmental pollutants with endocrine-disrupting abilities has been suggested as a possible explanation. The study[41] concluded that organochlorine levels were higher in Danish milk samples, suggesting a higher exposure for Danish boys as compared with their Scandinavian brethren.

The US Centers for Disease Control, in its report entitled 'Assisted reproductive technology ART surveillance – United States, 2004,'[42] published in June 2007 states that:

'Since 1978, assisted reproductive technology ART procedures have been used to overcome infertility. ART procedures include those infertility treatments in which both eggs and sperm are handled in the laboratory for the purpose of establishing a pregnancy (that is, in vitro fertilization [IVF] and related procedures). Since the birth of the first US infant conceived with ART in 1981, use of these treatments has increased dramatically. Each year, both the number of medical centers providing ART services and the total number of procedures performed have increased notably.'

There are, of course, other concurrent reasons for human reproductive decline, but the toxicity explanation is the most compelling. And yet, most of these women and men could reclaim their lost fertility simply by removing their toxins. It is a cheaper and less risky solution, and offers other health benefits as well – just think about it.

Regulatory agencies react slowly

Public health policy makers and regulatory agencies have been aware of the toxic mess for a long time now. The Swedish government, a pioneer in the public health policy field, banned mercury amalgam as a dental filling

---

[41] Damgaard IN, Skakkebaek NE, Toppari J, Virtanen HE, Shen H, Schramm KW, Petersen JH, Jensen TK, Main KM. Persistent pesticides in human breast milk and cryptorchidism. *Environ Health Perspect.* 114(7):1133-8, Jul 2006.
[42] Wright, VC., Chang, J., Jeng, G., Chen, M., Macaluso, M. Assisted reproductive technology ART surveillance – United States, 2004. *CDC Surveillance Summaries.* 56(SS06);1-22, June 2007.

material in 1994. The ban was based on research proving that the risks to dental patients' health and to the environment were serious. That same year, the German Federal Department of Health advised against using amalgam in all women of childbearing age, as there were great risks to the foetus. Recently, Norway banned the use of mercury totally as of January 2008.

Back in January 2005, the European Commission (EC) presented its Community Mercury Strategy, a comprehensive plan addressing mercury pollution regionally, as well as globally[43]. In the Strategy, the EC proposes further restrictions in the use of mercury, and an export ban for mercury from the EU. An important feature of the Strategy is support for, and promotion of, international actions to reduce global mercury supply, trade and demand. Strangely, this report does not go far enough on the use of dental mercury.

The US Food and Drug Administration (FDA) remain more complacent than its European counterparts about mercury and other toxicity issues. Regardless, even the FDA recommends those pregnant women and those who may become pregnant, avoid eating shark, swordfish, king mackerel and tile fish known to contain elevated mercury levels. Mercury accumulates in the food chain, so larger, longer-lived fish like the shark or swordfish contain the highest amounts of mercury and pose the greatest threat if eaten regularly.

The FDA also recommends the following fish as safe to eat: haddock, tilapia, wild Alaskan salmon and sole.[44] However, these are statistical averages. You cannot know the toxicity of the foods you eat unless you do individual testing. Sometimes, the toxins strike from where least expected: food, water, air, clothing, furniture, cosmetics, occupational exposure – and conventional dentistry and medicine are the prime suspects.

In January 2003, the European Union (EU) amended its cosmetics directive (76/768/EEC) to ban the use of chemicals known or strongly suspected of causing cancer, mutation or birth defects. The amendment went into force in September 2004 and bans carcinogens, reproductive toxins and mutagens from cosmetics. Companies are required to remove

---

43 Available at http://ec.europa.eu/environment/chemicals/mercury/mercury_strat.htm
44 www.fda.gov

these chemicals from cosmetic and personal care products sold in the EU. But don't be fooled that such Directives offer real protection.

RAPEX is the EU rapid alert system for all dangerous consumer products except food, medical devices, and pharmaceuticals. It allows for the rapid exchange of information between Member States and the Commission on measures taken to prevent or restrict the marketing or use of products posing a serious risk to the health and safety of consumers. Both measures ordered by national authorities and those undertaken voluntarily by producers and distributors are covered by RAPEX. Yet you will be amazed at the number of products being recalled because they violate even the most lax of the toxicity regulations.

The public health policy response to toxicity across the globe is too little, too late. The main reason for this is simple: these policies are influenced by powerful, industrial lobbies and other special interest groups. Human and environmental health carries a relative weight, and is always evaluated against apparently weightier considerations, such as corporate profits, donations to political parties and the overall focus by many governments on economic growth. Even if one does not want to take the cynical perspective, for every study showing a chemical's toxic impact on health, the industry produces a study claiming the opposite. Reading and interpreting science can be tricky these days. Even government agencies can be genuinely perplexed about what is valid and what is junk, or fraudulent science. Common sense and critical thinking are our last and only hope for survival. We cannot afford to be complacent if we wish to help ourselves and our families survive the toxic onslaught that we are bombarded with daily.

The toxic onslaught in a nutshell

The toxicological studies on pregnant and lactating women; infants, as well as young and old members of both genders, confirming that we are all toxic, are countless. How much more scientific evidence do we need, to be convinced of the obvious? The problem has been well identified. In a nutshell, it can be stated as follows: 'Even before we are born, we accumulate several toxins, which are passed on to us in the womb. After our birth, our bodies keep on accumulating and storing up all types of toxins. From the food we eat, the water we drink, the air we breathe and nearly everything we put in and on our bodies.

These include cigarettes, caffeine, medical drugs including over-the-counter drugs, alcohol, deodorants, shampoos, tap water, plastic-bottled water, plastic food containers, insecticides, pesticides, herbicides; ordinary food, junk food, fast food, processed food, gourmet food, 'Health' food; beauty creams, shaving creams; tin and lead-contaminated lipsticks; nickel ear/nose/nipple/etc rings; all artificial cleaning materials; swimming pools loaded with chemicals, dental mercury amalgams, other toxic dental restoration materials, root canals, dental implants and dentures; childhood vaccinations, adult vaccinations; food additives, flavour-enhancers, food preservatives, hormones, antibiotics and God only knows what else. We have converted our world into a toxic waste dump.'

Unfortunately, there is a lot of medical ignorance that could be exacerbating the situation. Despite the growing numbers of press reports linking chemicals with disease, and the increasing number of urgent warnings from scientists specializing in environmental medicine, the medical world appears to be oblivious to these warnings.

The problem begins in medical schools, as few doctors are taught about modern-day chemicals and their sources, let alone their health effects. Therefore during the taking of a medical history, the aspect of toxicity that often manifests itself in the patient's symptoms, and the reporting of it, are completely ignored. Maybe one of the reasons why none of this is taught in medical school is that there is no drug they can be given to remove these toxins and this is not good for the profits of the pharmaceutical companies who have a strong influence within the medical faculties. In addition, as many of these chemicals are present in foods, cosmetics, vaccinations, herbicides and the like – which involve large international corporations – then the topic is controversial if one does not want to stir the waters.

Toxins versus nutrients: the uneven battle

The body puts up a good fight for survival against the toxic onslaught. But the capacity of the body to deal with and eliminate these toxins is limited. It has several primary and secondary defense lines, namely its excretory and immune systems. These systems need 'ammunition' to keep up the fight, that is, a continuous intake of high-quality nutrients. Sadly, while the amounts and varieties of toxins are increasing, the nutrient intake in humans is declining. The nutrient content of the average modern meal has been on the decline for some decades now.

Only a small part of the globe's population has access to – and the inclination for – wholesome, nutrient dense, organic products. The rest of us struggle to survive on the conventional produce available in the typical grocery store. Even worse, a large percentage of the population feeds on junk, toxic, denatured and heavily-processed food – a recipe for a health catastrophe in itself. And the toxins are rising fast, while the nutrients (or antitoxins) are declining equally swiftly. Chronic degenerative diseases are largely the direct outcome of this uneven battle between nutrients and toxins.

The least one can do to help the imbalance is to try to eat a much organic food as possible, while supplementing with a good quality, high-potency multivitamin and mineral formula.

New 21st century theory of disease

Dr. Miller, of the Department of Family Practice, University of Texas Health Science Center at San Antonio, USA, believes that we are on the threshold of the new theory of disease – that is triggered by toxic chemicals. She states in one of her papers,[45] "In the late 1800's, physicians observed that certain illnesses spread from sick, feverish individuals to those contacting them, paving the way for the germ theory of disease. The germ theory served as a crude but elegant formulation that explained dozens of seemingly unrelated illnesses affecting literally every organ system."

She continues: "Today we are witnessing another medical anomaly – the unique pattern of illness involving chemically exposed people who subsequently report multisystem symptoms and new-onset chemical and food intolerances. These intolerances may be the hallmark for a new disease process, just as fever is a hallmark for infection."

I strongly agree with Dr Miller and believe that many of the new diseases that we are seeing today such as Gulf War Syndrome,[46] Chronic Fatigue Syndrome, Myalgic Encephalomyelitis (ME), fibromyalgia, childhood

---

[45] Miller C. Are We on the Threshold of a New Theory of Disease? Toxicant-induced Loss of Tolerance and its Relationship to Addiction and Abdiction. *Tox. Ind. Health*. 15:284-294, 1999.
[46] Miller, C. and Prihoda, TA Controlled Comparison of Symptoms and Chemical Intolerances Reported by Gulf War Veterans, Implant Recipients and Persons with Multiple Chemical Sensitivity. *Tox. Ind. Health* 15:386-397, 1999.

diabetes, attention deficit hyperactivity disorder and others are all chemically related disorders.[47]

How exposed are you to these chemicals?

Check out below how prone you are to developing a chemically-triggered 21st century disease, by checking off the various categories – the more of these that apply to you, the higher your risk if you:

- ❖ work with chemicals
- ❖ use pesticides around the house and garden such as fly spray, weed killer or flea powder
- ❖ use non-environmentally friendly cosmetics, toiletries and household cleaners
- ❖ you are responsible for disposal of chemicals used in medicines such as mercury preservatives in vaccines and flea shampoo
- ❖ eat nonorganic fruit, vegetables and meat products
- ❖ eat contaminated seafood, usually containing mercury
- ❖ eat too many processed foods, full of preservatives, colourings, flavourings and other additives
- ❖ drink unfiltered tap water containing aluminium and fluoride
- ❖ consume soft drinks from aluminium cans
- ❖ have mercury amalgam fillings in your mouth
- ❖ live in a major city with all the air pollution.

These chemicals are accumulative, so do not think that a little exposure will do you no harm – it simply takes longer to reach critical levels in the body, before symptoms appear. What are these signs and symptoms of chemical poisoning?

Signs and symptoms of chemical poisoning

In clinical practice I am often very vigilant in trying to detect symptoms that are related to chemical sensitivity and other toxicity issues. If the patient suddenly develops the following symptoms, then chemical exposure should be suspected:

---

[47] Miller, C. Prihoda, T. The Environmental Exposure and Sensitivity Inventory (EESI): A Standardized approach for measuring Chemical Intolerances for Research and Clinical Applications. *Tox. Ind. Health* 15:370-385, 1999.

❖ dark blue, black or pink circles under the eyes
❖ wrinkles or abnormally puffy bags under the eyes, as well as wrinkles on hands and knuckles
❖ bright red cheeks, nose tips or ear lobes
❖ unstable legs
❖ a spaced-out look and feeling
❖ itchy nose
❖ licking lips frequently
❖ fuzzy thinking, confusion; difficulty in concentrating, thinking clearly or remembering
❖ joint or arthritic pains
❖ runny nose or nasal congestion causing sinusitis and blocked nose
❖ extreme fatigue, even when rising in the morning
❖ headaches.

One study that tried to assess exposure to Bisphenol A (BPA) and 4-tertiary-octylphenol (tOP) in the American population found 92.6% and 57.4% of the persons, respectively had these chemicals in their urine.[48] These are industrial chemicals used in the manufacture of polycarbonate plastics and epoxy resins (BPA) and non-ionic surfactants (tOP). These products are in widespread use in the United States and the rest of the world.

Ways to address toxicity: the good, the bad and the ugly

Let us start with the ugly first: the typical misguided response to the toxicity onslaught is to visit the average doctor, who will note a few toxicity-induced symptoms, and come up with a superficial diagnosis. At first, a diagnosis appears simple: flu, sinusitis, eczema, tonsillitis, or otitis. Over time, diagnoses get complicated: asthma, arthritis, sacroiliatis, heart disease, renal disease, liver disease, cancer or any of the currently labelled chronic degenerative diseases which can strike. The ugly, symptom-based approach amounts to a classically wrong diagnosis.

The main causative factor, TOXICITY, remains undetected. Hardly anyone is searching for it, let alone finding it! Tragically, the ugly approach has become the norm, instead of the exception. Depending on the wrong diagnosis, which is typically a mere description of the symptom, the

---

[48] Calafat AM, Ye X, Wong LY, Reidy JA, Needham LL. Exposure of the U.S. Population to Bisphenol A and 4-*tertiary*-Octylphenol: 2003-2004. *Environ Health Perspect* Jan;116(1):39-44, 2008.

typical physician will prescribe chemical drugs to ingest, or refer you to other specialists who may contemplate removal of body parts (pardon the cynicism here, but this is the truth, as I experienced it from allopathic doctors – hopefully there will always be the exception among such practitioners).

With the ugly approach, the worse the disease, the worse the treatment gets. Cancer, the dreaded disease, is the perfect example. The reasoning goes: many toxins are proven carcinogens, so they could well be the cause of a person's cancer, right? Wrong! The ugly approach sees the world differently. Even at this advanced stage of body toxicity, when the body's immunity and vitality has been seriously compromised by carcinogens, the default medical intervention is to load the body with even more toxins: potent chemotherapeutic agents that are super-toxic, or cancer-causing radiation treatments to remove the original cancer. You also need additional drugs (Erythropoietin Stimulating Agents) to counter the decrease in red blood cell production caused by chemotherapy, which add their own serious side-effects. By then, the tumour is reduced, the cancer has metastasized and the patient is either dead or bankrupt – or likely both. 'Common sense' at its best!

What we should be doing, medics and patients alike, is exactly the opposite. Should we not be addressing the cause of the problem, the toxins, instead of chasing and suppressing the symptoms? We should be reducing the toxic load, not increasing it. We should be improving the tissue integrity, not cutting it apart. It seems evident to me that the common sense approach would dictate addressing the safe removal of the toxins, assuming our interest lies in achieving real, long-term relief for the patient.

Indeed, between the ugly and the good approach, there is also a bad way to address toxicity-caused illnesses. If you try to release toxins from the body too fast, or too clumsily, the body may be tipped over the edge. This is an issue that many well-meaning practitioners underestimate – either because of inadequate technical know-how, insufficient experience or poor judgment – with disastrous results vis-à-vis the recovery prospects of their patients. Unfortunately, there are plenty of bad ways out there to deal with toxicity-induced diseases, therefore sound and continuous research by the patient and practitioners to minimize such a risk is important.

Meanwhile, a growing group of medical practitioners have 'jumped on the bandwagon' so to speak, using their medical licenses to chelate people with various heavy metals – using more drugs such as EDTA, DMSA, DMPS and the like. This can often lead to disastrous consequences as these drugs mobilize metals quicker than the body can eliminate them, while stripping the body of the good minerals. In other words, the typical MD's knowledge of toxicology needs improvement, to say the least. There are natural, gentler ways of detoxifying the body of heavy metals and other xenobiotics. I hope that this book, based on extensive research, will provide food-for-thought to the many out there that are lost and confused about these complex issues.

Let's move now to the main detoxification treatments and protocols that I use at the DaVinci Centre, which effectively deal with the toxicity within my patients' bodies and are instrumental to the recovery of many diseases including chronic degenerative disorders.

The DaVinci Centre detoxification diet – clean, clean, clean!

The 15 day alkaline detoxification diet (15-DADD)

Most of the patients that come to me for a wide variety of health problems will be placed on the DaVinci Centre's 15-day Alkaline Detoxification Diet (15-DADD). This is a diet that I have put together through clinical experience, as well as studying the work of other practitioners[49,50,51,52] who are very well versed in the field of detoxification – which I believe will be a significant science in the future. Most of my patients can safely follow this 15-day detoxification programme except for a few who have other diseases such as diabetes, cancer, heart conditions, low blood pressure and some neurological diseases. There are modified protocols for all of the aforementioned, but these should be supervised by a qualified health practitioner.

These more complex patients need more thought and each detoxification regime can be tailored to suit each patient. This is why I take a careful history from each one, as well as examining all their clinical findings. These include blood tests, taking their blood pressure, as well as conducting an Iridology examination (looking at the iris, the coloured part

---

[49] Ballie-Hamilton, P. The Detox diet. UK: Penguin, 2002.
[50] Scrivner, J. Detox Yourself. UK: Judy Piatkus (Publishers) Ltd., 1998.
[51] Wade, C. Inner Cleansing: How to Free Yourself from the Joint-Muscle-Artery-Circulation Sludge. New York: Parker Publishing Co., 1992.
[52] Cabot, S. Juice Fasting Detoxification. USA: The Sprout House, 1992.

of the eye, using an iris microscope which gives me further health information), as well as other diagnostic instruments that I have at my disposal such as Live Blood Analysis, VEGA testing, Biological Terrain Analysis, heavy metal testing, Autonomic Response Testing, Thermography and more[53]. Generally, most patients will be able to tell me what their problem is, and its severity, as they have usually received a medical diagnosis before arriving on my doorstep.

Given that all is OK to begin the 15-day detox diet, I suggest that they eat only fresh fruit, salads, freshly squeezed juices, steamed vegetables and vegetable soups for 15 consecutive days. This means that they ONLY eat these foods for the duration, most of which will be rich in the live enzymes, which are the tools required to flush out the toxins from the body. You must be patient and put your mind to it, I cannot emphasize just how important the detoxification diet is to your success!

What will I be eating during the 15-DADD?

I strongly suggest that you try to eat as many raw fruits and vegetables as possible, including at least 1-3 fruit and vegetable juices daily. Carrot juice has a strong effect on the digestive system, provides energy, serves as an important source of minerals, promotes normal elimination, has diuretic properties and helps to build healthy tissue, skin and teeth. So I recommend as many carrot juices as they can handle, mixed with beetroot juice (about 1/3rd of a glass), which are powerful cleansing agents of the body. Beets are said to really cleanse the blood and kidneys – in nature, homogenous colours do not occur by accident – it is no coincidence that the red beetroot affects the blood!

I also encourage the use of a little 'green juice' mixed with each carrot juice. This can be anything from fresh parsley, lettuce, kale, collard greens, Swiss chard, alfalfa, cabbage, spinach, turnip greens, watercress, celery, cucumber, green pepper, scallions, coriander, or any other green vegetable in season. You can place a couple of inches of the green juice in the glass, and top up with carrot juice. All green vegetables contain chlorophyll, which is very oxygenating for the body. It is also an effective antiseptic, cell stimulator, red blood builder and rejuvenator – therefore helping to remove toxic sludge faster. Greens are also super-rich in live enzymes.

---

[53] www.docgeorge.com

I also suggest that each meal should begin with raw fruit or vegetables, seasoned with a little lemon, ginger, garlic, coconut or desired herbs. In this way, they are available for digesting the fat, protein, and carbohydrates from the meal that follows. These enzymes in vegetables control or restrict the amount of waste deposited on your adipocytes. Remember to chew all foods thoroughly.

These are the foods that I allow during the detoxification phase – no other family of foods is allowed. You may eat as many of the following foods as you wish, but it is best to eat only when you feel hungry. Wash all fruit and vegetables in a bowl of water with 4-5 tablespoons of grape vinegar added (not apple cider vinegar), to help wash away any pesticide/herbicide residues. Rinse afterwards with clean water. Here are the foods that you can eat in plenty – in fact, the more you eat and drink, the quicker you detoxify:

• SALADS – use any type of fresh vegetables you like, in any combination. Use organic vegetables when available, and include bean sprouts when in season. Salad dressings should be kept simple – a little virgin olive oil with fresh lemon or lime juice, or cider vinegar. Add plenty of fresh onion and garlic – these are very detoxifying!

• STEAMED VEGETABLES – eat any variety you like, including broccoli, cauliflower, potatoes, beetroot, carrots, etc. Steam as opposed to boil, and eat with a little herbal salt, lemon and a little virgin olive oil, with plenty of garlic. You may also have jacket potatoes with a little olive oil, garlic and parsley dressing.

• VEGETABLE/FRUIT JUICES – drink a minimum of 1-3 per day, and try to include one cocktail comprising one-third of a glass of raw green juice (spinach, parsley, cabbage and any other green vegetables), topped up with carrot juice. There is no limit to the amount of fresh vegetable and fruit juices that you may drink in a day.

• FRESH FRUIT – choose the fruit of your choice (preferably organic) and eat as much as you like, whenever you like. You could begin the day with 2-3 pieces of fruit, which are gentle on the digestive system. Make a tasty fruit salad.

• HERBAL TEAS – choose any of your choice. Chamomile is a good relaxant, aniseed and mint is good for the digestive system,

Kombucha, dandelion tea or 'coffee' (which is excellent for purifying the blood and detoxifying and stimulating liver function), Sage tea, (which is a blood cleanser), or Nettle tea, (which is excellent for driving away excess fluid out of the tissues and is a wonderful cleanser for all the detoxification organs). Drink as many as you like, with a little honey on the tip of a teaspoon if you like, but plain is best.

You will also need to drink at least 8-10 glasses per day of still mineral water to flush out the toxins – this is VERY IMPORTANT, so please take note!

When the 15 days are over, you should carry on eating the above for a couple more days while gently adding a little protein such as fresh steamed or grilled fish, organic chicken, pulses, a soft-boiled organic egg or a little cheese. Go gently on the protein for a couple of days before you begin eating normally again so that you do not overload your digestive system.

Lots of food and calories

This may appear to be an awful lot of calories, as there are no restrictions on the amount of such foods consumed over the 15-day period. The purpose of this diet, however, is to DETOXIFY – to remove the toxins from the fat cells and tissues as well as the organs, so that the body can return to its optimum level of functionality. I have yet to see anyone going through the 15-DADD actually put on any weight, so don't worry about counting calories – most people actually lose one or more kilos (2-4 lbs) over the 15 day period.

I had one gentleman weighing 150 kg (nearly 24 stone) who actually lost 10 kg (22 lbs) in 15 days, but I believe that most of this was accumulated fluid due to a drinking problem. On a biochemical and microbiological level there is much going on during the detoxification. The pH or acidity/alkalinity of the body is being adjusted back to normal, and any nasty pathogens in the body are encouraged to reverse their course, based upon the work of Enderlein, Neissens and Beauchamp who were proponents of pleomorphism as opposed to monomorphism. With our bad eating, smoking and drinking habits, body chemistry is unbalanced in the majority of people. This unbalanced body chemistry will be another metabolism blocker that will not allow the body to digest, assimilate, eliminate or get rid of fatty deposits optimally.

Detoxification symptoms – "The healing crisis"

When the body detoxifies it goes through various biochemical and physiological changes.[54] Generally, on the first day of fasting the blood sugar level is likely to drop below 65-70 mg/dl. The liver immediately compensates by converting glycogen to glucose and releasing it in the blood. After a few hours, the basal metabolic rate is likely to fall in order to conserve energy. This means that the heart, pulse and blood pressure will drop. More glycogen may be used from muscles, causing some weakness.

As the body requires more energy, some fat and fatty acids are broken down to release glycerol from the glyceride molecules and are converted to glucose. You may notice the skin becoming quite oily as these fatty acids and glycerol increase in the blood. The skin is one of the largest detoxification organs, so you may get some skin problems such as pimples, acnes or a pussy boil – this is all part of the body trying to cleanse. The complexion may become pallid for a day or two as the wastes accumulate in the blood.

The incomplete oxidation of fats may result in the formation of Ketones resulting in ketoacidosis. Combined with high levels of urea, resulting from protein metabolism, this state can cause a number of symptoms which may suppress appetite as they affect the satiety centre in the hypothalamus. Generally this takes a few days to happen and you may notice your appetite dwindling. You may get pains in different joints, or organs such as the lungs. There may be a considerable amount of yellow mucus released from the throat and expelled. The sinuses may also begin clearing with more mucus secreted.

Given that the body is releasing these toxins quickly during the first few days of the detoxification process, it should not surprise us to experience some changes in our bodies that may cause certain symptoms. Initially, for the first 2-3 days these symptoms can be a little unpleasant, SO BE WARNED! A fair number of people will have headaches, nervousness, diarrhoea, upset stomach, energy loss, furry tongue, halitosis (bad breath), as well as acne or other skin rashes, a general feeling of malaise, frequent urination due to the toxins irritating the bladder and some of their existing

---

54 Salloum, TK. Fasting Signs and Symptoms: A Clinical Guide. USA: Buckeye Naturopathic Press, 1992.

symptoms may be exacerbated. When the toxic residues enter the blood, they affect mind and body functions.

These may be unpleasant symptoms for the first couple of days, but they are a NORMAL part of the detoxification process, and in natural medicine we call this the HEALING CRISIS. All these symptoms indicate that the DETOX IS WORKING! This is a temporary and transient crisis, it will pass – so hang on in there and don't worry that there is something wrong with you.

There was always something wrong with you, and now you are doing something about it – you are reversing this toxic process that your body has adapted to, but that is not healthy. If you are a coffee drinker, then the symptoms will be more pronounced, as your body will be in a state of withdrawal. Yes, coffee is a drug and when you come off it you go into withdrawal, meaning that your body will start asking for a dose of what it is addicted to. When it doesn't get it, then it screams for it louder and louder, usually in the form of headaches, migraines, muscle pains, general weakness and lack of concentration.

Enduring a cleansing crisis is the hardest part of the healing process. To stop feeling bad, most people want to eat, but do not eat during a cleansing crisis. The body is overloaded with the work of removing toxins. Digestion makes matters worse. Drinking one or two glasses of sodium bicarbonate (baking soda) – one teaspoon in each glass drunk twice daily, will help to neutralize the ketoacidosis.

Helter skelter rides are common – the 'downward slope' is when the body is vigorously cleansing and the blood gets swamped with toxins causing you to feel down, moody, depressed, achy – like having a bad cold. You feel weak and lethargic. The mind rationalizes: 'I feel horrible: this can't be working.' You can maintain a normal routine of work on a dip but it requires willpower and determination. It also helps to know that the longer the down period, the greater the fasting high.

Phases of Detoxification

There is a lot going on in the body during the detoxification process – most of the work is happening in the largest detoxification organ of the body – the liver. The detoxification phases in the liver are composed of two phases, known as Phase I and Phase II. These phases chemically biotransform toxins into progressively more water-soluble substances through a series of chemical reactions so that they can be excreted from the body.

Phase I detoxification

This phase of detoxification usually involve oxidation, reduction, or hydrolysis. A family of enzymes commonly referred to as cytochrome P450 mixed-function oxidases perform the most important processes – detoxifying xenobiotics and endogenous substances.[55]

At least 50 enzymes in 10 families governed by 35 different genes allow Phase I to take place. Many forms of cytochrome P-450 enzymes are involved in Phase I reactions. The highest concentration of cytochrome P-450 occurs in the liver, which is the most active site of metabolism. The lungs and the kidneys are secondary organs of biotransformation, with about one-third of the liver's detoxification capacity. Cytochrome P-450 has also been found in the intestines, adrenal cortex, testes, spleen, heart, muscles, brain, and skin.

Our understanding of these detoxification pathways over the last couple of decades has helped clinicians understand how they can help patients overcome toxic effects.[56] Sluggish, imbalanced, or impaired detoxification systems can result in the accumulation and deposition of metabolic toxins, increased free radical production and its ensuing pathology, impaired oxidative phosphorylation, and reduced energy.

The action of detoxification enzymes in both Phase I and Phase II detoxification pathways depends on the presence of various nutrients.[57,58] For example, alcohol dehydrogenase, an enzyme that converts alcohols (such as ethanol) to aldehydes in an oxidation reaction, depends on an adequate supply of zinc to function properly. In the next metabolic step, the enzyme aldehyde oxidase changes the aldehyde into an acid that can be

---

55 Grant DM. Detoxification pathways of the liver. *J Inher Metab Dis.* 14;421-430, 1991.

56 Davies MH, Gough A, Sorhi RS, Hassel A, Warning R, Emery P. Sulphoxidation and sulphation capacity in patients with primary biliary cirrhosis. *J Hepatol.* 22(5):551-560, May 1995.

57 Anderson KE, Kappas A. Dietary regulation of cytochrome P-450. *Annu Rev Nutr.* 11:141-167, 1991.

58 Bland JS, Bralley JA. Nutritoinal upregulation of hepatic detoxification enzymes. *J Appl Nutr.* 44(3&4):2-15, 1992.

excreted in the urine. Aldehyde oxidase depends on an adequate supply of molybdenum and iron. Other minerals that are required by enzymes include manganese, magnesium, sulfur, selenium, and copper.

Other supporting nutrients involved in cytochrome P-450 enzymes include vitamins B2, B3, B6, B12 and folic acid. The tripeptide glutathione and the branched-chain amino acids leucine, glycine, isoleucine, and valine are also required. Flavonoids and phospholipids are supportive as well.

Protective antioxidant support is required for handling reactive oxygen intermediates produced during Phase I activity. Antioxidant support requires the carotonoids, including beta-carotene, vitamin C and E and coenzyme Q10.

Usually, the enzymatic reactions in Phase I decrease chemical toxicity. However, toxic or reactive chemicals can form during Phase I that are more toxic than the original compound. This is known as bioactivation. When Phase II detoxification proceeds normally, these chemicals are then rendered harmless and excreted. However, if there is an imbalance in the active levels of Phase I and II detoxification, these toxins will remain in the body. Imbalance between Phase I and Phase II is associated with increased symptoms of nervous, immune, and endocrine system toxicity.

Toxic chemicals produced during Phase I include teratogens (causing fetus malformation), mutagens (causing cell mutation), and carcinogens (causing cancer). For example, benzo[a]pyrene, a chemical found in coal tar and cigarette side stream smoke, is biologically inert until it is converted by the mixed-function amine oxidase system into a metabolite that can then initiate cancer causing activity. During Phase I, many compounds also form dangerous reactive free radicals -chemicals with an unpaired electron that can cause tissue damage. A buildup of free radicals can increase the risk of cancer.

The level of functioning of Phase I can be measured with a simple caffeine metabolism test. A known quantity of caffeine is ingested, and saliva samples are taken twice at specified intervals. The efficiency of caffeine clearance is directly related to the efficiency of Phase I detoxification. Rapid clearance of caffeine shows enzyme induction (increased production), either from xenobiotic exposure or toxins within the body. A slow rate of caffeine clearance indicates that cytochrome P-450 activity in the liver is abnormal. Patients with slow caffeine clearance have difficulty eliminating xenobiotics and other toxins.

The function of Phase II can be evaluated through the ingestion of both acetaminophen and aspirin. This test measures the recovery of the products of glutathione conjugation, sulfur conjugation, glucuronidation, and glycine conjugation (acylation) in the urine. Comparison to normal values allows evaluation of the efficiency of Phase II. A high ratio between Phase I and any of the Phase II pathways implies imbalanced detoxification in the body.

The detoxification process requires large amounts of caloric energy, which comes mainly from the food we eat. If we do not eat enough protein, the body breaks down vital tissue protein to produce the energy it needs. This decreases the available amounts of Phase I and Phase II enzymes, amino acids, and peptides, because the body breaks down protein to amino acids and peptides. The greater the toxic burden of the body, the higher the need for protein, carbohydrate, fat, and micronutrient intake.

Supplements that help the detoxification pathways

Some of the nutrients required for the proper functioning of the detoxification pathways have already been mentioned above. To reiterate, it is strongly advised that you drink at least 10 glasses of mineral or reverse osmosis water daily, so that you can flush out the toxins quicker. It is also wise to take a multivitamin formula to help optimize your levels of vitamins and minerals, which are crucial raw materials for many of the detoxification pathways of the body. Choose one that has high levels of vitamins and minerals, not just the RDA levels.

Taking between 1-2 grams of vitamin C daily during the detoxification process will also help as vitamin C will also help to absorb certain toxins, as well as helping the immune system cope with a heavy burden of toxins that it needs to get rid of. I usually recommend a Calcium/Magnesium Ascorbate in powder form, which is an alkaline form of vitamin C, and is much gentler on the stomach and gut than plain ascorbic acid.

Stay with the detoxification process, and allow yourself time to rest, particularly during the first few days. This is why it is best starting on a Friday, given that you will have the weekend at home to get organized and rest when you need to. I do not recommend vigorous exercise during this initial period, but a 20-30 minute walk with a friend or loved one in some open-air park is fine. You need to conserve your energy levels for the detoxification process. Under normal circumstances, the body uses 80% of its energy for detoxification, which is a substantial amount, and this will increase during the 15 days of this intensive detox programme.

The good news!

The good news is that after the initial healing crisis you WILL FEEL A LOT BETTER. This is literally a guarantee that I can give you personally, as I have witnessed this hundreds of times with my patients, as well as myself. I personally detoxify twice a year for 15 days, and another 7 days in the summer when fruit and juices are plentiful here in Cyprus. I KNOW how it feels when your body begins to get rid of the toxins and you are over the healing crisis – a clarity of mind that is crystal clear, increased concentration, increased energy levels, better sleep, calmer, more reflective state of being, increased awareness of your environment, better digestion, your constipation improves, body pains dwindle or melt away, arthritis improves, chests and throats clear, skin colour and tone greatly improves and I have had many clients who cut down or actually stopped smoking, as the body rebels harder during a detox programme.

These are all benefits that you will experience, so STICK WITH THE PROGRAMME and achieve OPTIMUM HEALTH. Once you experience this state of optimum health you will wonder what the hell you were doing when you had moderate health, just like the majority of people walking the planet today. The Alkaline Detox Diet is one of the most positive steps you can take and should be treated and enjoyed that way – treat yourself for 15 days, eat as much as you like, whenever you like, of the foods that you are allowed during the detox.

Before starting the detox programme

There are a few indications which would exclude some people from starting the detox programme and they should not do so if any of the following apply:

• You are pregnant – the toxins released during the detoxification process can harm the embryo, as the embryo's capacity to detoxify is limited due to its poor organ functionality at such early stages of development.

122

• You are breastfeeding – toxins released into the mother's blood will travel to the milk, so the baby will get a dose of toxic milk that will not help them in any way. Wait until after the baby is weaned off the breast and meanwhile you could start eating healthily.

• You are presently being treated for an illness or condition such as diabetes or heart problems without medical supervision. It is important for your doctor or health practitioner to know what you are doing, as with diabetics, for example, it is possible that you might go into a hypoglycaemic episode where your blood sugar levels fall below normal, due to the increased insulin production by the pancreas. I have seen this a number of times – as the pancreas begins to clear of toxic overloads, it begins to function better, so it can begin to produce MORE insulin than before, resulting in a sudden decrease of blood sugar levels. This is fine as long as a health practitioner is aware of what is going on, and can adjust the dosage of drugs to suit.

• You are recovering from a serious illness without expert medical supervision – if you are recovering from cancer, any type of operation, an accident or other serious disease, then you should be extremely careful of detoxifying by yourself, as the toxins released in the body could upset the healing process and period of convalescence. Seek guidance from an experienced health practitioner who has experience in detoxifying. It is pointless asking a doctor who has no idea of detoxifying, as you are more than likely going to get a negative report, just from pure ignorance. Seek the help of an experienced person in these matters, and take note that not many medical doctors are knowledgeable of the detoxification process, nor have experience in these matters. Only very few do, so do not take it for granted that all are knowledgeable because they are doctors.

• You are taking any prescribed or non-prescribed medication – again, the toxins mixed with the drugs could exacerbate further the healing crisis and cause more symptoms than are necessary.

• You are not ready at this moment in time to begin – the detox programme does require a little discipline and organization so would not be suited to a person who is travelling continuously, or eating out continuously with business associates, or who is under a particular stress from marital or domestic problems. We need to prepare ourselves psychologically and emotionally as well before we begin. If you feel that this is not the right time for you, then postpone it for another time when you are.

Preparing for the detox

Preparing for the detox is not difficult, nor is it costly, but should be done some time BEFORE you decide to begin. There are a number of things that you need to gather before you start. A checklist of essentials is outlined below:

• A large stock of fresh vegetables and fruit in season – kept in the fridge for freshness. If you have access to ORGANIC FRUIT and VEGETABLES then this should be your obvious first choice. Organic produce is free from the pesticides and chemical fertilizers that are harmful to the body, but are also richer in nutrients due to the organic fertilizers that are used. One famous doctor, Dr. Gerson, said that 'The soil is our second metabolism.' What he meant by this profound statement was that the nutrient quantity and quality of the soil is going to determine the quality of our bodily functioning or metabolism. Organic produce has been 'fed' the right ingredients of minerals, trace elements and vitamins that our bodies require to function optimally. I sincerely wish I had a steady supply of organic produce at my disposal here in Cyprus, where I work and live, but unfortunately we are not that health conscious as a nation to begin organic farming as yet.

• A good thermos flask – you can use this for transporting freshly squeezed fruit or vegetable juices to and from work. It is important to remember, however, that the live enzymes and vital energy in freshly squeezed juices has a life-span of ONLY THREE HOURS. So it is crucial that you drink the juice within these 3 hours, and try to keep the juice as cool as possible – heat can destroy these very vulnerable enzymes. You may also use the flask to transport herbal teas, either hot or cold (with ice cubes) if you wish.

• A good quality juicer – there are many different types of juicers on the market, and it is a true science to choose the right one. Most of the juicers on the market for domestic use are centrifugal juicers. If you are buying one try to find the best that money will buy as this is going to be a sound health investment that will see you through many years of life. There are cheaper ones at half the price that will probably only last a year or less, so choose carefully. You could pick up a good one for less than

$100, but if you can pay to buy the Rolls Royce of juicers, go for something like a Champion juicer (about $300), which will extract 25% more nutrients from vegetables and juices than the centrifugal juicer. The Champion juicer is a masticating juicer – it grinds the fruit or vegetable into a paste before spinning at high speed, to squeeze the juice through a screen set into the juicer bottom. The ultimate in juicers is the Health Stream Press which can extract up to 50% more juice than a centrifugal juicer, but can cost from $500 to over $2,000 for the automated press.

•   A steamer – metal (stainless steel) or bamboo – the type you place over or in the pan of hot water to steam vegetables. Steaming is far preferable to boiling as when you boil vegetables in water they lose minerals such as potassium, which is crucial to health. Steaming vegetables decreases the losses of these important minerals.

•   Olive oil – use extra virgin olive oil – this is extracted using a cold press method from whole, ripe, undamaged olives. It is made without heat and is unrefined, as compared with olive oil that is not virgin or extra virgin. It still contains many of the natural factors unique to olives, which are normally lost through degumming, refining, bleaching and deodorizing. Virgin olive oils do not suffer nutrient losses and molecular changes that negatively affect human health. Choose this oil over ones that do not have the word 'virgin' or 'extra virgin' on the label.

•   Fresh garlic – have plenty of fresh garlic at hand - it would be wise to eat one clove a day as this contains more than 200 chemical compounds, most of them having therapeutic qualities. Eating fresh parsley and lemon juice, or sucking on a whole clove can help to neutralize garlic odour on the breath. Garlic can inhibit and kill bacteria, fungi, parasites; lower blood pressure, blood cholesterol and blood sugar; prevent blood clotting, protect the liver and contains anti-tumour properties. It can also boost the immune system to fight off potential disease and maintain health.

Regarding detoxification, which particularly interests us here, garlic can stimulate the lymphatic system, which expedites the removal of waste from the body. In the meantime it can nourish most of the organs such as the heart, stomach, circulation and lungs, as well as protect the cells from damage by nasty free radicals (molecules that harm the body). The sulphur elements in garlic also help to stimulate certain enzyme systems that are beneficial for detoxifying such as the liver's glutathione pathways, which help to remove toxins from the body, and there are going to be plenty of these passing through the liver in the next 15 days. So, now you understand why garlic is so important – it is one of the true wonders of nature, and I cannot understand why people dismiss it because of its odour, yet we accept so many other disgusting smells such as smokers smelling like ashtrays!

• A brush made of natural fibre – this is going to be used for SKIN BRUSHING (see details below).

• Water – you will need a large supply of either mineral or distilled water throughout the detoxification process. I suggest that you drink at least 10 glasses daily – this may mean having a glass next to you at home and the workplace and keeping it topped up. You will be surprised how many glasses you can drink in a day if you do this systematically. It really is a matter of habit, but what I have found is that if you don't have the water to hand, you will not remember to drink. Water is absolutely crucial to detoxification, as it is part of the flushing process, in order to get the toxins that are released by the cells out of the body. After a lot of research regarding water filters, I have personally settled for the reverse osmosis unit with a vortex energizer in circuit to put the proper right-spin quality back – there are many companies now that can fit the unit under your sink and add a separate small tap specifically for the drinking water. This is connected to your tap water, but the reverse osmosis filter will eliminate literally everything from chlorine, fluoride, heavy metals, pesticide residues as well as micro-organisms – it is squeaky clean water that you can drink and cook with.

• Fresh lemons or cider vinegar – what you use is really a matter of taste, but both are excellent and healthy condiments. Cider vinegar made from apples is very rich in potassium, a mineral that is required by all cells during metabolism. In his book 'Cider Vinegar' by Cyril Scott, he talks about how cider vinegar can help overweight people, citing a number of case histories. He recommends two teaspoonsful of cider vinegar in a tumbler of water, to be taken on rising in the morning. Exactly how it works is an enigma, but even if it does not work for weight loss, it will certainly help to alkalize the blood, which is normally acidic in most people, and will help to clean it.

• Herbal teas – there are a number of herbal teas that you could drink every day throughout the detox programme. Green tea is excellent, and apart from being rich in vitamin A, E, C, calcium and iron, it contains healthy phytonutrients called Epigallocatechin Gallate (EGCG), which inhibits the growth of cancer and lowers cholesterol levels. Dandelion 'coffee' is also excellent, as this herb purifies the blood, detoxifies and stimulates the function of the liver and is a natural diuretic. It is good to drink teas that help to drain the detoxification organs and get rid of the toxins. Another good one is stinging nettle tea, which helps to drive away excess fluid out of the tissues and helps with metabolism by increasing the elimination through the kidneys. Other goodies are chamomile, peppermint, rosehip, blackcurrant, elder flower, strawberry and Melissa. Most of these can be found in good health food shops – either in tea bags, or loose.

Major detoxification centres of the body

The toxins will be released through four major detoxification centres of the body – the more you can help these detoxification pathways to open up, the less detox symptoms you will have. The major detoxification organs/centres of the body are:

1. Skin – excretes toxins such as DDT, heavy metals and lead through sweat. Skin brushing and saunas, as well as infrared saunas, are good ways of opening up the skin pores in order for toxins to be released.

2. Liver – filters the blood to rid it of bacteria; secretes bile to rid the blood of cholesterol, haemoglobin breakdown products and excess calcium. It also gets rid of prescription drugs from amphetamines, digitalis, nicotine, sulphonamides, acetaminophens, morphine and diazepam. There are good herbs that can open up the detox channels in the liver such as dandelion (Taraxacum officinale), milk thistle (Silybum marianum), Green tea (Camellia sinensis), Artichoke (Cynara scolymus), Methionine, N-Acetyl Cysteine and Alpha lipoic acid and others.

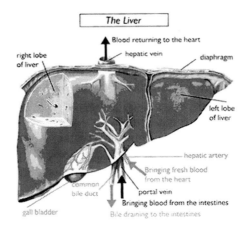

3. Intestine – mucosal detoxification to rid toxins from bowel bacteria; and excretion through faeces of fat-soluble toxins excreted in the bile.

4. Kidneys – excretion through urine of toxins after they are made water-soluble by the liver.

Food enzymes and detoxification

In order to remove the sludge and harmful waste from the body cells and tissues, it is important that you eat foods rich in live enzymes such as fresh fruits and vegetables and their fresh juices. These are dynamic catalytic substances that have the power to break down the fatty wastes stubbornly clinging to your fat cells, and wash them out of the body. Food enzymes scrub your cells clean and therefore slim them down, and consequently slimming you down too.

Thorough chewing is a unique way of detoxifying the sludge from the mucous membranes of the gastrointestinal tract (GI). Whenever we chew, an enzyme called *urogastrone* is released which can help digest sludge present on the mucous membranes as well as offering a protective coating of the GI to protect against erosion.

Initially, science thought of enzymes as dead chemicals that merely acted as catalysts – making things work faster. Since then, the works of people like Dr. Edward Howell: 'Enzyme nutrition' and Anthony Cichoke: 'Enzymes and enzyme therapy,' has shown that enzymes are indeed very much alive and have lots of stored potential energy. As Dr. Howell states in his book, 'They are protein carriers charged with vital energy factors, just as your car battery consists of metal plates charged with electrical energy.'

These enzymes help you to digest your food, to absorb nutrients into your bloodstream and to dispatch nutrients to every part of your body. Without enzymes there would be no life! These live enzymes with this vital energy come only from raw, live foods or their juices. Since good health depends on all metabolic enzymes doing an excellent job, we must make sure that nothing interferes with the body making enough of them. One of the problems with maintaining the level of these enzymes is that they are very sensitive to heat – they are intolerant of heat. If water is hot enough to feel uncomfortable to the hand, it will injure enzymes in food. Nearly all of the food that we eat is cooked – most of it is cooked to death! Cooked food is deficient in enzymes with their vital energy. This means that you are also deficient in enzymes, which will lead to incompletely metabolized food (which is stored as waste in your adipocytes), giving you excess weight.

It is therefore crucially important to attack the stored-up sludge in your adipose tissue mass. So how do we get a good source of live enzymes? – we eat live, raw foods.

If there are digestive problems such as bowel distension, bloating, flatulence and wind, pain after eating – it would be wise to supplement a digestive enzyme with your food. You will find that as the food is digested your bloating will be a thing of the past in 15-20 days, but carry on taking the digestive enzymes for at least 3 months.

If there are also a difficulty digesting protein concentrates such as meat and pulses, then this is an indication of hypochlorhydria or an insufficient production of hydrochloric acid by the stomach. This will cause stomach bloating, a feeling of heaviness after eating protein foods that will last many hours. This is because the stomach has to keep the food there for many hours in order to digest it correctly and you are likely to get fermentation, and wind will be expelled by mouth. In this case you will also need to take Betaine hydrochloric acid and Pepsin capsules with food.

The infamous coffee enema – the detox secret!

If you are feeling really lousy during the 15-DADD, there is one thing that can give immediate relief even though you will be surprised and maybe shocked to hear it. It's a coffee enema – yes, that's having a cup of coffee but not by mouth!

The use of coffee in enemas for detoxification purposes is well known. It is a common remedy that has been used by holistic and alternative medicine professionals for many years. It is commonly used in cancer clinics that treat cancer using natural methods. But why does it work?

How does the coffee enema work?

The effects of a coffee enema are different than a saline or herbal enema. The caffeine, theophylline and theobromine – which are all phytonutrients found in coffee beans – combine to stimulate the relaxation of smooth muscles, causing dilatation of blood vessels and bile ducts, as I go on to explain. The effects of having a coffee enema are not the same as drinking coffee. In terms of their physiological effect, studies have shown that the rectal instillation of fluids will stimulate gallbladder contraction and emptying, with the elimination of the many toxins that the bile contains. This was reported as far back as 1929 by Garbat and Jacobi.[59]

There is a direct communication of veins from the rectal area to the liver called the enterohepatic circulation or Portal Vein system. This means that the coffee is absorbed into the haemorrhoidal vein, then taken up to the liver by the portal vein where it stimulates the liver to produce more bile with all its processed toxins, and moves this bile out toward the small intestine for elimination.

---

[59] Garbat and Jacobi. Secretion of bile in response to rectal installations. *Archives of Internal Medicine*, Volume 44, pp. 455-462, 1929.

Portal Venous System

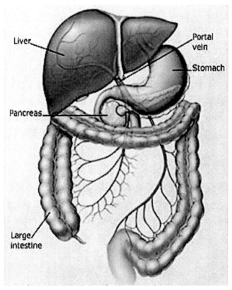

The coffee also contains certain alkaloids, which stimulate the production of glutathione-S-transferase (GT) in the gut, one of the main detoxification enzymes produced by the liver. Research has shown that the levels of GT can increase by about 600% when coffee enemas are administered. Moreover, the enzymes in coffee known as palmitates further help the liver to eliminate the toxins contained in bile acid. With the bile ducts dilated, bile carries toxins away to the gastro-intestinal tract. Simultaneously, peristaltic activity is encouraged because of the flooding of the lower colon – further eliminating toxic loads.

The benefits of increasing quantities of GT in the gut are:

- ❖ GT binds bilirubin and its glucuronides so that they can be eliminated from the liver cells.
- ❖ GT blocks and detoxifies carcinogens, which require oxidation or reduction to be activated. Its catalytic function produces a protective effect against many chemical carcinogens.
- ❖ GT forms a covalent bond with nearly all free radical substances which is the precondition for their elimination from the body. The intermediate products of potential liver poisons also belong to this category of forming free radical pathology.

In 1981, for instance, Dr. Lee Wattenberg and his colleagues were able to show that substances found in coffee - kahweol and cafestol palmitate - promote the activity of a key enzyme system, glutathione S-transferase, above the norm. This system detoxifies a vast array of electrophiles from the bloodstream and, according to Gar Hildenbrand of the Gerson Institute, "must be regarded as an important mechanism for carcinogen detoxification." This enzyme group is responsible for neutralizing free radicals, the harmful chemicals now commonly implicated in the initiation of cancer. In mice, for example, these systems are enhanced 600% in the liver and 700% in the bowel when coffee beans are added to the mice's diet.

Dr. Peter Lechner, who is investigating the Gerson method at the Landeskrankenhaus of Graz, Austria, has reported that "coffee enemas have a definite effect on the colon which can be observed with an endoscope."

As many of you have never had an enema in your life, let alone a coffee enema, here are a few guidelines to follow to make the experience a pleasant one.

Preparing the coffee enema formula

It's really quite simple to prepare a coffee enema – it's probably better to make a certain quantity for say 8 enemas and store this in a glass bottle in the refrigerator – this is how to make the coffee concentrate, enough for 8 enemas:

1. Boil 2 litres of purified water.

2. Add 340 grams of ground organic coffee.

3. Simmer for 1/2 hour.

4. Cool, then strain.

5. Reconstitute to 2 litres.

6. Put into 2 x 1-litre glass bottles (ex milk or juice bottles) and mark bottles at 250mls with marker!

Instructions for a coffee enema

How do you use a coffee enema?

1. Take 250mls of coffee concentrate.
2. Add enough warm purified water to make up to one litre.
3. Hang the enema kit (usually a plastic bag of 1-1 ½ litres with a narrow hose attached with a rubber insert at the end and a tap or clip to control the flow) on a tap or door with the douche bag approximately 40-60 cm (1-2 feet) above where your body will be. You could try hanging it on a window or door knob – use a metal hanger or improvise by tying a length of string onto the enema bag and tying this somewhere.
4. Make sure the valve tap is closed.
5. Pour the 1 litre diluted coffee enema into the douche container.
6. Open the tap to clear all air out of the tubing, being careful not to lose coffee, then turn the valve off.
7. Place a blanket and towel on the floor.
8. Lubricate the tip of the catheter with KY-Jelly or similar gel-lubricant (do not use Vaseline).
9. Lie on your right side, insert the tip of the catheter (approx 2-3 inches) with both legs drawn close to the abdomen to allow the fluid to run into the bowel slowly. You can also try lying on your back - see below for other positions.

Use the tap to turn off during use (i.e. if you get cramping or the feeling that you are full).

It's important to try to retain the fluid for as long as possible up to 15 minutes – it may be that initially you cannot hold the fluid for longer than 2-3 minutes. This is OK, but try every time to hold it for longer periods of time to get the maximum absorption and maximal benefits.

Do this once a day after your normal bowel motion throughout the 15-day ADD. Remember you are using the coffee enema as a way of cleaning the liver and toxic gallbladder, not as a means of stimulating peristalsis and bowel evacuation, even though it can have this advantage as well.

What position should you use?

You have a few choices as far as positions are concerned. Here are some examples:

- ❖ The left side position: Lie on your left side. Bend your right leg (upper leg) toward your chest. Keep your left leg straight. This position should be fairly comfortable while giving good access to your anus.
- ❖ Doggie style (knee chest) position: Kneel on your elbows and knees with your head down and you buttocks high in the air. You might even want to put your chest to the floor.
- ❖ On your back: Lie on your back with your knees bent. Your knees should be together while your feet are separate. This should allow good access to your anus from below.

Note: It is possible to undergo an enema on a toilet, however in this position the body is almost forced to expel. You will most likely have trouble holding an enema while seated.

Temperature is important when administering an enema – 102 degrees Fahrenheit or 37 degrees centigrade is about body temperature. If the water is colder or hotter than this then it may cause spasms and cramping of the intestine, leading to rapid expulsion and pain.

Administering your first enema

Prepare your enema, hang it in the appropriate position (about 1-2 feet above your anus) and take up your chosen position. The clamp should be on the enema tubing close to your hand so you can have easy control over it with one hand.

Lubricate your anus with the KY Jelly or similar – you don't need too much, but it would be good to apply a little lubricant to the tip of the enema tube too.

Now push down in order to relax and open the sphincter muscle at the anus – take a deep breath if this helps. You should not really feel the tube entering when the anus is relaxed and there should certainly be no pain.

Once the tube is inside, turn on the flow slowly and begin filling the colon. Stay calm and concentrate on the water filling your colon. Once you feel pressure then see how much you can feel comfortable with and then turn off the flow. Stay in this position for as long as you can so that the coffee can be fully absorbed.

If you feel the need to evacuate, try and stay still for a few seconds – usually the feeling goes away as the colon relaxes.

When it is time to evacuate, simply get up slowly with the tube intact and sit on the toilet – remove the tube slowly and evacuate.

As soon as you have evacuated, take up position again and refill your colon and again hold the coffee in for as long as you can.

Repeat this procedure until all the coffee has been used up.

After completing your enema you can use some hydrogen peroxide in water to sanitize your equipment or any other antiseptic that you may have available. When you have completed washing the bag simply hang it up to dry to avoid any mould growth.

Note: Enema bags should be used only by one person and should not be shared, much like a toothbrush.

Other detoxification techniques

There are many other techniques to help the body expel toxin. I will outline some here that you can easily implement during the 15-day Alkaline Detoxification Diet – if you use all of these during the 15 days you will be squeaky clean by the end of it!

Skin brushing

The body is much like a large lake with many tiny streams running from it, and in the human the 'streams' help to drain the toxins from the body. These tiny 'streams' join up to form what is known as the lymphatic system of the body, and it does just that – removes toxins. One of the best and simplest ways of stimulating lymphatic drainage is with a technique called SKIN BRUSHING. It stimulates the movement of lymphatic fluid in the lymph vessels, and helps to break down congestion in areas where the lymph flow has become sluggish and toxins have collected.

This is also an excellent technique to remove unsightly cellulite in women – a condition in which stasis of lymph fluid has accumulated excess proteins, fats and waste materials in certain areas of the body. This eventually results in puckered skin, alterations to connective tissue and distortions of the natural body shape.

You must put aside 5 minutes of your day and practice this wonderful technique, particularly during the 15-day detoxification programme. Before your bathe in the morning and evening, brush your skin all over with a natural-fibre brush – looks like a clothes brush but made of natural as opposed to synthetic fibres). You can begin from the shoulders and work down over the whole body, except the head. Use long, smooth strokes and work from the shoulders downwards to the waist, and then from the feet upwards to the waist. You only need to go over the skin once, every time you do it. Press as firmly as you feel comfortable with – as you become fitter you will be able to use more pressure.

You will be utterly amazed at how much junk and toxins are eliminated through the pores of skin, using this method. After all, the skin is one of the largest detoxification organs of the body, spreading out over 2 square metres – which is a large organ. If the other detoxification organs are congested, such as the liver, kidneys and gut (constipation), then you can bet your life that the skin will be working overtime.

To test the efficacy of this method, every time you skin brush simply wipe your skin with a flannel and hang it up in the bathroom. After a few days of doing this, the smell of the flannel will be quite revolting, from the quantity of waste products that have come directly through the skin's surface.

Detox-breathing exercise

This powerful breathing exercise will help you eliminate the toxins you are releasing, and strengthen and tone your entire system.

CAUTION: Do not use if you have a heart condition, high blood pressure, epilepsy, a hernia or if you have any ear, nose or eye problems.

1. Inhale slowly and deeply. Don't overstrain in any way.
2. Exhale briskly, as if you were sneezing. As you do, become aware of your abdomen, which will naturally tighten and flatten as you exhale.
3. Inhale naturally and exhale briskly again.

Continue this cycle for as long as you feel comfortable. It is very energetic so you may not be able to manage more than a minute to begin with. Do it regularly throughout your weekend and notice how you improve.

When you finish, return to normal breathing. Take notice of how you feel.

Carry out this exercise if you can take a sauna or go swimming. You could also try a good massage session: manual lymphatic drainage is particularly useful while detoxing as it supports the lymphatic system. But any massage will do you good (ask your therapist to use detoxing oils if you're having aromatherapy).

Detox 'visualization'

Repeat the detox-breathing from this afternoon and then spend some time doing some visualization exercises.

Sit either on a straight-backed chair or on the floor.

Check your body to ensure you aren't holding on to tension, especially in the jaws, shoulders, legs and buttocks.

Now focus on your breathing. Don't try to change it – just be aware of it. Notice how you breathe in and how you hold your breath for a moment before exhaling. Then pause again before you inhale. It's a four-step process.

Continue breathing breath like this and if your mind starts to wander, don't get annoyed with yourself – just gently bring it back.

Imagine you're exhaling toxic thoughts and emotions from your body and mind, and inhaling new, exciting energy and possibilities.

When you feel ready, return your focus to your breathing.

Now become aware of your body – of your buttocks sitting on the floor or chair; of your head balancing on your neck; of your shoulders relaxed and heavy.

Now become aware of the world around you: the sounds, the temperature. Slowly and gently open your eyes and return to normal consciousness.

Sit for a few minutes. Drink some water before getting up. You should now be in a very relaxed and tranquil state.

Epsom salts bath

Before turning in for an early night, you're going to have a thorough skin-brushing session and then take an Epsom-salts bath. This induces alot of perspiration so you can sweat out lots of the toxins you are starting to release.

CAUTION: Avoid taking this bath if you have heart trouble, are diabetic or feel tired and weak. Instead, you can substitute with a mineral bath or the cider vinegar bath described below.

Dissolve about 16oz (450g) of Epsom salts into a warm bath – which shouldn't be too hot.

Get in and relax for about 20 minutes. Visualise all the toxins coming out from your pores and dissolving in the water. Drink a hot herbal tea (thyme or peppermint) to increase the sweating and replace any fluids you lose. You can prepare this in a flask before you get into the bath or have your partner bring it in.

Get out carefully as you may feel light-headed. Don't rub your body; just swathe yourself in large, warm towels and go to bed, making sure your feet are wrapped up warmly. You'll probably go straight to sleep.

Cider vinegar bath

Again, plan to get to bed early. Skin brush thoroughly (you should be expert by now). Add two cups of apple cider vinegar to a warm bath. Make sure that the water is not too hot. Get in and relax for about 15 minutes. This bath is deeply detoxifying. Pat yourself dry and go to bed.

Sauna or steam bath

This may be considered an optional luxury as opposed to an essential, but if you have access to a sauna or steam room at your local leisure centre or health club, then take advantage of it during your 15 day detox.

If you have serious health problems such as diabetes, valvular heart disease, high blood pressure or advanced arteriosclerosis, seek medical advice first before you march off to the sauna – you do not want it to exacerbate existing health problems.

Saunas are excellent for opening up the pores of the skin and allowing toxins to leave the body quickly. It is recommended that you take a short warm shower followed by 10 - 15 minutes in the sauna, then a 30-second cool or cold plunge or shower. It is a good idea to take a few minutes' rest at this time while the body's physiology returns to normal after the initial 'shock'. Take another 10-15 minutes in the sauna once you are used to the process, followed by a cool shower or plunge, then a rest. If you can afford a massage at this time, you will really be indulging yourself, your skin and your health.

When in the sauna, stay on the bottom bench first until your body acclimatises, then you can think about moving to the upper bench. Drink plenty of mineral water, as your body needs it. And do not eat for an hour before or after the sauna.

Deeper cleansing

There are also other levels of cleansing that you can use to really clear toxins of various kinds from different parts of the body. You can cleanse your bowel, clear heavy metals, the lymphatic system, lungs, kidneys and blood. This is quite a major subject in itself but we will touch on individual topics for those who are really interested in doing a thorough cleanse – I can guarantee you that you will never look back as your begin to regain your health!

The theory of autointoxication

The compelling suspicion that a stagnant bowel filled with putrefying matter can leak out and become a source of infection for the rest of the body, was first suggested by the ancient Egyptians. In the 19th century this became known as 'The theory of autointoxication – self poisoning from one's own retained wastes.' This idea has been enthusiastically embraced by every subsequent generation. One of the main causes is constipation.

Constipation

Constipation has done more to provide the health profession with an obvious solution to undiagnosable ailments than any other simple complaint. It is defined as 'The difficult or infrequent passage of faeces' and it is associated with the presence of dry, hardened stools.

Constipation is a national pastime and slow bowels are more common today than years previous. For one thing, people not only ate better 100 years ago, they were more active and got out doors more. When the bowels slow down, toxins are not eliminated but are reabsorbed and carried back to the liver for recycling and elimination. Reabsorbed bile salts have been linked to increased cholesterol levels – therefore, high cholesterol is a major precursor of constipation. Also, when the bowels get slow and toxin levels increase, the pathogenic microorganisms grow to out-number the normal flora, causing dysbiosis. Although friendly bowel flora such as Acidophilus (small intestine) and Bifidobacteria (colon) are needed to correct this, it is the clogged bowels that are the major problem. When the bowels move again, everything else will fall into order.

Our endocrine glands, which control metabolism, are also involved since it is our thyroid that controls metabolism and metabolism affects how our bowels are functioning. In this way, constipation can be seen as a symptom of hypothyroidism. Low body temperatures (a symptom of hypothyroidism) are very common today –although they are not 'normal' – as many authors have reported.

Intestinal toxaemia, which is a form of blood poisoning, is caused by the absorption of bacteria and their toxins through the intestinal wall.

The large intestine (colon) is the most prolific source of bacterial contamination in the entire body. Thirty-six toxic substances have been isolated from the human colon, including such compounds as indole, skatole, phenol and cresol. When these kinds of toxins are passing through the intestinal wall, they can enter the lymphatic or portal system and be directly transported to the liver. Temporary increases in the toxic load of the liver occur during periods of stagnation in the colon. Any prolongation of this state will impede the detoxification and bacteria killing function of the liver. The importance of this function cannot be overlooked when one realizes that blood from the intestinal tract enters the liver before it is delivered to the tissues of the body.

An overburdened liver, which cannot handle the toxic load from the intestine, transfers the task of detoxification onto another organ, the kidney. Unfortunately, the kidney is not able to reduce the amount and kind of toxins that enter the liver or to detoxify them as efficiently as the liver. The toxins that the kidneys do not remove from the blood, adversely affect the kidneys and increase circulating body-toxin levels.

The Oxford Dictionary defines constipation as 'Irregular and difficult defecation.' The question is, 'What is a regular bowel movement when there is no norm, and regularity becomes a meaningless expression when some people have a bowel movement regularly every Sunday morning, while others regularly empty their bowels after every meal?'

Defecation is a reflex action, stimulated by distension of the rectum with faeces, but it is under voluntary control in adults and normally takes place only when time and circumstances are suitable. The presence of food in the stomach stimulates a reflex action called peristalsis, which moves food residue into and along the colon. Mass peristalsis gives us the feeling that we need to empty our bowels. This reflex action usually occurs after the first meal of the day but can also be stimulated by only drinking some liquid on rising.

If the call to defecate is persistently neglected, the reflex mechanism becomes less sensitive and constipation can result. This is likely to happen when there are time constraints causing hurry and stress (stress ceases peristaltic action in the colon). Also when there are insufficient toilets or they are cold, dirty or inaccessible.

Some healthy people do not defecate every day and do not have any discomfort, and many others open their bowels every day with excruciating agony – passing dark, rock hard, compacted stools – and both cases would be considered constipated.

Ideally one should defecate as many times as we have a proper meal, usually 3 times per day, the main rule still being that we have a bowel movement at least once a day. The stool should be fibrous, light in colour, float in the water, break up easily and cause no pain or discomfort to pass – in fact no toilet paper should be needed. Pain or discomfort whilst passing hard or dry stool at less than daily intervals can be considered as constipation. Many people have suffered heart attacks as a result of vigorous efforts to have a bowel movement as continuous efforts to evacuate material from the rectum increases the heart rate, blood pressure and respiration.

Referred to essentially as a Western disease, constipation is virtually unheard of among third world people adhering to traditional fibre-rich diets. Constipation is implicated in many Western diseases such as diverticulosis, obesity, varicose veins, cancer of the colon and rectum, appendicitis and haemorrhoids are very rare in the undeveloped countries.

Nature needs some help and urgently

In the U.S. approximately 80 million people suffer from bowel problems. 100-120.000 a year lose their lives – usually from bowel cancer. Colon cancer is the second leading killer in the Western World. Behind these statistics are also those saved by colostomies (surgical removal of the large intestine) – in the US only approximately 250.000 people a year. In UK and the rest of Europe, the numbers are more or less the same.

Bowel disorders, especially colon cancer, was unknown to our grandparents and bowels experts all over the world now agree that poor bowel management is the root of most health problems. The faulty Western, commercialized diet is the focal point of the problem. A diet high in meat, white sugar, white flour, fat and low in dietary fibre and plain water (dehydration) is believed to be connected with constipation.

The root of the problem is clearly indicated by laxative sales, estimated at 600 – 800 million dollars a year. Statistics from the US and Europe are corresponding.

Laxatives aggravate the problem of constipation by interfering with the colon's ability to eliminate normally on its own. The chemicals within laxatives irritate and stimulate the colon to abnormally contract, in order to expel the irritating substances. In addition the oral route of administration is the least optimal method for evacuation of the colon because crucial digestive processes occurring in the stomach and small intestine are interfered with. Most laxatives and purgatives precipitate dehydration. Hippocrates took the view of not disturbing and messing up the entire peptic system with harsh laxatives, as the problem lies at the extreme end of this same system. Standard enemas, even highly recommended as first aid, only cleanse the rectum and last portion of the colon, missing out most of the large intestine.

Colon Hydrotherapy is an extended and more complete form of an enema. This method extends beyond the rectum to cleanse the entire colon and offers greater therapeutic benefits. It addresses the cause or source of the constipation problem. Other methods treat only the symptoms and provide temporary relief of the problem. See below for further details.

The prevention of constipation may not seem of vital importance, except perhaps to the sufferer. However, there is substantial evidence to show that eating enough dietary fibre helps to prevent many bowel diseases as well as reducing the risk of heart disease, lowering cholesterol and blood pressure, improving blood sugar balance and maintaining a healthy gut flora.

Why constipated? – the biggest reasons? Dietary (lack of natural dietary fibre and consumption of devitalized foods, especially white sugar, white flour and all their by-products; neglecting the urge to eliminate; dehydration (too little water); stress; too little exercise (sitting for long hours); abuse of stimulants and drugs; irregular hours (work – rest, awake – asleep) and pathological conditions.

The most common signs and symptoms due to an impacted, constipated colon are:

* ❖ infrequent or difficult bowel movements; hard compacted stools and low stool weight;
* ❖ tiredness, fatigue, lethargy, lack of energy, poor concentration and irritability;
* ❖ bloating and flatulence; headaches, mental depression or dullness; Irritable Bowel Syndrome – IBS, diverticulosis, colitis, leaky gut, cancer of the bowel, Crohns Disease, appendicitis, hiatus hernia; malabsorption – nutrient deficiency; bad breath and a coated tongue; haemorrhoids, varicose veins, obesity and cellulite.

Colon Hydrotherapy

Colon Hydrotherapy is one of the most powerful and effective ways of cleansing and detoxifying our entire system. The mucous membrane of the large intestine is the first and most important defense system against toxic substances (followed by the liver, the lymph system, lungs and the skin), thus a very important part of the body's immune system. As I outlined above, nearly all doctors and practitioners of natural medicine take the view that most disease originates in an unhealthy colon.

Exogenous toxins such as poor nutrition, sterilized and denatured foods, environmental toxins and poisons, abuse of medicines and narcotics as well endogenous toxins from emotional conflicts and stress, clog detoxifying channels on an on-going basis.

Having three bowel movements a day does not negate the fact that after years of dietary indiscretion, a gradual build-up of mucus and undigested foods begin to form in the lining of the colon. Dehydration and stagnation occur. Our bodies are being poisoned by these toxic substances which can cause inflammation, damage the intestinal wall and cells; and intoxicate the nerves and glands. These toxins can also be absorbed through the walls of the colon into the blood and lymph and ultimately to into the cells and tissues. The resulting toxaemia can become a chronic condition but for most of us it creates erratic conditions in the body that we call disease.

Indications for Colon Hydrotherapy

Colon Hydrotherapy may be undertaken with the approval of a physician or health care professional for: acute faecal impaction, Crohn's disease, diverticulitis, mucous colitis and during the first four months of pregnancy when it may alleviate morning sickness. Other indications include: abdominal discomfort, acne, bad breath, constipation, candida overgrowth (yeast syndrome), carbohydrate indigestion, celiac disease, cellulite, diarrhoea, digestive problems, diverticulosis, eczema, excessive mucus, flatulence (gas), IBS (irritable bowel syndrome), nausea, stomach bloating, sluggish atonic colon, mild to moderate haemorrhoids, intestinal toxaemia, parasites and worms, spastic colon, shingles, systemic toxicity, thrush and varicose veins.

Colon Hydrotherapy can also be a part of a holistic approach and supportive in conditions where the immune system is compromised, such as: allergies, arthritis, cancer, chronic fatigue, Epstein-Barre, gout, lupus, migraine headaches, MS (multiple sclerosis), psoriasis, rheumatoid arthritis, sciatica, sinusitis etc…

Colon Hydrotherapy is also found to be beneficial in conjunction with medical procedures such as: pre-and post surgery, barium x-ray, bowel and stomach examinations. It can be used as a preventative measure: athletes have opted for colon therapy to improve metabolic efficiency; it can be very beneficial when suffering from colds and influenza, life-style change, weight loss programmes and travelling. It is of utmost importance for elderly and handicapped persons, in fasting and cleansing programmes; and when working through emotional issues.

However, it is contraindicated for any of the following conditions: gastrointestinal bleeding, cancer of the colon or rectum, anal fissure or fistula, abdominal hernia, acute haemorrhoids, severe cardiac disease, renal insufficiency, pregnancy after four months; up to six months after colon or rectal surgery.

So what is Colon Hydrotherapy?

Colon Hydrotherapy is a gentle and safe method of cleansing the large intestine (colon) from toxic waste material, including gas, accumulated faecal matter, parasites and mucus deposits. This is achieved by introducing a continuous flow of purified water into the colon, accompanied by abdominal massage – which helps to break up impaction, remove collected, stagnating stool throughout the colon – and thereby stimulating the channels of elimination into removing stored toxins from different areas of the body.

This process is painless, easy and odourless. The water and waste are run out through a transparent waste tube so that the amount, form and type can be observed and judged. Contrary to traditional enemas the treatment is thorough and cleanses the entire colon. The treatment lasts about 45 minutes to one hour and is totally hygienic – all equipment is disposable and the cleansing is always performed by a qualified colon hydrotherapist. The physical goals of each session are to hydrate the system, remove waste, stimulate peristalsis, and rehabilitate nerves, muscles, glands, circulatory and immune systems.

Before Colon Hydrotherapy: eat lightly during the previous day. On the day of the cleanse do not consume any food or water (liquid) for at least 2 hours before the treatment. Your abdomen will be massaged and you will need to urinate less, if at all, during the session. Bring a t-shirt so that you feel comfortable.

Heavy metal detoxification

As I have mentioned in some depth at the beginning of this chapter, heavy metals such as arsenic, aluminium, antimony, cadmium, lead, mercury and uranium are insidious in today's world. There is probably not a person on this planet that does not have some or all of these in their system, leading to heavy metal toxicity, which is the cause of many illnesses.

The early signs of heavy metal poisoning are vague or often attributed to other diseases. These include headaches, fatigue, muscle pain, indigestion, tremors, constipation, anemia, indigestion and tremors. Mild toxicity symptoms include impaired memory and distorted thinking ability. Severe toxicity can lead to death.

Hair mineral analysis is a convenient but often unreliable screening test. The most accurate measurement is by blood analysis of actual toxin levels within the red blood cells. Many toxic metals have a tendency to accumulate inside the cell, where most of the damage is done. Serum toxic metal levels do not correlate well with intracellular toxic metal levels.

Much more will be said about heavy metals and other toxins in Chapter 7 but here is a brief solution to this problem. One of the safest and most effective ways is to use a natural heavy metal chelating therapy named 'The HMD Ultimate Detox Protocol'[60]. The main formulation that mobilizes the metals is called HMD™ – you will need to take 50 drops, three times a day shortly before meals, in some water or juice.

In addition, there are two other drainage remedies that can be taken along with the HMD™, and are part of the HMD Ultimate Detox:

Chlorella (500mg) for absorbing the stray heavy metals that may get reabsorbed from the gut. Recommended adult dosage: 2 tabs three times per day.

---

[60] www.detoxmetals.com

'Organic Lavage,' another drainage remedy, which combines a number of organic herbs that help to clean the blood and help the kidneys, liver and lymphatic system to open up and drain the toxins out of the body. Recommended adult dosage: 25 drops x 3 daily for 3-6 months, along with the HMD™ and chlorella.

Lung & Lymphatic Cleanse

The lymphatic system is the garbage collector, the internal vacuum cleaner sucking up metabolic garbage, toxins and excess fluid from the extracellular fluid of every organ. If this flow is impaired, the fluid becomes thick and toxic. The parts of the body that rely on it for elimination become less efficient and sluggish as they fill with their own waste. This otherwise life-sustaining system now becomes a breeding ground for infection. When the fluid enters the bloodstream, as is part of the normal process, infection can now spread to any organ or part of the body. Many viruses, bacteria and parasites stay locked within the lymphatic system when these conditions are present. The result: physical ailments, degenerative disease, the hastening of the aging process and even death!

The lymphatic system acts as a secondary circulatory system, except that it collaborates with white blood cells in the lymph nodes to protect the body from being infected by cancer cells, fungi, viruses or bacteria. It is a system of thin tubes that runs throughout the body, called 'lymph vessels.'

Unlike the circulatory system, the lymphatic system is not closed and has no central pump. It is not under pressure and only moves because of exercise or muscle contraction. When the lymphatic system is congested, the cells become deprived of oxygen, affecting the body's ability to rid itself of its own waste material. Over time, other body systems that rely on the lymphatic system for waste removal will also become compromised, setting the stage for pain and disease.

Swollen glands, with which most of us are familiar, are symptomatic of blocked lymph nodes, which indicate a breakdown in the mechanical functioning of the lymphatic system.

Other Symptoms/Diseases of Congested Lymphatics				
Allergies	Chronic sinusitis	Heart disease	Eczema & other skin conditions	Loss of energy
Prostatitis	Fibrocystic disease	Chronic fatigue	Repetitive parasitic infections	MS
Oedema	Lupus erythromatosis	Inflammation	High blood pressure	Viral infections
Puffy eyes	Bacterial infections	Low back pain	Loss of energy	Cancer
Ear or balance problems	Arthritis	Headaches	Cellulite	Excessive sweating

Detoxification exercises

Rebound exercise, using a small rebounder or trampoline is so efficient in stimulating the lymph flow that Dr. C. Samuel West calls it 'Lymphocizing.' This is truly a fabulous way to move the lymphatic fluid, as well as exercise the lungs and other systems of the body. Every house should have a rebounder! The up and down rhythmic bouncing causes all of the one-way valves to open and close simultaneously, increasing lymph flow as much as fifteen times! Rebounding does that.

Aerobics exercise, which is widely associated with cardiovascular health, also helps cleanse the lungs. During active and intense exercise, forced expiratory volume of the lungs' oxygen exchange capacity is increased, and 'dead air' normally trapped within the small alveoli of the lungs is expelled in exchange for fresh air. It is important to exercise in non-polluted areas.

Breathing exercises combined with physical activity increase the action of lymphatic cleansing. Like jumping jacks – jumping in the air with arms and legs splayed out like an X and then the next jump bringing your feet to the middle and arms by your sides. This can be done when you synchronize your breathing with the movement of your legs and arms. For example, when you are walking, or jumping on a trampoline, inhale four times and exhale four times – one breath with each jump but slowly. Move your arms and legs each time you take a small breath. Inhale through your nose and exhale through your nose or mouth - swing your arms forward and back in time with each pace and breathe with each step.

Kidney & blood cleanse

To optimize kidney cleansing: drinking one quart of pure filtered water per day for every 50 pounds of body weight is one of the absolute basic foundations for anti-aging. If you are in good health, try drinking 10 to15 glasses of water daily. It is best to limit your intake to filtered or bottled water.

The right kind of water is especially important. Distillation is the process in which water is boiled, evaporated and the vapour condensed. Distilled water is devoid of dissolved minerals and is thus able to actively absorb toxic substances from the body and eliminate them. Drinking distilled water during detoxification for a short period of time (less than 4 weeks), helps the body to eliminate unwanted minerals. Once this is accomplished, distilled water consumption should be discontinued.

Long term use of distilled water can be dangerous because of the rapid loss of sodium, potassium, chloride and trace minerals which can inevitably lead to multiple mineral deficiencies. Furthermore, distilled water can potentially over-acidify the body. When exposed to air, distilled water absorbs the atmospheric carbon dioxide, which becomes acidic with a pH of 5.8. – normal drinking water should be slightly alkaline with a pH of 7.2-7.4.

The ideal water for long-term human consumption should be slightly alkaline and contain minerals such as calcium and magnesium. Water filtered through reverse osmosis tends to be neutral and is recommended for long term consumption. Water filtered through a solid charcoal filter is slightly alkaline. Make sure that the filter you choose is of good quality and removes pollutants and parasites such as cryptosporidium. The best type of filter to do this is a reverse osmosis filter.

Some of the herbs which can help cleanse and support the kidneys include Juniper berries, Parsley root, Marshmallow root, Golden Seal root, Uva Ursi leaves, Lobelia herb, Dandelion, Gravel root and Ginger root.

Killing Uninvited Guests

Schmidt and Roberts in their 1989 'Foundations of parasitology'[61] book noted that 25% – 30% of people living in the southeastern US – mainly children – were infected with whip worm (the trichuris species)[62]. Meanwhile, the Centers of Disease Control also stress that parasitic infections affect persons living in developed countries, including America. Zoonotic diseases, i.e. those transmitted from animals, are often caused by parasites, and infected people can even experience symptoms so severe as to be life-threatening. Food can become contaminated if livestock, i.e. cows and pigs, are infected with parasites such as cryptosporidium and trichinella. People can acquire trichinellosis by ingesting trichinella-infected, undercooked meats. Cryptosporidiosis can be passed to humans if orchards or water sources near cow pastures become contaminated by infected bovine faeces; or if tainted fruit is consumed without being washed adequately beforehand.

In addition, pets too can act as parasite hosts and pass them on to humans. Young animals, such as puppies and kittens, are more likely to be infected with ascarids and hookworms. According to official CDC data:

'Trichomonas is the most common parasitic infection in the USA, accounting for an estimated 7.4 million cases per year. Giardia and cryptosporidium are estimated to cause two million and 300,000 infections respectively in the US annually. Cryptosporidiosis is the most frequent cause of recreational water-related disease outbreaks in the US, causing multiple outbreaks each year. There are an estimated 1.5 million new toxoplasma infections and 400 to 4,000 cases of congenital toxoplasmosis in the US each year; 1.26 million persons in this country [US] have ocular involvement due to toxoplasmosis; and toxoplasmosis is the third leading cause of deaths due to food-borne illnesses (375+ deaths).[63,]

---

[61] Schmidt, GD and Roberts, LS., Foundations of Parasitology (4th ed). USA: Times Mirror/Mosby College Publishers, 1989.

[62] For a brief history of human parasitology, visit the site: http://cmr.asm.org/cgi/content/full/15/4/595. Further information can also be found at: http://www.alternative-doctor.com/allergies/parasites.htm

[63] The CDC's A-Z index listing of Parasitic diseases can be accessed at: http://www.cdc.gov/ncidod/dpd/parasites/index.htm

In the EU, the European Food Safety Authority (EFSA) was set up in January 2002 following a series of food crises, which have hardly subsided since then: mad cow/ sheep/goat disease, foot-and-mouth disease, bird flu and so on. In its latest report, the EFSA says the most commonly reported zoonotic infections in humans in the EU are, by far:

'... those caused by bacterial zoonotic agents that can be shed by asymptomatic farm animals: the 2004 data indicates salmonellosis (192,703 reported cases) and campylobacterosis (183.961) – followed by yersiniosis (10,381), human listeriosis (1,267), parasitic zoonoses is 2,349 (trichinellosis, toxoplasmosis and echinococcosis put together). Compared to the main bacterial food-borne infections mentioned above (395,455 put together), reported human cases of 'classic' zoonoses are relatively low: brucellosis (1,337), tuberculosis due to M. bovis (86) and rabies (two imported).'

It is important to bear in mind that official reports give only an indication of the situation in the European Community or the US due to serious under-detection and under-reporting, which varies by country or state.

But perhaps even harder to accept is that the parasites within you are infected by their own parasites in turn – parasites within parasites! The story is endless. For an enlightening exposition on the nature of symbiotic, as well as parasitic endobiotic relationships, (microorganisms living within other organisms) Dr Peter Schneider's article: 'Prof. Enderlein's research in today's view. Can his research results be confirmed with modern techniques?'[64] is enlightening.

Parasites, thus, are everywhere and in their most pathogenic states cause havoc in body, mind and spirit, with doctors responding with a range of treatments intended to suppress the symptoms, while failing to attack their source – the parasites themselves.

So, what can we do about these parasites we carry? Dr. Hulda Clark, Ph.D., N.D., a naturopathic physician, has brought the issue of parasitically-caused diseases and other types of toxicity back into the spotlight in recent years, dealing with this subject at length in her book:

---

[64] Schneider, P. Prof. Enderlein's Research in Today's View: Can his research results be confirmed with modern techniques? First published in the German language in the *SANUM-Post magazine* (56/2001) Semmelweis-Institut, Germany, 2001.

'The cure for all diseases.'[65] Clark describes various methodologies and procedures to cleanse the body from these nasty creatures. This is not the only herbal parasite cleanse that is used at the DaVinci Centre, as sometimes other therapies are combined using Sanum remedies, homeopathics, other herbal formulas and bioresonance therapy. The cleansing program itself is an easy therapeutic protocol to follow, and is laid out below – this is an adapted version of Hulda Clark's protocol which is the actual one used at the DaVinci Centre.

The herbal parasite cleanse

There are a number of herbs that can be used to eliminate parasites – this protocol developed by Dr. Hulda Clarke has worked well in clinical practice, even though there are occasions when it needs to be repeated more than once.

Ingredients:

1. Black walnut hull tincture – to be taken in water or juice before meals on an empty stomach. Day 1 – day 14: take two teaspoons of the walnut tincture in a half-cup of water shortly before meals, once daily.

2. Wormwood capsules – take the following before dinner with water or juice. Take all the capsules for a day together, as a single dose.

Day 1 – one capsule	Day 8 – four capsules
Day 2 – one capsule	Day 9 – five capsules
Day 3 – two capsules	Day 10 – five capsules
Day 4 – two capsules	Day 11 – six capsules
Day 5 – three capsules	Day 12 – six capsules
Day 6 – three capsules	Day 13 – seven capsules
Day 7 – four capsules	Day 14 – seven capsules

---

[65] Clark, HR. The Cure for All Diseases. San Diego, CA: New Century Press, 1995.

3. Cloves capsules – take before meals. Day 1 – take one capsule three times in the day before food. Day 2 – take two capsules three times in the day before food. Days 3–14 take three capsules three times daily.

It is a simple and effective program that is complete in only 14 days. It is probably good to repeat this every six months when you repeat the 15-day alkaline detoxification diet. They can run in parallel so they both start and finish together.

The liver and gallbladder flush

The liver is the gateway to the body and in this chemical age its detoxification systems are easily overloaded. Thousands of chemicals are added to food and over 700 have been identified in drinking water. Plants are sprayed with toxic chemicals, animals are injected with potent hormones and antibiotics, and a significant amount of our food is genetically engineered, processed, refined, frozen or cooked. All this can lead to destruction of delicate vitamins and minerals, which are needed for the detoxification pathways in the liver. The liver must try to cope with every toxic chemical in our environment, as well as damaged fats that are present in processed and fried foods.

This is why it is crucially important to cleanse your liver, much like you clean your house, bedroom, car and external self. Probably cleansing at least once per year is a good thing. When the liver gets overloaded it cannot metabolize fats and cholesterol so easily, and this is when your cholesterol level start increasing and gall stones form , but also the liver itself becomes 'fatty.' Fatty livers are usually found in about 50% of people over the age of 50 – this is often seen by radiologists over time when examining patients routinely. Any imbalances in the liver will have a direct effect on the gallbladder, as it is the liver that produces the bile and gallstones.

Let's look at the gallbladder and how this organ can be easily cleansed, with amazing health benefits.

The gallbladder is a pear-shaped organ that stores about 50 ml of bile until the body needs it for digestion. Bile is a bitter, yellow or green alkaline fluid secreted by hepatoacytes (special cells) in the liver – the human liver can produce close to one litre of bile per day. The bile stored in the gallbladder is between 5-10 times more concentrated and potent that the bile secreted directly by the liver. This bile is discharged into the duodenum (the first part of the small intestine) mainly for the emulsification (breakdown) of fats during digestion – this is why people who have had their gallbladder removed are likely to have a tough time digesting fatty foods.

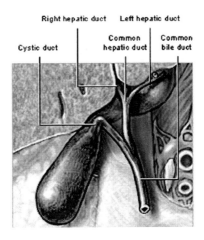

Gallbladder Anatomy

Gallstones

If the tubing of the gallbladder is filled with gallstones, then this can cause a number of health problems including allergies or hives, but some people have no symptoms. These stones cannot be seen by ultrasound scan or X-rays as they are not actually in the gallbladder but in the ducts – they may also not be calcified stones. There are many types of gallstones, most of which have cholesterol crystals in them. They can be black, red, white, green or tan coloured.

As the stones grow and become more numerous the back-pressure on the liver causes it to make less bile. This is also thought to slow the flow of lymphatic fluid. Imagine the situation if your garden hose had small stones in it – the result would be that much less water would flow. When there are gallstones present, much less cholesterol leaves the body, resulting in elevated cholesterol levels.

Moreover, gallstones are porous so can pick up all the bacteria, cysts, viruses and parasites that are passing through the liver. These masses or 'nests' of infectious material hang around the liver and supply the blood flowing through it with lots of fresh bugs daily. This is one way that parasites are circulated and reproduce. These parasites and infectious nests must be removed, and the simplest way of doing that is to remove the gallstones.

The pathogenesis of gallstones

Gallstone prevalence is especially high in certain populations and regions of the world. The stones consist mainly of cholesterol, bilirubin and calcium salts, with smaller amounts of protein and other materials. In Western countries essentially all gallstones, whether cholesterol or pigmented, arise in the gallbladder, while in Asia a significant fraction of pigmented stones originate in the bile ducts. In Western countries cholesterol is the principal constituent of more than three quarters of gallstones.

In the simplest sense, cholesterol gallstones form when the cholesterol concentration in bile exceeds the ability of bile to hold cholesterol in solution. Non-cholesterol stones are categorized as black or brown pigment stones, consisting of calcium salts of bilirubin.

Most of the stones are made of cholesterol (75-80%), with bilirubin stones (also called black pigment stones) being rarer and consisting of calcium bilirubinate, with large amounts of mucoprotein. Brown pigment stones are usually the hardest and smallest of the stones and these are usually made of calcium salts of unconjugated bilirubin, with variable amounts of protein and cholesterol.

Gallstones affect many millions of people

It is estimated that 20% of the world's population will develop gallstones in the gall bladder at some stage in their lives. This figure does not take account of the numerous stones that accumulate in the liver and its ducts, given that the liver produces them in the first place, and they then travel down to the gall bladder.

In the United States over 10% of the total population has gallstones. Each year 1,000,000 new patients are diagnosed. Performance of 500,000 cholecystectomies (gallbladder removal) leads to an annual expense of more than $5 billion in direct costs. Gallstone prevalence varies with age, sex and ethnic group. Ultrasound surveys show a female: male ratio of 2:1 in the younger population and an increasing prevalence in both sexes with age. After the age of 60, 10-15% of men and 20-40% of women have gallstones. Childbearing, oestrogen-replacement therapy and oral contraceptives increase the risk of developing gallstones.

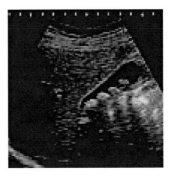

Ultrasound scan of gallstones

How do we remove gallstones without resorting to surgery?

Cleansing the liver of gallstones dramatically improves digestion, which is the basis of your whole health. You can expect your allergies to disappear, too, more with each cleanse you do! Incredibly, it also eliminates shoulder, upper arm, and upper back pain. You have more energy and an increased sense of well-being.

I have personally witnessed the removal of gallstones from hundreds of patients – some of them with gallbladder symptoms expelled many stones that did not even appear on ultrasound, probably because they were trapped in the liver and gallbladder ducts and were not sitting in the gallbladder where the radiologists usually look.

Most, however, did not have any symptoms at all, yet would flush out literally hundreds of stones – no exaggeration! One woman in her 50's had three scans and the radiologists found nothing. She had pains in the gallbladder region for 20 years. When she did the gall bladder flush she removed 280 stones the first time around, and about 200 the second time! Here's her first flush with the gallstones – the coins are there to indicate size ratios and are Cypriot.

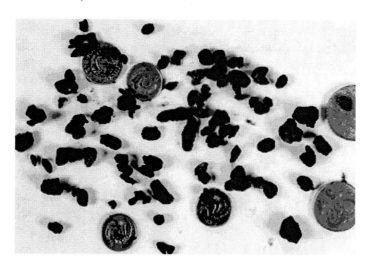

Gallbladder stones flushed naturally

About a week before I did my first gall bladder flush (on myself) I went to see a friend who is an ultrasound specialist. He checked my gall bladder and found it as clean as a whistle. When I flushed a week later I removed 5 LARGE stones (about the size of a walnut), and about 150 smaller stones, including gravel – here is a photo of some of them:

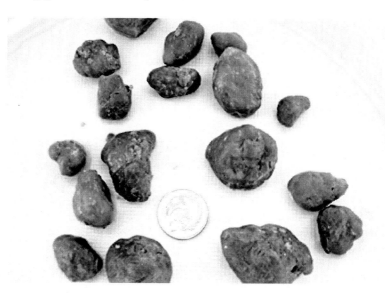

The authors stones on his first gallbladder flush

It is believed by many naturopathic doctors that EVERYONE has gallstones, even children, with all the junk food that they eat these days (but some less than others), and I have validated this many times in clinical practice.

The cleanse that I recommend below takes place within a period of less than 14 hours and can be done at home over the weekend. It is a harmless, pain-free and natural way of removing stones, without requiring invasive procedures such as surgery, laser, etc. Now that is a statement that will not be believed by the majority of general surgeons performing their gallbladder removals!

I had a personal experience of a 78-year old nun from a local convent here in Cyprus who was under my care for various health problems, including gallstones. She collected her stones in a jam jar after her flush and took them to the surgeon at the local hospital here in Larnaca. His first reaction was, 'But that's impossible; you can only remove gallstones surgically or with a laser!' The nun looked at him in amazement and said, 'But Doctor, do you think I am lying to you?' whilst holding her rosary beads. The surgeon adamantly persisted in his point of view whereby the nun said, 'OK Doctor, you scanned me about 3 weeks ago and you found stones and said that I require an operation. Is it possible that these stones disappeared by themselves?' He replied, 'No, this is not possible, once they are in the gallbladder they will stay there until they are removed, and yours were quite large, too.' The nun wisely replied, 'OK Doctor, if this is the case, then why don't you scan me again and let's see if they are in the gallbladder or in the jam jar?' So off they went to the ultrasound room, where he performed another scan – they emerged 30 minutes later after a thorough examination.

There were absolutely NO STONES in the gallbladder at all and now the surgeon looked really surprised. After a short silence he perked up and said, 'I cannot see any stones now so this may have been a wrong diagnosis, but you certainly have quite a lot of sludge, so the operation should proceed.' The nun was flabbergasted and did not know what to say, but before leaving, they agreed to have the stones analyzed in the hospital lab – the results came back: 'GALLBLADDER STONES!'

The moral of this interesting story is: do not try to persuade your doctors and surgeons as there is a mindset akin to brainwashing where it is difficult for them to accept new concepts and treatments, particularly when they are based on the principles of Nature, who they are not too friendly with! Just keep the information to yourself – it is your health that you are trying to optimize, so why go through all the hassle of creating enemies with your doctor, who you may need on other occasions. Remember that many years ago people and scientists were convinced that the world was flat, and it's ironic that there are still these believers in the 21st Century!

Preparations for the gallbladder flush

OK, enough of little stories, let's proceed with the details of the gallbladder flush, beginning with the ingredients that you should first collect:

Apple juice (which is high in Malic acid and pectin); it acts as a solvent in the bile to weaken adhesions between solid globules, while softening the stones. This is crucial to the success of the procedure as it enables them to pass HARMLESSLY through the gall ducts.

The apple juice should be coarse, unfiltered and free of additives and preservatives – you will need to drink close to ONE LITRE (3-4 GLASSES) DAILY FOR 14 DAYS PRIOR TO THE FLUSH. In the worst case scenario, if you cannot find fresh apples to juice, then you can use packaged apple juice, which would still contain these ingredients, but see if you can pick up some organic ones. (An alternative to apple juice, which is just as effective, is taking Malic Acid in capsule form (magnesium malate) – you will need to take one capsule, three times daily for 14 days before attempting the flush).

Four tablespoons of Epsom salts (magnesium sulphate). This allows magnesium to be absorbed into the bloodstream, therefore relaxing smooth muscles that surround the gallbladder ducts. This enables larger stones that may otherwise create spasms to pass through a relaxed bile duct. This also is a very crucial part of the therapy and you CANNOT do the flush without taking these salts, which are freely available in most pharmacies – ask for the B.P. variety for internal use, not those used for soaking in the bath – you will require about 70 grams per flush.

Half a cup of Extra Virgin Olive Oil, which stimulates the gall bladder and bile duct to contract powerfully, thus expelling the stones into the duodenum or small intestine. Once you drink the cup of olive oil and citrus fruits it enters the gut and the gallbladder – which, detecting huge quantities of fat or oil, begins to go into spasm, expelling all the waste rubbish that has been stored for years.

At least a couple of large grapefruits (oranges will do if there are no grapefruits) mixed together with the juice of two fresh lemons or limes. The more acidic the juice, the faster the transit of the olive oil through the stomach and into the duodenum, which helps prevent or minimize nausea.

I have supervised hundreds of such cleanses using exactly this protocol that I am recommending here, without one patient suffering any harm whatsoever. But please follow the instructions carefully, and it must be said that you have ultimate responsibility, given that none of you are actual patients of mine.

On the day of the gallbladder flush there are some rules to follow:

1. Take no medications, vitamins or pills that you can do without on the day of the flush. They could prevent success.
2. Eat a NO-FAT breakfast and lunch such as cooked cereal with fruit, fruit juice, brown bread with a little honey (no butter, milk or margarine), baked potato or other vegetables with salt only.
3. 2:00 PM – Do NOT drink or eat anything after 2:00 PM – only mineral water is fine, non fizzy.
4. 6:00 PM – Drink one serving (3/4 cup) of ice cold Epsom salts. Mix one tablespoon Epsom salts into 3/4 cup cold water and stir well. You may add 1/8 teaspoon of vitamin C powder to improve the taste. You may drink a little water afterwards, or rinse your mouth out. Epsom salts can also be mixed in with apple juice to make it taste nicer, or a few drops of lemon or lime can be added; or a little orange juice.
5. 8:00 PM – Repeat the Epsom salt drink as above.
6. 9:45 PM – Pour 1/2 mug (a large 10 oz. mug) of olive oil and squeeze 1/2 cup of orange or grapefruit juice into this, with the juice of two whole fresh lemons. Shake or stir hard until the oil and fruit juice mix thoroughly. Visit the bathroom now, shower, brush your teeth, go to the toilet etc. so that you are ready to lie down as soon as you have taken the olive oil mixture.
7. 10:00 – PM Drink the olive oil and juice you have mixed. Drinking through a plastic straw helps it go down easier. Drink it standing up, not sitting or lying. You may use a little honey

between sips to help it down. Try to drink it as quickly as you can, within 5 minutes.

TIPS: If you find it difficult drinking the olive oil mixture by itself it is possible to mix it with prune juice or grape juice with a tablespoon of honey and put it in a blender for a minute of so.

If you can obtain ozonated olive oil – maybe your naturopath has an ozonator and can make some ozonated olive oil for you – it may be better to use this as it will kill off any bacteria, parasites or other micro-organisms that may be lingering in the bile when it enters the intestine.

LIE DOWN IMMEDIATELY, ON YOUR RIGHT SIDE! You may fail to get stones out if you don't. The sooner you lie down, the more stones you will get out. Try to keep perfectly still for 20 minutes as the more you move the less stones your gallbladder will expel. You may feel a train of stones travelling along the bile ducts like marbles. There is no pain because the bile duct valves are open, thanks to the Epsom salts. GO TO SLEEP.

NEXT MORNING – upon awakening take another dose of Epsom salts. Drink 3/4 cup of the mixture. You may go back to bed. Don't drink this before 6:00 a.m.

2 HOURS LATER – take your 4th and last dose of Epsom salts. Drink 3/4 cup. You may again go back to bed and rest if you wish. Between the first and this dosage of Epsom salts expect to frequent the toilet more often with diarrhoea.

AFTER 2 MORE HOURS – you may begin to eat. Start with fruit juice or a carrot juice. Half an hour later eat some fruit. One hour later you may eat regular food but keep it light – salads, steamed vegetables, fruit, juices, etc. Its probably a good idea to drink some prune juice too as this will help to clear the gut.

BY SUPPER you should feel well. There are occasions when you may feel a little unwell for a couple of days, particularly when you have not done a liver flush before the gallbladder flush. Parasites in the liver can also cause symptoms to linger. Other times this may be due to stones and debris remaining in the colon and causing irritation and inflammation. Colon hydrotherapy or a good, deep enema can help this problem.

IN THE MORNING expect diarrhoea. Try to catch the gallstones in a sieve placed on the toilet pan so that you can see them. If any of you have a digital camera please take photos and send me a copy for my clinical archives – info@docgeorge.com.

Most of the stones will be SOFT and green, breaking easily, or even dissolving. All these green stones are as soft as putty thanks to the malic acid in the apple juice, and are mostly made of cholesterol. Some stones may be dark, near black in colour because of the bilirubin they contain. Other stones may be small and hard, made of calcium and oxalates (see image below). You may see all these types in one flush, but most of them will be the soft green ones made of cholesterol as about 80% of the stones in the gallbladder are made of these.

A few days after the flush (maybe 10-15 days) stones from the rear of the liver will have travelled 'forward' towards the main bile ducts leaving the liver, and fill the gall bladder again! This is why it is sometimes necessary to do up to 6 cleanses (perhaps one each month) in order to get rid of all the stones. If a cleanse produces no more stones, your liver can be considered to be in excellent condition!

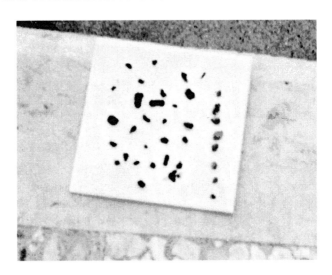

Small hard stones on the right of image

Helpful hints

On rare occasions some people may feel nauseous – this is related to the toxic bile leaving the gallbladder and causing discomfort and the feeling of wanting to vomit. There are a few things that may help in such cases:

Taking one hydrochloric acid tablet at bedtime will help reduce any nausea during the night – these are sold in health food stores.

If you have a tendency to get nauseated from the oil, take 2 tablespoons of Aloe Vera juice after your doses of oil and citrus juice.

Placing a hot water bottle over the liver area (under the right ribcage) during the night also helps relieve nausea.

Many people complete this procedure with minimal discomfort, and nearly everyone feels much better after completing it. Flushing the liver and gall bladder in the manner described (if the gall bladder is present) stimulates and cleans these organs as no other process does.

Oftentimes, people suffering for years from gallstones, lack of appetite, biliousness, backaches, nausea, and a host of other complaints, will find gallstone-type objects in the stool the day following the flush. These objects are light to dark green in colour, very irregular in shape, gelatinous in texture, and of sizes varying from 'grape seed' size to 'cherry' size. If there seems to be a large number of these objects in the stool, the flush should be repeated in 2-4 weeks.

Infrared Heat Therapy

Infrared rays are energy waves produced by the sun and are part of the electromagnetic spectrum, each section of which has energy of different wavelengths. Other waves include visible light (the rainbow colours), microwaves, ultraviolet rays and X-rays.

Infrared energy is a radiant form of heat – it heats objects directly through conversion, without having to heat the airspace between. This infrared heat, in the form of special lamps, pads or mats, is routinely used by physical and massage therapists and chiropractors.

The benefits of infrared therapy are numerous: improvements in microvascular circulation of blood and lymph, enhancement of tissue fluid exchange, relaxation of muscles, improvement in flexibility, deep cleansing of soft tissues with efficient removal of toxins and waste products, the improvement of fibroblast functions for connective tissue repair, acceleration of cellular metabolism, stimulation and support of immune system functions, as well as the reduction of physical and psychological stress and fatigue. In fact, there are hardly any medical conditions that do not benefit from infrared heat therapy and, in particular, infrared sauna therapy.

In an infrared sauna, our bodies absorb most of the infrared radiation directed onto our skin. The heat here produces more than three times the sweat volume produced by conventional saunas – at much lower temperatures. Additionally, infrared saunas can be used by heart-disease patients because they operate at a relatively low temperature and humidity, allowing easier toleration of the treatment.

The sweat produced from an infrared sauna is also fattier (oily) because the heat penetrates deeply into the fat layers of the body. This property allows for the removal of heavy metal toxins that accumulate because of sluggish elimination or high exposure. Many clinics' detoxification programs, including the DaVinci Natural Health Centre, use an infrared sauna for mercury and other toxin elimination – heavy metals are mobilized and eliminated through sweat, stool, urine, and hair.

The Sauna Experience

Before a sauna session - avoid heavy meals two hours before a sauna session. Drink four ounces of water before entering a sauna and eight or more ounces afterwards. Add sea salt to your diet, and two tablespoons (or about 10 tablets) of kelp daily, especially if your water is mineral-free. Remove metal jewelry before entering a sauna, as it may become very hot.

Preheat an infrared electric light sauna for 10-15 minutes, or you may enter as soon as you turn it on. It need not become hotter than $115f$. When it reaches $115f$, open the door slightly so the sauna stays at this temperature.

Preheat a traditional sauna to $150f$. With a far infrared sauna, enter as soon as you turn it on, or preheat for 10-15 minutes. A far infrared sauna need not be hotter than about 130f. When it reaches 130f, open the door slightly to continue receiving the rays without it getting any hotter.

During a session. You may wear light clothing in a traditional sauna. Clothing is not used in infrared or far infrared saunas. The beneficial rays are best received directly on the skin.

Use a small towel to wipe off sweat. Sit on another small towel. Have a third towel on the floor to avoid slipping. Meditate or relax. Talking or working are not recommended while in a sauna.

To enhance the effects of a sauna session, you may visualize absorbing the heat and energy through every pore. You may also visualize releasing toxins as you sweat. Deep, slow breathing and sitting up straight are also helpful. Sound therapy, such as listening to low tones, is also excellent.

In an infrared electric light sauna, with lamps on one side, turn every few minutes to heat the body evenly. Sit on a stool or a chair without a back. Face the lamps, turn to the side and around to the back. Avoid touching the hot lamps. Looking at the lamps is not harmful, but is not recommended. Do not let water, a towel or clothing touch the hot lamps. One will not get a tan in an infrared sauna, though the skin may redden for an hour afterwards.

Finishing Up. How long you remain in a sauna depends on your health condition and how long you have used saunas. Body temperature should not increase more than four degrees. Your pulse should not increase more than 50% of your resting pulse. Begin with 15 minutes if one is ill. If your heart begins to race, sweating stops or you feel very faint, end the session immediately. Sixty minutes is a maximum time.

When finished, take a shower. It may be warm or cool, but not hot. Clean the body with a skin brush or loofa in the shower. Brush all over, even face and hair. It may be painful at first. However, it soon feels wonderful. Skin brushing enhances the cleansing effect of the sauna.

Avoid soap, if possible, as you should be very clean. Soap can leave a film and clog the pores. Use shampoo and conditioner only if needed. Most contain chemicals toxic to the body. Also skip most oils, lotions and creams. These also contain chemicals that may clog the pores. Rinse out the towels used in the sauna so they will be ready for your next sauna session.

After showering, drink eight or more ounces of water. Sit for at least 10 minutes. These simple steps allow the body to reap the full benefit of the sauna experience.

Supervision and Safety. Supervision during a sauna therapy program is always best, and essential if one has a chronic condition. The presence of an attendant or friend is also most helpful.

Removing drugs from tissue storage may cause flashbacks or temporary drug effects, the same as when you took the drug. If you have used LSD or other psychotropic drugs, have an attendant close by, as a few have experienced flashbacks or even full-blown LSD trips.

However, saunas are quite safe for most people, providing one follows the procedures above. If debilitated or very heat sensitive, begin with less time in the sauna. Always consult a health professional if one has multiple sclerosis, a serious heart condition or other chronic illness.

Pregnant women and children under five should avoid saunas. Young children must be accompanied by an adult. Continue prescribed medication while taking saunas, unless directed otherwise.

Use a sauna twice a week to twice a day. If one is very debilitated, begin with once a week. Work up to daily use as you are able to do so. When beginning, stay inside only 20-25 minutes. Many people do not sweat easily. Instead, their bodies overheat and they tolerate less time in the sauna.

In a few weeks to a few months, most people acclimate to sweating and can more easily regulate their body temperature. Sweating often increases a lot over a few months. Also, the more one relaxes, the more one will sweat.

Healing Reactions. Healing reactions are temporary symptoms that occur as toxic substances are eliminated and chronic infections heal. Symptoms vary from mild odors, tastes or rashes to periods of fatigue, bowel changes, aches, pains or headaches.

Almost everyone has some chronic infections. These may flare up as they are healed due to repeated sauna use. Usually only rest and natural remedies are needed to help infections resolve faster.

Emotional healing also takes place, especially with the use of infrared electric light saunas. Memories may arise consciously or, at times, in dreams. Temporary anxiety or other emotional states may occur and usually pass quickly. Some are directly related to the elimination of toxic substances. Others are associated with emotional clearing.

Almost all healing symptoms are benign and will pass quickly. Consult a knowledgeable practitioner if any cause concern.

An Integrated Healing Program. A healthful lifestyle and an integrated healing program greatly enhance the results of sauna therapy. Rest several times during the day, eat natural foods, breathe deeply and exercise a little each day.

Reduce your exposure to toxic chemicals at home and at work. Toxic products range from pesticides and insecticides to solvents, body care products, paints, cleaners, new carpeting and toxic building materials.

A specific diet for your metabolic type and a supplementary nutrient program based on a properly performed hair mineral analysis are also most helpful, and essential when body chemistry is far out of balance.

Ionic footbath therapy

This mode of therapy uses an electrical device for external detoxification. At the DaVinci Natural Health Centre we use the Focus Ionic Footbath (http://hymbas.com) How do these devices work? Firstly, you need to know what an ion is: a charged atom or molecule that has gained or lost an electron, thus creating an electromagnetic field capable of neutralizing opposingly-charged particles, such as toxins, in the human body. With a foot spa, the main control unit delivers an electrical current through the ionizer probe placed in the water of the footbath.

The low-level direct current to the probe causes the water and salt to generate positively and negatively-charged ions by separating the oxygen and hydrogen components of water. The Bio-Body Cleanser allows the positive and negative ions to travel through the body (ion channels) and attach themselves to toxic substances with the opposite charge. Since most toxins in our bodies are in the form of positive ions, they will be neutralized and cleansed by the negative ions produced by the ionic footbath therapy.

With a constant flow of negative ions being produced in the water, this also raises the user's pH to a more alkaline state. This is important because most people live in an acid state – their bodies contain an excess of hydrogen ions, and their pH is lower than 7.45 – a normal value. Such individuals need exposure to higher concentrations of negatively-charged ions, to shift their pH to a more balanced acid-alkaline state.

There are many other types of detoxification protocols that can be used, but this chapter hopefully has provided the main ones for a healthier life.

In the next chapter we will be discussing how systemic Candidiasis can adversely affect our health, and what we can do to successfully eradicate it.

PART B

Chapter 5

Systemic Candidiasis

Elimination using the DaVinci Candida Protocol

As you probably remember from my introduction, one of the health challenges that I was facing many years ago was Candida, also known as Systemic Candidiasis; systemic means 'all the body.' It took me over 11 years to finally rid myself of Candida, after pursuing many different therapies from experts who had written books on the subject. I will share with you the secrets that I discovered while formulating the DaVinci Candida Protocol – which has now been published in peer-reviewed journals.[1, 2]

While rapaciously reading the literature on Candida, as well as attending lectures, I discovered that many practitioners were trying to kill off the pathogenic, mycelial form of Candida using natural substances, without making any attempt to convert the pleomorphic, pathogenic Candida back to the normal, budding form. It is also critically important to change the internal milieu[3] using the detoxification protocols that were mentioned in Chapter 4 – this is another deficit of many Candida protocols out there.

Candida is a real scourge of the 21st century, fuelled by a toxic body and an abuse of antibiotics and sugar-laden products. The prevalence of Candida in the general population is difficult to determine as there are no epidemiological studies that I am aware of, but generally I am picking up about 25% - 30% of my patients who fit the picture of systemic Candidiasis. People suffering chronic diseases are more likely to have Candida, both related to the imbalance of their internal mileau, but also the number of drugs that they have been treated with – I would go as far as to say that all patients with cancer have systemic Candidiasis.

---

1 Georgiou, G.J. *British Naturopathic Journal*, Vol. 25., No. 1 & 2, 2008.
2 Georgiou, G.J. *Explore!* Volume 14, No. 6, 2005.
3 Internal mileu – a nutrient-filled fluid matrix, which bathes all the cells of the body – an important   factor for keeping various bacteria alive and spreading. See Chapter 2 for more details.

Indeed, one Italian oncologist, Dr. Tullio Simoncini, has gone as far as to say that "cancer is Candida."

There have been a number of other books written on systemic Candidiasis which have been considered as classics as they set the path for thinking about this systemic disease with so many symptoms that the diagnosis is often confusing – it was termed by Dr. Truss as "The Missing Diagnosis".[4,5,6,7]

What is Candida?

Traditionally, fungi are considered plants, but they contain no chlorophyll and cannot make their own food. Fungi tend to inhabit cool to tropical climates and are found in the air we breathe as well as in moist and shady soil, water, manure, dead leaves, fruit, leftover food and a wide variety of places and circumstances.

Candida albicans is a yeast that lives in the mouth, throat, intestines and genito-urinary tract of most humans, and is usually considered to be a normal part of the bowel flora (the organisms that coexist with us in our lower digestive tract). It is actually a member of a broader classification of organisms known as 'fungi.' Candida are unicellular yeasts, somewhat larger than bacteria. They divide mostly asexually, can switch between a yeast and a pseudohyphal or hyphal form, and, like other yeasts, flourish in habitats where there is an abundance of sugar.

The normal budding forms can be cultured from faeces in up to 80% of healthy adults.[8] Candida numbers increase significantly following antibacterial therapy,[9] but seem to be unaffected by a refined carbohydrate

---

4 Trowbridge JP and Walker M. The Yeast Syndrome Bantam Books, New York, New York 1986.
5 Truss C: The Missing Diagnosis Birmingham Alabama (The author), 1983.
6 Crook, WG. The Yeast Connection and the Woman. Professional Books, Jackson TN 1987.
7 Crook WG: The Yeast Connection, A Medical Breakthrough 2nd Addition Professional Books, Jackson, TN, 1984.
8 Bernhardt H, Knoke M. Mycological aspects of gastrointestinal microflora. *Scand. J Gastroenterol* 32(suppl 222): 102–106, 1997.
9 Seelig MS. Mechanisms by which antibiotics increase the incidence and severity of candidiasis and alter the immunological defences. *Bacteriol Rev* 1 30:4442–4459, 1966.

diet.[10] It seems likely that intestinal Candida numbers are regulated in a similar way to intestinal bacteria.[11]

There are 81 different types of Candida species such as C. albicans, C. glabrata, krusei, lusitaniae, parapsilosis, tropicalis and more. Candida albicans and C. glabrata are the two most common Candida species that cause systemic Candidiasis in humans but the other species may also be responsible.

C. albicans is a diploid organism which has eight sets of chromosome pairs. Interestingly, Candida is one of the few microorganisms that has a diploid gene controlling the same protein – this means that it is capable of pleomorphic activity: being able to mutate forms from the budding form to the mycelial (fungal), pathogenic form. Its genome size is about 16 Mb (haploid) – about 30% greater than S. cerevisiae (baker's yeast).

The pathogenesis of disease associated with Candida in humans is driven by host factors. Some strains of Candida produce gliotoxin, which may impair neutrophil function.[12] However, Candida is a polyantigenic organism containing up to 178 different antigens,[13] which might explain the number of cross-reactions to yeasts (Malassezia, bread/brewers yeast) moulds[14] and even human tissue.[15]

It was shown recently that there is a potential cross reactivity with gluten because of several amino acid sequences that are highly homologous to alpha-gliadin and gamma-gliadin. Such a mechanism might lead to wheat intolerance with its accompanying symptoms, and even trigger Coeliac disease in genetically susceptible people.[16] Furthermore, a placebo-

---

10 Weig M, Werner E, Frosh M, Kasper H. Limited effect of refined carbohydrate dietary supplementation on colonization of the gastrointestinal tract of healthy subjects by Candida albicans. *Am J Clin Nutr* 69:1170–1173, 1999.

11 Fitzsimmons N, Berry DR. Inhibition of Candida albicans by Lactobacillus acidophilus: evidence for the involvement of a peroxidase system. *Microbios* 80: 125–133, 1994.

12 Shah DT, Jackman S, Engle J, Larsen B. Effect of gliotoxin on human polymorphonuclear neutrophils. *Inf Dis Obstet Gynecol* 6 : 168–175, 1998.

13 Poulain D, Hopwood V, Vernes A. Antigenic variability of Candida albicans. *CRC Crit. Rev Microbiol* 12:223-70, 1985.

14 Koivikko A, et al. Allergenic cross-reactivity of yeasts. *Allergy* 43:192-200, 1988.

15 Vojdani A, Rahimian P, Kalhor H and Mordechai E. Immunological cross reactivity between Candida albicans and human tissue. *J. Clin Lab Immunol* 48:1-15, 1996.

16 Nieuwenhuizen WF, Pieters RH, Knippels LM, Jansen MC, Koppelman GJ. Is Candida albicans a trigger for the onset of coeliac disease? *Lancet* 361: 152–2154, 2003.

controlled crossover study has revealed that dietary yeast may affect the activity of Crohn's disease.[17]

Candida produces alcohol and contains glycoproteins, which have the potential to stimulate mast cells to release histamine, and apparently prostaglandin (PGE2) –inflammatory substances which could cause IBS-like symptoms.[18,19] Other circumstantial evidence supports the theory of yeasts as a trigger for IBS: Secretory immunoglobulin A (SIgA) is front line in the defence of mucous membranes, especially in the intestine where it is active against infectious agents and certain antigens.[20] At least three different Candida species are able to produce proteases which can degrade: IgA1, IgA2 and SigA.[21] This protease activity can induce polyclonal B-cell response and inflammation. An infection of the intestinal mucosa with Candida might lead to an inactivating of SigA, and inflammation within subgroups of patients with IBS symptoms.

Candida is sensitive to a number of antifungal agents, such as nystatin, which is not absorbed from the gastrointestinal tract after oral administration. It destroys Candida by binding to sterols in the cell membrane, and thereby increasing permeability with loss of cellular contents.

The problem begins when the normal, budding Candida species that we have in our gut – which 90% of babies are born with – actually change forms to the mycelial or hyphae form, which is pathogenic or disease-causing. This only happens when the internal mileau of the gut and other tissues becomes more acidic, either through taking a variety of drugs such as antibiotics – that wipe out the friendly flora of the gut – or through eating very acidic foods such as sugar and other refined products.

17 Barclay GR, McKenzie H, Pennington J, Parratt D, Pennington CR. The effect of dietary yeast on the activity of stable chronic Crohn's disease. *Scand. J Gastroenterol* 27 :196–200, 1992.
[18] Romani L, Bistoni F, Puccetti P. Initiation of T-helper cell immunity to Candida albicans by IL-12: the role of neutrophils. *Chem Immunol.* 68:110-35, 1997.
19 Kanda N, Tani K, Enomoto U, Nakai K & Watanabe S. The skin fungus-induced Th1- and Th2-related cytokine, chemokine and prostaglandin E2 production in peripheral blood mononuclear cells from patients with atopic dermatitis and psoriasis vulgaris. *Clinical & Experimental Allergy*; 32(8): 1243-50.
20 Brandtzaeg P. The mucosal B cell and its functions. In: Brostoff J, Challacombe S (eds): Food allergy and intolerance. London: Saunders; 127-171, 2002.
21 Reinholdt J, Krogh P, Holmstrup P. Degradation of IgA1, IgA2, and S-IgA by Candida and torulopsis species. *Acta Path Microbiol Immunol Scand.* Sect C 95:65-74, 1987.

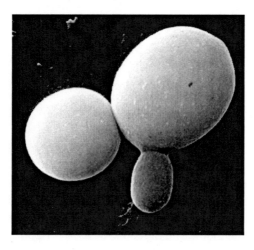

Normal, budding Candida

It appears that this change in pH can trigger genes in the Candida to begin a pleomorphic change into a stealth organism that is very virulent – if fed with sugar, it can increase itself from 1 to 100 cells in 24 hours. These 100 cells can then produce 100 each in the next 24 hours, and so on. And so by the 4th day we will have 100 million Candida cells – this is really exponential, explosive growth!

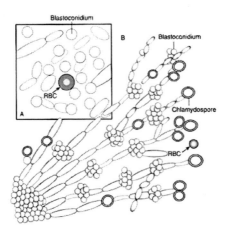

Mycelial, pathogenic form: Pseudohyphae with chlamydospores
(grape-like spores) making up the clusters of blastoconidia

What is the role of Candida?

Candida has two parasitic functions:

To gobble up any putrefied food matter in our digestive system (mostly caused by improper digestion, due to low stomach acid).

After we die, Candida acts to decompose the body, feeding off our corpses and returning us to Mother Earth!

When conditions are right, they transform their 'bud' form into the mycelial state, where filament-like roots invade deep into the mucosa in search of nourishment. The mycelia release phospholipase, an enzyme that attacks cell membranes of the mucosa: splitting fatty acids, generating free radicals and causing inflammation in the intestine and other tissues.

Wherever the yeast colonize they cause symptoms, whether an itchy anus or vagina, diarrhoea, heartburn or sore throat. The mycelial forms release 79 different toxic by-products that damage specific tissues and organs, and will determine which symptoms will occur. These toxins, such as acetaldehyde, can also compete with hormone receptor sites and cause hypothyroidism, hypoestrogenism as well as binding cortisone, progesterone and other hormones for its own use and causing endocrine deficiency states. [22]

How do you get it?

Candida albicans prefers people. Candida enters newborn infants during or shortly after birth. Usually, the growth of the yeast is kept in check by the infant's immune system and thus produces no overt symptoms. But, should the immune response weaken, the condition known as oral thrush can occur as a result. By six months of age, 90% of all babies test positive for Candida and by adulthood, virtually all humans play host to Candida albicans and are thus engaged in a life-long relationship.

Candida coexists in our bodies with many species of bacteria in a competitive balance. Other bacteria act in part to keep Candida growth in check in our body ecology, unless that balance is upset. When health is

---

[22] Calderone, R. A., and R. L. Cihlar (ed.). Fungal pathogenesis: principles and clinical applications. Marcel Dekker, Inc., New York, N.Y, 2002.

present, the immune system keeps Candida proliferation under control, but when the immune response is weakened, Candida growth can proceed unhindered. It is an 'opportunistic organism,' one which – when given the opportunity – will attempt to colonize all bodily tissues. The uncontrolled growth of Candida is known as 'Candida overgrowth' or 'Candidiasis.'

Unfortunately, there are many factors in our modern society that can upset the ecological balance of the body, weaken the immune system and thus allow the yeast to overgrow. Of these, the major risk factors which may predispose one to the proliferation of Candida are:

❖ Steroid Hormones, Immunosuppressant Drugs such as cortisone, which treat severe allergic problems by paralyzing the immune system's ability to react.
❖ Pregnancy and Birth Control Pills which upset the body's hormonal balance.
❖ Diets High in Carbohydrate and Sugar Intake, Yeast and Yeast Products, as well as Moulds and Fermented Foods
❖ Prolonged Exposure to Environmental Moulds
❖ Antibiotics and Sulpha Drugs – probably the chief culprit of all: antibiotics kill all bacteria. They do not distinguish good bacteria from bad. Antibiotics kill the 'good' flora which normally keeps the Candida under control. This allows for the unchecked growth of Candida in the intestinal tract. It is normally difficult to recover a yeast culture from bodily surfaces. However, after 48 hours of taking tetracycline, yeast can be cultured easily from anyone.

The prevalence today of Candida may be most directly related to the widespread societal exposure to antibiotics – from prescriptions for colds, infections and acne; and from additional consumption of antibiotic-treated foods such as meats, dairy, poultry and eggs. Notably, antibiotics do not kill viruses; they only destroy bacteria. Yet, they are universally prescribed for all colds, flu and other viral problems. Such indiscriminate and extensive use of antibiotics is not only considered a primary cause of Candida overgrowth, but is recently being found to be responsible for the unbridled development of 'killer bacteria.'

The rapid and direct proliferation of the yeast following antibiotic use strongly suggests that the problem of Candida is one which stems from an inner state of imbalance, rather than from an outside attack by a microbe or disease. This is a very important point to understand if one wishes to get rid of an overgrowth problem, suggesting that Candida is not so much a problem as is the body's own failure to control it!

Why is it a serious problem?

Once begun, if not recognized and treated appropriately, Candida overgrowth can result in a self-perpetuating, negative cycle. Large numbers of yeast germs can weaken the immune system, which normally protects the body from harmful invaders. Even though Candida is part of the ecological balance in the body since birth, it is still recognized by the immune system as a foreign body that needs to be controlled.

So, when overgrowth occurs, a chronic stimulation of the immune system results – every second, every minute, every hour, every day, every month, every year – in an attempt to regain control. In time, it is believed that this can exhaust the immune system, predisposing one to more serious degenerative processes. Many believe chronic drains on the immune system such as Candida and parasites can play a direct role in the development of cancer and AIDS. Seen in this light, Candida overgrowth should not be taken lightly.

Candida produces its effects by two routes. Firstly, there is a direct route initially by invasion of the gut and the vagina – Candida is capable of spreading along the entire length of the gut. The presence of chronic vaginitis can often indicate widespread Candidiasis. Secondly, there can be indirect effects caused by the spread of toxins through the bloodstream to other sites in the body.

Candida can alter its form from a simple yeast organism to a 'mycelial fungal form' with a network of root-like fibres called rhizoids. These can penetrate and damage the gut lining, allowing foreign food proteins to be absorbed into the bloodstream and to challenge the immune system, so that multiple food allergies or intolerances may result.

Toxic waste - acetaldehyde

Toxic waste from mycotoxins[23] from Candida infestations can also be absorbed into the bloodstream causing 'Yeast Toxin Hypersensitivity'

---

23 Hussein, H. S., and J. M. Brasel. Toxicity, metabolism, and impact of mycotoxins on humans and animals. Toxicology 167:101-134, 2001.

leading to many symptoms such as anxiety, depression and impaired intellectual functioning. The main toxin implicated here is acetaldehyde, which is a normal by-product of metabolism, produced in small amounts and rendered harmless by the liver. If, however, there is excess production of this by Candida, particularly in low-oxygen environments, and a lack of the appropriate liver enzymes – which tend to be deficient in 5 per cent of the general population – the acetaldehyde will become bound strongly to human tissue. This may cause impaired neuro-transmission in the brain, resulting in anxiety, depression, defective memory and cloudy thinking.

Acetaldehyde intermediates cause a good part of the cellular damage that occurs. Acetaldehyde in the intestinal wall and liver will disrupt intestinal absorptive processes, as well as impairing the function of lymphocytes and red blood cells.[24] Acetaldehyde damages host cells by attacking them with free radical and peroxidative mechanisms. When yeast cells are deficient in oxygen, they are also more resistant to immune defenses and so patient hypoxia is a major contributing factor to yeast susceptibility for these two reasons.

Adequate amounts of glutamine, selenium, niacin, folic acid, B6, B12, iron, and molybdenum will allow the acetaldehydes to be metabolized into acetic acid, which can be excreted, or converted further into acetyl coenzyme A. Supplementing with these nutrients during the treatment of Candida will help to reduce unpleasant symptoms related to acetaldehydes.

Effects on immunity

Some 40 to 60% of all the immune cells in our body are in the gut. The immune system may also concurrently be adversely affected by poor nutrition, heavy exposure to moulds in the air, as well as an increasing number of chemicals in our food, water and air, including: petrochemicals, formaldehyde, perfumes, cleaning fluids, insecticides, tobacco and other indoor and outdoor pollutants. Over 10,000 chemicals have been added to our food supplies alone that were not there just a hundred years ago! We do not have the genetic recognition of these substances as foods or as useful additions to our bodies.

---

24 Truss, CO. Metabolic abnormalities in patients with chronic candidiasis – the acetaldehyde hypothesis, *Journal of Orthomolecular Medicine*, 13:63-93, 1984.

Specifically, yeasts tend to secrete a toxin called Gliotoxin,[25] which can disrupt the immune system by inactivating enzyme systems and producing free radicals, thus interfering with the DNA of leukocytes. It is also cytotoxic.

The resulting lowered resistance may not only cause an overall sense of ill health, but may also allow for the development of respiratory, digestive and other systemic symptoms. One may also become predisposed to developing sensitivities to foods and chemicals in the environment. Such 'allergies' may in turn cause the membranes of the nose, throat, ear, bladder and intestinal tract to swell and develop infection.

Such conditions may lead the physician to prescribe a 'broad spectrum' antibiotic . . . which may then further promote the overgrowth of Candida and strengthen the existing negative chain of events, leading to further stress on the immune system and increased Candida-related problems. This I have seen happen in clinical practice many times. If only physicians could think laterally for a minute, many hundreds of thousands of superfluous antibiotic prescriptions could be done away with to the benefit of the patient as opposed to the pharmaceutical industry.

Heavy metals such as mercury and others are found in higher amounts when Candida is present as the Candida yeasts actually store the metals in their cells – these metals are then released when the Candida die during treatment. It is therefore wise to begin a heavy metal chelating programme concomitantly with the Candida protocol.[26]

Occupational exposure studies have found that mercury impairs the body's ability to kill Candida albicans by impairment of the lytic activity of neutrophils and myeloperoxidase in workers whose mercury excretion levels are within current safety limits. Such levels of mercury exposure were also found to inhibit cellular respiratory burst, thus encouraging the proliferation of Candida. Immune Th1 cells inhibit Candida by cytokine related activation of macrophages and neutrophils.

---

25 Iwata, K.; Yamamoto, Y 'Glycoprotein toxins produced by Candida albicans.' Proceedings of the Fourth international conference on the mycoses, PAHO scientific publication #356, June 1977.
26 See www.detoxmetals.com for such a programme, using a scientifically-tested natural toxic metal chelating agent called HMD®.

Development of Th2 type immune responses deactivates such defences. Mercury inhibits macrophage and neutrophil defence against Candida by its affects on Th1 and Th2 cytokine effects. Candida overgrowth results in production of the highly toxic canditoxin and ethanol which are known to cause fatigue, toxicity and depressive symptoms. Another study found such impairment of neutrophils decreases the body's ability to combat viruses such as those that cause heart damage, resulting in more inflammatory damage.

The main components of the immune system are:

B-lymphocytes: these produce proteins called immunoglobulins, which bind with antigenic substances and render them harmless. An antigen is a substance which the body recognizes as being alien and therefore potentially harmful. An immunoglobulin is a particular kind of protein which coats the antigen and by being made harmless; the antigen can then be digested by other cells.

T-lymphocytes: there are three types:

a) The killer cells: these attack and destroy substances by using enzymes and hormones.
b) The helper cells: these help B cells to make the immunoglobulins.
c) The suppressor cells: these protect the body from the excesses of its defense system by opposing B-cell antibody production.

Chronic candidiasis caused by the opportunistic pathogen Candida albicans is characterized by a depressed cellular immune response.[27,28] Lymphocytes from many patients with chronic candidiasis fail to proliferate in vitro in response to mitogens and/or Candida antigens.[29] In addition, a high percentage of these patients often fail to mount delayed-type hypersensitivity reactions to Candida antigens.[30] Evidence exists which suggests that the organism itself may be responsible for inducing a

---

27 Rogers, T.J., Balish, E. Immunity to Candida albicans. *Microbiol. Rev.* 44, 660, 1980.
28 Kirkpatrick, C.H. Host factors in defense against fungal infections. *Am. J. Med.* 77(D), 1, 1984.
29 Kirkpatrick, C.H., Rich, R. & Bennett, J. Chronic mucocutaneous candidiasis: model building in cellular immunity. *Ann. Int. Med.* 74, 955, 1971.
30 Cahill, L., Ainbender, E. & Glade, P. Chronic mucocutaneous candidiasis: T-cell deficiency associated with B-cell dysfunction in man. *Cell. Immunol.* 14, 215, 1974.

state of immunological non-responsiveness.[31] It has been reported that treatment of the infection with anti-fungal agents may lead to a restoration of immune function.[32] More recently, Candida-specific suppressor cells have been identified in patients with chronic candidiasis.[33] In addition, extracts of Candida have been shown to induce suppressor cell activity in normal human lymphocytes.[34] This Candida-associated immunosuppression may be an important factor in exacerbation of the disease.

It is largely the suppressors which are involved in fighting the Candida challenge, partly because Candida's adaptability allows it to produce disguising antigens, which deter the immune system from recognizing it as foreign and harmful. In this way the immune system may eventually become non-responsive to the presence of Candida albicans. Candida toxins will then circulate virtually unchallenged, and Candida will grow in a range of tissues either as a yeast or a mycelial fungus.

This apparent tolerance of Candida by the immune system can only be reversed in the long term by ending exposure of the body to yeast antigens and toxins. A high percentage of serum from symptomless people has been found to contain yeast toxin immunoglobulins. This indicates that the B-cell immune defenses must be constantly counteracting Candida toxins. When alive, yeasts are able to invade the immune system to a certain degree. When they are killed, proteins making up the yeast cell wall are absorbed through the lining of the intestine and can cause heightened allergic reactions, resulting in a phenomenon called 'Die off' or the 'Herxheimer reaction.[35]' This may in fact signal a good response to treatment.

---

31 Durandy, A., Fischer, A., Ledeist, F., Drouhet, E. & Griscelli, C. Mannan-specific and mannan-induced T-cell suppression activity in patients with chronic mucocutaneous candidiasis. *J. Clin. Immunol.* 7, 400, 1987.

32 Budtz-Jorgensen, E. Cellular immunity in acquired candidiasis of the palate. *Scand. J. Dent. Res.* 81, 372, 1973.

33 Gupta, S. Autologous mixed lymphocyte reaction in man. XI. Deficiency of autologous mixed lymphocyte reaction and abnormalities of monoclonal antibody-defined T-cell subsets in chronic mucocutaneous candidiasis. *Scand. J. Immunol.* 21, 525, 1985.

34 Damle, N., Childs, A. & Doyle, L. Immunoregulatory T-lymphocytes in man: soluble antigen specific suppressor inducer T-lymphocytes are derived from the CD4+, CD45R-, p80+ subpopulation. *J. Immunol.* 139, 1501, 1987.

35 The Herxheimer reaction is explained in more detail later in this chapter.

The diagram below clearly shows how Candida is known to impair immune functioning by directly and negatively impacting the helper-suppresser ratio of T- lymphocytes.

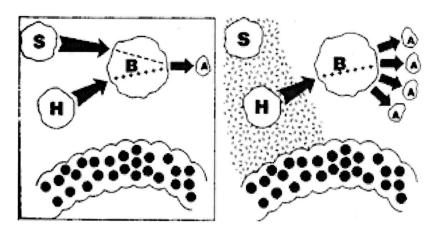

Diagram 1: How yeast toxins (black dots) injure the immune system
S = Suppressor cell; H = Helper cell; B = B-cell; A=Antigens

First diagram: Yeast and intestinal lactobacilli bacteria in balance = normal immune function. A balance between intestinal lactobacilli bacteria and yeast allow for normal immune lymphocyte function: helper cells stimulate the B-cells to make antibodies, whereas suppressor cells appropriately oppose B-cell antibody production. Antibody production is in balance.

Second diagram: Overgrowth of intestinal yeast, release of toxins into the bloodstream, and altered immune function. Intestinal yeast overgrowth and yeast toxins released into the bloodstream inhibit suppressor cell function. Stimulation of antibody production by helper cells is now unopposed, and inappropriate antibody production occurs. Here we have a heightened state of allergy, as well as an increased susceptibility to autoimmune conditions.

Occupational exposure studies have found mercury impairs the body's ability to kill Candida albicans by impairment of the lytic activity of neutrophils and myeloperoxidase in workers whose mercury excretion levels are within current safety limits. Development of Th2 type immune responses deactivates such defenses. Mercury inhibits macrophage and neutrophil defense against candida by its affects on Th1 and Th2 cytokine effects. Candida overgrowth results in production of the highly toxic canditoxin and ethanol which are known to cause fatigue, toxicity, and depressive symptoms. Another study found such impairment of neutrophils decreases the body's ability to combat viruses such as those that cause heart damage, resulting in more inflammatory damage.

What are the signs of Candida infection?

The result of heightened Candida overgrowth is a list of adverse symptoms of considerable length. Basically, the characteristics of Candida overgrowth fall under three categories, those affecting:

- ❖ The gastrointestinal and genitourinary tracts
- ❖ Allergic responses
- ❖ Mental/emotional manifestations.

Initially the signs will show near the sites of the original yeast colonies. Most often the first signs are seen in conditions such as nasal congestion and discharge, nasal itching, blisters in the mouth, sore or dry throat, abdominal pain, belching, bloating, heartburn, constipation, diarrhoea, rectal burning or itching, vaginal discharge, vaginal itching or burning, increasingly worsening symptoms of PMS, prostatitis, impotence, frequent urination, burning on urination, bladder infections.

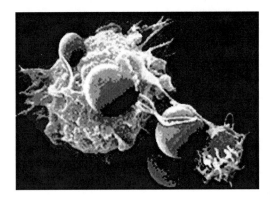

White blood cell killing Candida

But, if the immune system remains weak long enough, Candida can spread to all parts of the body causing an additional plethora of problems such as fatigue, drowsiness, uncoordination, lack of concentration, mood swings, dizziness, headaches, bad breath, coughing, wheezing, joint swelling, arthritis, failing vision, spots in front of the eyes, ear pain, deafness, burning or tearing eyes, muscle aches, depression, irritability, sweet cravings, increasing food and chemical sensitivities, numbness and tingling, cold hands and feet, asthma, hay fever, multiple allergies, hives and rashes, eczema, psoriasis, chronic fungal infections like athlete's foot, ringworm and fingernail/ toenail infections.

In addition, 79 different toxic products are released by Candida, which in itself places a considerable burden on the immune system. These get into the bloodstream and travel to all parts of the body where they may give rise to a host of adverse symptoms. As mentioned above, yeasts in the body produce a by-product called acetaldehyde, a toxic substance resulting in several health consequences. In fact, acetaldehyde is the compound that produces the symptoms in an alcohol 'hang-over.'

Molybdenum plays a role as a co-factor in helping break down acetaldehyde to a form that actually provides us with energy and also plays a large role in the detoxification pathway for acetaldehyde in the human body. There are dozens of known toxins released by yeast in the body. This damages and overworks both the liver and the immune system as the body tries to detoxify these poisons.

In Candida overgrowth, the yeast colonies can dig deep into intestinal walls, damaging the bowel wall in their colonization. The invasive Candida filaments produce disease affecting the entire body in a number of ways:[36]

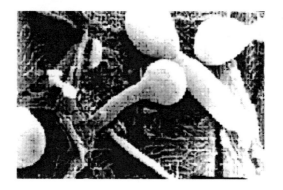

Candida penetrating human tissue

---

[36] Crandall M. The pathogenetic significance of intestinal Candida colonization. *Int J Hyg Environ Health* 207; 79-81, 2004.

Destruction of the intestinal membrane, allowing for:

a) Severe leaks of toxins from activity of undesirable microorganisms within the layers of encrusted faecal matter into the bloodstream, causing a variety of symptoms and aggravating many pre-existing conditions. Under the anaerobic conditions of the colon, Candida itself will produce a number of toxins by fermenting sugars.

b) Absorption of incompletely digested dietary proteins. These are extremely allergenic and may produce a large spectrum of allergic reactions. Food allergies are very common with Candidiasis, as is environmental hypersensitivity (to smoke, auto exhaust, natural gas, perfumes, air pollutants), probably due to Candida filaments infiltrating lung and sinus membranes.

c) Migration of Candida itself into the bloodstream. Once in the blood, it has access to all body tissues and may cause various gland or organ dysfunctions, weakening the entire system and further lowering resistance to other diseases.

Candida can also attack the immune system, causing suppressor cell disease, in which the immune system produces antibodies to everything at the slightest provocation, resulting in extreme sensitivities.

Finally, Candida overgrowth can be dangerous if not controlled. The persistent, constant challenge to the immune system by an ever-increasing, long-term overgrowth of Candida, can eventually serve to wear down the immune system and cause a seriously weakened capacity for resistance to disease.

Women are more likely to get Candida overgrowth than are men. This is related to the female sex hormone progesterone, which is elevated in the last half of the menstrual cycle. Progesterone increases the amount of glycogen (animal starch, easily converted to sugar) in the vaginal tissues, which provides an ideal growth medium for Candida. Progesterone levels also elevate during pregnancy. Men are affected less frequently but are by no means invulnerable.

Recurrent vulvovaginal infections of Candidiasis can be effectively eradicated using the Davinci Candida Protocol (DCP) described below, along with boric acid suppositories. In one study of 100 women with chronic resistant yeast infections, who had failed extensive and prolonged conventional therapy, were treated with 600mg boric acid vaginal suppositories twice a day for two or four weeks. This regimen was effective in curing 98% of the women who had previously failed to respond to the most commonly used antifungal agents.

Clinical effectiveness doesn't really get any better than this: The DaVinci Candida Protocol (DCP) works most of the time, it's relatively inexpensive and it's easy to use. The only down side I have observed apart for the initial die-off reactions which can be uncomfortable, is that the boric acid can cause some burning as the capsule melts. Using vitamin E oil or lanolin, or even vaseline on the external genitalia to protect it from the boric acid seems to avert any significant discomfort.

How do you know you have it?

Currently, diagnosis is primarily clinical, as well as the use of biodermal screening devices such as the VEGA EXPERT which I use in clinical practice. Since almost everyone has Candida in their bodies, tests for its presence are useless. Confirmation of overgrowth is very difficult through laboratory tests as it is difficult to culture and identify the pathogenic, mycelial form of Candida. Since what it does is to paralyze the immune system against it, allergy tests to determine the system's reaction to it are also ineffectual.

Furthermore, the results of the yeast imbalance and the combined effects of different hormones, as well as mycotoxins generated and released by the yeast into the bloodstream and the confusion created in the immune system – produces such a wide variety of symptoms, which are seemingly so unrelated (such as wheezing, depression and fungus infection under fingernails), that a definite diagnosis cannot be made from any specific pattern of signs and symptoms.

Signs and symptoms

There are a wide variety of signs and symptoms that are prevalent in Systemic Candidiasis – being able to score these systematically provides a good, overall picture. The patient's history and symptoms are usually the key to arriving at a diagnosis. Dr. Crook's Candida Questionnaire is also extremely helpful as it enables the patient to score their symptoms and arrive at a number – anything above 180 for women, and 140 for men is highly significant and represents the majority of symptoms that relate to this condition.[37]

Laboratory tests

Conclusive laboratory tests have not yet been developed, even though there are a number of tests appearing on the market that can help in the diagnosis of Candida, but they all have their advantages and disadvantages.

An easy-to-use diagnostics platform rapidly identifies *Candida* yeast species directly from positive blood cultures. The new assay, peptide nucleic acid fluorescence in situ hybridization (PNA FISH), is a highly sensitive, and specific assay that uses PNA probes to target species-specific ribosomal RNA (rRNA) in bacteria and yeasts.

Called the 'Yeast Traffic Light,' the assay is one of the latest molecular-based PNA FISH diagnostics platforms that provides rapid identification of bloodstream pathogens in hours instead of days. Laboratories can identify, in a single Yeast Traffic Light test, up to five Candida species – directly from positive blood cultures – including: C. albicans and/or C. parapsilosis, C. tropicalis, C. glabrata and/or C. krusei – in hours instead of days – enabling clinicians to provide early, effective and appropriate antifungal therapy for patients afflicted with Candidemia.

The results of the test indicate the yeast responsible for the infection: green fluorescing cells indicate C. albicans and/or C. parapsilosis; yellow fluorescing cells indicate C. tropicalis and red fluorescing cells indicate C. glabrata and/or C. krusei.

Other laboratory tests that can be used are:

CECA (CandiSphere Enzyme Immuno Assay Test) which diagnoses Candida by detecting antibodies against cytoplasmic proteins of the invasive fungal yeasts. This test is claimed to be 95% sensitive and 92% specific for Candidiasis.[38]

---

[37] Please see Appendix B.
[38] The Chronic Candidiasis Syndrome: Intestinal Candida and its relation to chronic illness OAM 1996-1997, 16. Gutierrez, J; Maroto, C. et al: Circulating Candida antigens and

Direct stool examinations for chronic intestinal Candidiasis. A gram stain for yeast along with direct microscopic examination is a very accurate diagnostic tool for Candida. This method avoids quantification inaccuracies that appear with cultures.

Serum or urine Darabinitol levels[39]. This is a Candida carbohydrate metabolite, which is also a neurotoxin. You may have difficulty finding a lab that will do this test.

A Candida culture may be considered if there is the presence of oral thrush/white coating on the tongue. Excessive growth may be an indication, especially if it increases with your symptoms. The culture may take at least a week or more to grow correctly and the sample must be taken using proper protocols.

Serum Candida antibody levels (IgG, IgM, and IgA). These will not be definitive since the body's ability to defend itself against Candida is limited due to its location in the gastrointestinal tract. Positive or negative responses are difficult to interpret. Candida IgE may be helpful. However, a test of IgG blood antibodies to Candida albicans in conjunction with a direct yeast culture stool sample evaluation is recommended.

Biodermal screening

There are other testing procedures that I use in clinical practice, but mainly bio-dermal screening, using the VEGA Biodermal screening.

When an ampoule of pathogenic Candida is placed in the honeycomb of the VEGA EXPERT and the probe placed on an acupoint of a finger, it is very clear when a patient 'resists' as the conductivity drops. What I have also found time and time again in over 2,000 Candida patients that I have tested to date, is that not only do they register positive on the VEGA to Candida, but also all other yeast families such as yeast, mushrooms and fermented products involving yeast such as wine, beer and vinegar products. I personally find the VEGA a very useful diagnostic device that

---

antibodies: useful markers of candidemia. *Journal of Clinical Microbiolog*, 31(9): 25502, 1993.
[39] Walsh, TJ, Lee JW et al: Serum Darabinitol measured by automated quantitative enzymatic assay for detection and therapeutic monitoring of experimental disseminated candidiasis: correlation with tissue concentrations of Candida albicans. *Journal of Medical & Veterinary Mycology*. 32(3):20515, 1994.

can answer a lot of questions that more traditional laboratory testing cannot.

Autonomic response testing (ART)

Another method of testing for Candida is to use a form of Kinesiological muscle testing called Autonomic Response Testing (ART) invented by a German neurologist Dr. Dietrich Klinghardt, M.D. Ph.D. Both of these tests are described in more detail in chapter 2.

The secrets to success

It is my opinion that if one wants to be successful in eradicating this pathogen, you must kill it using natural anti-fungal remedies, while at the same time cleaning up the internal mileau. One must also try to convert the pathogenic, mycelial Candida back to the normal budding yeasts – this is a **crucially important step** often missed by many practitioners of natural medicine. The only remedies that can do this successfully are the Sanum isopathic fungal remedies invented by Professor Enderlein,[40] after many years of experimentation using darkfield microscopy. See below for further details. Many physicians now believe that as an interim measure before embarking on a treatment protocol for Candida overgrowth, these remedies possess such minor risk and expense that they should be considered in any chronic illness.

One clinical trial a person may attempt is to avoid certain foods for five days which are known to facilitate the growth of yeast. Such foods include the following:

a) **Sugar and Simple Carbohydrates** such as those found in all sweetened food, including the use of honey, molasses, sorghum, maple syrup, sugar, fructose, maltose, dextrose, corn syrup, etc.

b) **Yeast Products** such as beer, wine, yeast leavened bread, natural B vitamins, brewer's yeast.

c) **Fermented and Mould-Producing Foods** such as mushrooms, cheese, vinegar, mustard, ketchup, relish and other condiments made with vinegar.

---

40 Referred to in Chapter 2 – Live Blood Analysis.

After avoiding these foods for 5 days, try adding them back individually into the diet in large quantities. By observing how one feels while off these foods, in comparison to any adverse affects experienced when going back on the foods, one may get a clue as to any possible yeast involvement as a causative factor for any adverse symptoms.

If adverse symptoms are provoked by a return to the yeast enhancing foods, your physician may feel that there is at least a possible reason to suspect Candida overgrowth, which may then warrant more definitive action. This may not be the best method and personally I do not use it as I would use VEGA screening and ART to determine whether there is pathogenic Candidiasis, backed up by the signs and symptoms, using Dr. Crook's Candida Questionniare (see Appendix B). However, if you are not a VEGA practitioner or use any other form of ANS testing, then this may be a good way to begin.

Having had Candida myself and spent many years trying to find a comprehensive cure for this systemic condition, I eventually discovered a successful treatment protocol which not only cured my own Candidiasis but has also helped over 2,000 patients who have been through this protocol at my DaVinci Centre. I have thus called it the DaVinci Candida Protocol (DCP). So, let us examine in more detail the premise of this protocol.

The DaVinci Candida Protocol (DCP)

I hear from practitioners and patients the same story when it comes to treating Candida – that the patient feels better initially while they are on the treatment programme, but when they complete it they find that many of the old symptoms will return after a few weeks or months. Why is this the case? In my experience, I believe that it is literally impossible to kill ALL the pathogenic Candida organisms in the body tissues and organs – remember these are the mycelial or rhizoid forms, not the normal budding forms which are asymptomatic.

As we take the various antifungal herbs, certainly some of these pathogenic forms will be killed off, but even if a small percentage were to remain – say 5% – then they would quickly proliferate as soon as we go back to a normal diet. It will only be a matter of a few weeks before symptoms return again in force. This is classically what happens with cases of vaginal thrush as well as many cases of systemic Candidiasis. I am certain that there will be many people and practitioners who will relate to this, as I hear it often from both groups.

One of the factors that I consider unique in the DaVinci Candida Protocol, that took me more than 10 years to develop, is the use of the Sanum Isopathic remedies that can actually alter the pathogenic forms of Candida back to their normal, budding forms. This is based on the work of Prof. Enderlein many years ago, who developed what are now called the Sanum isopathic remedies, who I mentioned above.

The DaVinci Candida Protocol has five basic objectives:

1. Starve the Candida by eliminating the foods mentioned above that feed it.
2. Kill the Candida through the use of anti-Candida products mentioned below.
3. Repopulate the bowel flora with a high-potency GG-probiotic such as Culturelle that contains 30 billion live bacteria and has been well researched in university trials.
4. Regulate the dysbiosis and convert the pathological, mycelial form of Candida back to the normal form by the use of the Sanum remedies.
5. Restore biochemical balance to the body and strength to the immune system. This will allow the body once again to regain and maintain control over Candida growth by optimizing the diet – this would involve avoiding food intolerances and following the Metabolic Type Diet by Wolcott[41]. Also kill off other parasites using Hulda Clark's parasite cleanse[42] or similar, and begin chelating heavy metals out of the system.

None of these objectives are mutually exclusive, nor can they be addressed in a serial way – they all need to be looked at concomitantly for the treatment protocol to be successful. Incidentally, if the DaVinci Candida Protocol is followed diligently by the patient and practitioner, the success rate of eliminating the Candida approaches 100%. It is only those very rare cases where we have a case of antifungal-resistant Candida that there is a problem – this usually happens when the patient has been treated time and time again with medicinal anti-fungals and the Candida have now become

---

41 For details, please refer back to the section entitled Nutritional testing for metabolic typing in chapter 2.
42 For details, please refer back to the Herbal parasite cleanse in chapter 4.

a 'super Candida' – this again can be eliminated using this protocol but the time required will be stretched from three months to 4-5 months. I have never had an antifungal-resistant case that was not cured in a maximum of 5 months, but as I said earlier, these are very rare occurrences.

Phase 1 - starving the candida

I have found that it is literally impossible to treat Candida if one does not cut out **ALL** forms of sugar for a period of 3 months. The foods that should be strictly **AVOIDED** during that time include:

Sugar – and all foods that contain sugar. These include white and brown sugar, honey, syrups, liquor, lactose, fructose, all confectionary and sweet cakes, chocolates, ice-creams, home-made sweets and cakes, biscuits, fizzy beverages and all fruit drinks.

Yeast – and all foods that contain yeast including breads, vinegar, ketchups, mayonnaise and pickles.

Mushrooms – all types, including Chinese mushrooms such as Shitake.

Refined Foods – all white flours, white rice, white pasta products, cornflour, custard and refined cereal products, unless they are wholemeal or organic.

Fermented Products – all alcoholic beverages, vinegar and all vinegar products such as ketchup, mayonnaise and pickles, beer.

Nuts – all types of nuts that are cleaned and packaged without their shells – these have a tendency to collect fungal spores and moulds from the atmosphere, which will antagonize the Candida. Nuts that are fresh with their shells are OK.

Fresh and Dried Fruit – all fresh fruit should be avoided for the initial **six weeks only** as again, the fructose they contain will feed the Candida and make it extremely difficult to eliminate.

All other fruit that is not fresh such as cooked, tinned or dried and fruit juices should be avoided for the full 3 months – your health practitioner will advise you when to begin eating fruit again. Obviously this includes fresh fruit juices (vegetable juices are OK), as well as marmalades. There are book written about the "anti-Candida diet" that may be worth reading.[43]

Phase 2 – killing the candida

There are a number of herbal formulas, homeopathics and probiotics that are used in the DaVinci Candida Protocol – they have been carefully selected after years of experimentation, and the fact that they have worked time and time again with hundreds of people. The aim of using these supplements is to kill off the Candida. Here are the supplements in order:

1. **Kandidaplex** – a doctor-formulated compound that contains Berberine, undecylenic acid, biotin, sorbic acid, citrus seed extract and Pau D'Arco. Dosage: 2 caps x 3 daily.

2. **Horopito** (practitioner-strength) – a New Zealand herbal product that contains two powerful anti-fungal agents that have been shown to kill Candida – Pseudowinterata colorata and the synergistic herb Aniseed, that boosts effectiveness 6 fold. Dosage: 1 cap twice daily.

3. **Caprylic Acid** (600mg) – a derivative of coconut that stops the Candida reproducing, as well as killing the Candida. Dosage: 1 tab x 3 daily.

4. **Candida 30c:** homeopathic – freely available in most pharmacies. Dosage: 2 pillules or 1 cap x 3 daily for 2 weeks only. These are stopped just as the Sanum remedies are begun.

Phase 3 – repopulating the friendly bacteria

This phase runs parallel with phase 2 and uses good quality, human strain probiotics such as the high-potency GG strain of probiotics – one well-researched brand that we use is Culturelle but there are others too.

Culturelle contains 30 billion live bacteria per capsule, in order to repopulate the deficient flora of the gut. Dosage: 1 capsule per day.

To these supplements we add a good-quality multivitamin such as OPTIMUM 6 to provide all the vitamins and minerals that the immune system requires for optimal functioning.[44]

---

43 Burton, G. Candida Control Cookbook. New York: NAL, 1989.

Phase 4 – using isopathic remedies to normalize pathogenic candida

All the above must be taken for the full 90 days of the protocol, with the exception of the Candida 30c. After two weeks of the anti-Candida diet, certain specialized isopathic remedies are introduced, known as Sanum remedies from Germany, after the work of Prof. Enderlein, as follows. See Table 1 regimen below. Each of these isopathic remedies is only taken a couple of times per week, as follows:

1. **Mucokehl D5 tabs** - 1 tab twice weekly.
2. **Pefrakehl D4 caps** - 1 cap twice weekly.
3. **Notakehl D5 tabs** - 1 tab twice weekly.
4. **Fortakehl D5 tabs** - 1 tab twice weekly.
5. **Nigersan D5 tabs** - 1 tab twice weekly.
6. **Albicansan D4 caps** - 1 cap every second day.

If there is vaginal discharge, or anal Candida, then vaginal or anal pessaries of Albicansan D3 must also be used to eliminate this topical infection. These can be used every second day last thing at night, after sex.

These Sanum remedies mentioned above are continued for 10 weeks until the end of the Candida protocol. It is wise to begin the Sanum remedies TWO WEEKS after beginning the general protocol in order to allow a considerable portion of the Candida to die off, and to reduce the severity of the Herxheimer reaction.

Fruit can be re-introduced back into the diet FOUR WEEKS after the beginning of the Sanum remedies.

All capsules and tablets should be taken at different times from food and should not be taken together, as they clash. Follow this simple table of how and when to take your Sanum remedies. These remedies are taken BEFORE or SEPARATE from food.

Open the capsules and pour the powder that they contain under the tongue and allow it to dissolve and absorb for a few minutes.

---

44 All the abovementioned supplements are available from www.worldwidehealthcenter.net (USA customers) or www.seeknatural.co.uk (UK and European customers).

	M am	M pm	Tue a.m.	Tue p.m.	W a.m.	W p.m.	Thu a.m.	Thu p.m.	Fri a.m.	Fri p.m.	Sat a.m.	Sat p.m	Sun a.m.	Sun p.m.
Albican	■				■				■				■	
Mucok		■					■							
Pefrake				■						■				
Nigersa					■						■			
Fortake						■								■
Notake			■								■			

Table 1 – Protocol for the Sanum Remedies

Prof. Enderlein's Sanum remedies work by changing the harmful microorganisms in the body fluids into non-aggressive forms, probably by changing the pH and electrical conductivity[45]. Harmful bacteria and toxins are broken down and excreted through natural processes. They also help to alleviate the dysbiosis and bring the internal mileau of the intestine back into balance.

Phase 5 – balancing the body chemistry

It is a commonly recognized and accepted fact that immune system efficiency is highly dependent on the proper biochemical balance in the body. This of course, is dependent on proper and adequate nutrition to supply the body with all the required biochemical constituents (vitamins, minerals, enzymes, intrinsic factors, etc).

Different people require different amounts and balances of nutrients for optimum health. The criteria for the determination of these differing nutritional requirements lies within the definition of one's metabolic type, i.e., the genetically determined metabolic and nutritional parameters that define each person's individuality on every level.

It is precisely because different people have different metabolic types, and therefore different needs for nutrition, that the allopathic, symptom-treatment approach in nutrition is baseless and so often ineffective. This further explains why what (nutritionally) helps make one person better, may have little or no effect on another, or even make a third person worse.

I have not tried to modify this protocol as I have found it to be so

---

45 Georgiou, G.J. The physics behind live blood analysis and zeta potentials, *Explore!* Vol. 14, No. 5., September 2005.

successful in the treatment of over 1,500 patients to date, that I dare not juggle with it in case it loses its effectiveness. I'm sure that it can be improved upon, and would welcome comments from other practitioners working with Candida. It is only through sharing that we will grow and become better practitioners.[46, 47]

Herxheimer reactions

Depending on the severity of Candida overgrowth and the amount of the agents taken, the Candida can be killed off in vast numbers in a very short period of time. As they are killed, they release substances that are toxic to the body – these are called mycotoxins. If the elimination organs such as the kidneys, liver, lymphatics, gut and skin cannot clear these mycotoxins quickly and they accumulate in the tissues, then a temporary toxic or allergic-type reaction can occur. The technical name for this experience is a Herxheimer reaction but it is more commonly referred to as 'die off.'

Usually die-off lasts only a few hours, though it can last several days. It can usually be controlled by reducing the dosage of the remedies used to kill the Candida, as well as taking drainage herbs and homeopathics that your practitioner will advise you on.

Signs of Herxheimer reaction can be many and varied but generally involve such discomfort as aching, bloating, dizziness, nausea, and overall 'goopy sick' feeling, or a worsening of original symptoms. Fortunately, die-off is generally short in duration, and although uncomfortable, is at least a confirmation of the presence of Candida and that something 'good' is happening.

Exercise as well as insuring proper, daily bowel evacuation has been reported as being helpful in countering the adversities of die-off. Maintaining a high daily intake of pure water is also important to keep the channels of elimination open. Sometimes taking a teaspoon of baking soda (sodium bicarbonate) in a glass of water can help to quickly neutralize acidic reactions in the body that lead to inflammation and pain.

---

46 Georgiou, G.J. Scourge of the 21st Century: Systemic Candidiasis – (Part 1). *British Naturopathic Journal*, Vol. 25, No. 1, 2008.
47 Georgiou, G.J. Treatment of Systemic Candidaisis – (Part 2). *British Naturopathic Journal*, Vol. 25, No. 1, 2008.

It may be possible to slow down these symptoms, many of which are caused by acetaldehyde, one of the main toxins produced by yeast. Taking Molybdenum can break down this toxin into something far less harmful. From examining the biochemical pathway of Acetaldehyde into acetic acid, (Threonine to acetaldehyde to acetic acid to acetyl coenzyme A), both Niacine amide (NAD) and aldehyde oxidase are required for these chemical pathways. Both of these are dependent on certain nutrients such as riboflavin, iron, and molybdenum – it may be worth considering adding these to the Candida protocol if Herxheimer reactions are bad.

Case studies

There is still a lot of controversy surrounding the topic of Candida, and I am the first to agree that we do not have all the answers. One thing that I have witnessed in clinical practice, however, is the astounding recovery that many of these so-called Candidiasis patients make when placed on the DaVinci Candida Protocol (DCP).

Personally, I have seen many different skin problems clear when the systemic Candidiasis is treated, including: psoriasis, as well as chronic sinusitis, joint pains, cheloid or scar formations, cracked hands, chronic coughs and sore throats of many years standing, chronic thrush and vaginal discharge, headaches and migraines, chronic fatigue or myalgic encephalomyelitis (ME) and many other rather atypical symptoms that were labelled as 'Idiopathic' which basically means 'unknown aetiology.' Here are a few case histories for your interest.

Case 1 – This is the case of a woman who went in for a D & C scrape of the uterus. During the surgery, the gynaecologist ruptured the uterus and she required emergency surgery due to heavy internal haemorrhage. During that time, she received a number of IV antibiotics and a couple of months after being discharged, she suffered from splitting hands along with chronic thrush, fatigue and other skin rashes of unknown origin. She made a dramatic improvement in all of these symptoms after completing the DaVinci Candida Protocol.

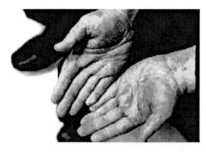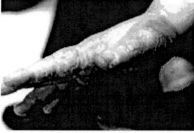

Case 1: Bad case of splitting hands after IV antibiotics

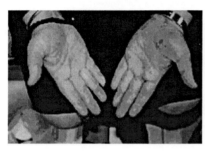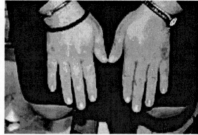

Case 1: Two months into the DaVinci Candida Treatment

Case 2 – This is a lady who had suffered from chronic psoriasis for over 20 years – this had spread to most of her torso as well as the limbs. One of the underlying problems of the skin problem was systemic Candidiasis, which cleared after three months of the DaVinci Candida Protocol.

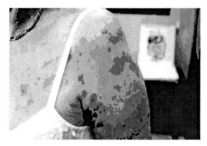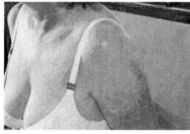

Case 2: Chronic psoriasis (left) and 3 months after completion of DaVinci Candida Treatment

Case 3 - **A** complex case of an idiopathic skin problem of 20 years' duration. Using the Candida Treatment Protocol resulted in over 75% improvement, but there was a bacterial element that needed further treatment to completely eliminate it

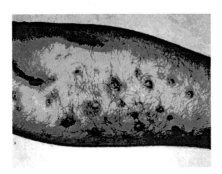 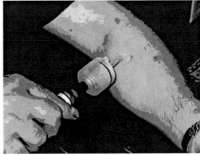

Case 3: Idiopathic skin problems of 20 years' duration (left) and after treatment (right)

Chapter 6

Parasites: the uninvited guests!

It always amuses me when I tell a patient that they are a suspect for parasites, based on their symptomatology and other screening tests. They are usually aghast with disgust at how 'dirty' they must be! Little do they know that they are in the majority, as it is estimated that about 80% of most populations in the Western world have some sort of parasites. So, what about you? To check whether you may have parasites, answer the questionnaire found in Appendix A at the end of the book.

I am including this chapter here as parasites can cause a lot of health problems and appear to be one of the underlying causes of many chronic degenerative diseases, including cancers. My intention is not to discuss the details of parasitology, as that would require a book in itself – but to touch on the subject with some examples of the more common parasites, and end with some natural remedies that will help to clear these parasites from the body. There are combinations of natural remedies that can remove literally hundreds of parasites concomitantly – these are powerful combinations that have been tried and tested in clinical practice by many practitioners around the world.

What is a parasite?

The word parasite comes from the Greek word *para* meaning 'beside' and *sitos* meaning 'food.' A parasite is any organism that derives its food, nutrition and shelter by living in or on another organism.[1]

Circulated worldwide, the Journal of the American Medical Association (JAMA) reported in 1984 that more than one-half of the 8.3 billion people on Earth were infected with parasitic disease. Parasites generally live and breed in the mucous layers of the body – there are over 100 kinds of parasites that can live in the human body.

---

[1] Parasitism is a type of symbiotic relationship between two different organisms of different species where one organism, the parasite, benefits at the expense of the host.

All parasites generally prevent the absorption of nutrients from food and irritate the intestinal lining while entering the bloodstream, and causing toxicity in the body tissues.

In November 1993 the National Institute of Allergy and Infectious Disease (NIAID) reported that parasites in the US affect millions of Americans. The Centers for Disease Control (CDC) estimates that between 100,000 and 1,000.000 cases of Giardia lamblia occur each year. In the Spring of 1993, 100 people died and 400,000 became seriously ill because of contamination of the water supply in Milwaukee by the parasite Cryptosporidium. A nationwide survey by the CDC in 1976 estimated that one in every six people, selected at random, had one or more parasites.

One person can pass millions of Giardia lamblia cysts each day, and most infections probably result from ingestion of water or food contaminated with human sewage. Open sewers in city streets and contamination of drinking water with this sewage undoubtedly results in many infections.

Many cases of 'travelers' diarrhoea' are caused by Giardia. Even in developed countries potable (drinking) water can be contaminated with small amounts of sewage, especially when septic systems are built too close to wells. Thus, it is not surprising that G. lamblia is found throughout the world.

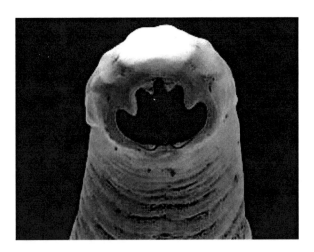

Parasitic infections cause a tremendous burden of disease in both the tropics and subtropics as well as in more temperate climates. Of all parasitic diseases, malaria causes the most deaths globally. Malaria[2] kills approximately 1 million people each year, most of them young children in sub-Saharan Africa.

Nasty consequences!

Some parasitic worms have the ability to fool our bodies into thinking that they are a normal part of the tissues and organs – this tricks the immune system and prevents it from attacking these intruders. When parasites are established in our bodies, they do several things:[3]

Some worm infections can cause physical trauma by perforating (burrowing) into the intestines, the circulatory system, the lungs, the liver and many other organs – this will make organs and tissues look like Emmental Cheese!

They can block and damage certain organs by lumping together into balls – which can be mistaken for cancer tumours – they will travel into the brain, heart, lungs and other organs.

They absorb nutrients such as vitamins and minerals; and amino acids needed for digestion. This can often lead to anaemia and cause drowsiness after meals.

They excrete metabolic waste products (toxic waste) that poison our bodies. This particular condition is called *Verminous Intoxification*. This can overburden our detoxification systems leading to an accumulation of toxins that could open the door to more serious disease.

Parasites can severely depress the immune system, opening more doors to the development of further degeneration, fatigue and illness.

Parasites can destroy tissues and organs much faster than they can regenerate, leading to degeneration.

---

2 http://www.cdc.gov/Malaria/biology/life_cycle.htm
3 Leventhal, R., Cheadle, RF. Medical Parasitology: A Self-Instructional Text. USA: FA Davis Company, 2002.

So who are these uninvited 'guests?'

Just briefly, let us examine some of the more common parasites found in humans in order to get some idea of what we are up against. By no means is this a comprehensive coverage of the subject, just a brief glimpse into this fascinating world that lives inside most of us.

Parasites that live inside the body of the host are called *endoparasites* (e.g. hookworms, that live in the host's gut), and those that live on the outside are called *ectoparasites* (e.g. fleas and mites).

Categories of parasites

Parasites are generally separated into different categories or groups as follows:

1. Nematodes (Nematoda) include roundworms, pinworms and hookworms.
2. Protozoa are single-celled organisms that include Toxoplasma, Giardia, Cryptosporidium and amoeba.
3. Tapeworms (Cestoda).
4. Flukes (Trematoda).

The most common gastrointestinal parasites are roundworms, pinworms and tapeworms.

Worms

Roundworms (Ascaris lumbricoides)

Roundworms[4] are the most common intestinal parasites in the world – they are more prevalent in tropical and subtropical areas, especially in Asian countries which practice crop fertilization with 'night soil' (raw human sewage). About 1 billion people are currently infected with this organism. This creature is spread directly

to humans from soil or from food contaminated with faeces. Children are very prone to roundworm infection. These worms are mobile and can

---

4 Crompton, DW, et al (eds). Ascaris and its public health significance. Taylor and Francis, Philadelphia, 1989.

travel up into the liver, heart and lungs, growing up to 35 cm in length.[5] People with this infection suffer from malnutrition due to competition for food and the inhibition of absorption of proteins, fats and carbohydrates; as well as diseases such as pneumonia, jaundice and seizures. Roundworms are diagnosed when their eggs are found in a stool specimen.[6]

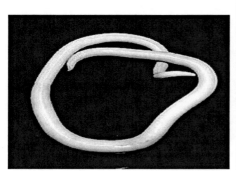 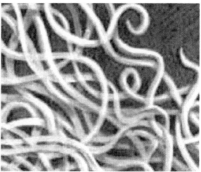

Adult Ascaris (left) and Ascaris worms (right)

Pinworms (Enterobius vermicularis)

This is one of the most common parasitic worms found in the Western, Industrialized World, and is particularly common in children. It is estimated that pinworms infect more than 10% of the population of North America and Europe. Pinworm infestation is picked up through contact with contaminated food, water, house dust, as well as through human contact.

Adult pinworms live in the large intestine (colon) and after copulation the male dies. The female moves outside the anus and lays her eggs on the perianal skin (a single female can produce more than 10,000 eggs), and they are then transferred from the itching anal area to the mouth. After laying the eggs the female also dies. In one month the egg has grown to a sexually mature worm.

---

5 Bethony J, Brooker S, Albonico M, Geiger Stefan M, Loukas A, Diement D, Hotez PJ. Soil-transmitted helminth infections: ascariasis, trichuriasis, and hookworm. *Lancet.* 367:1521-32, 2006.
6 Crompton, DW. Ascaris and ascariasis. *Adv Parasitol* 48:285-375, 2001.

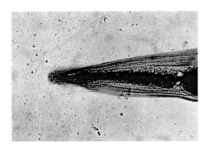 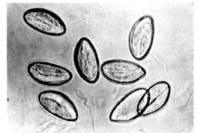

Adult pinworm head (left) and eggs (right)

Pinworms can quickly transmit to the entire family through the bathtub, toilet and bed clothes. Perianal itching is the most common symptom. A ten-year study of 2,000 cases of pinworm in children linked seemingly unrelated symptoms, i.e. epilepsy, hyperactivity and visual problems. The conventional treatment for pinworms is the prescription drug, Vermox, which is chewable.

People infected with pinworms:

- ❖ can be asymptomatic
- ❖ can have mild gastrointestinal upsets
- ❖ suffer from perianal itching
- ❖ may have behavioural changes
- ❖ can be restless and irritable
- ❖ can suffer with insomnia
- ❖ in women the pinworms can enter the vagina and cause additional irritation.

Pinworms are HIGHLY CONTAGIOUS. The eggs are infective within a few hours of being laid and can infest bed linen, clothing, carpets, hands and can cause nail biting.

Tapeworms (Taenia species)

There are several species of tapeworms (taenia)[7] that can live in the human body, usually derived from pork and beef, but also from fish and pets. Eating poorly cooked foods is one way of getting infected. Tapeworms can grow up to 7 meters long but they rarely cause symptoms, unless they grow very large and block the intestinal tract.

---

7 Schmidt, GD. Handbook of Tapeworm Identification. CRC Press, Boca Raton, Fla, 1986.

Tapeworms are found in three types of meats - each a different species and all treated the same. They are the beef tapeworm (Taenia saginata), pork tapeworm (Taenia solium) and fish tapeworm (Diphyllobothrium latum).

Despite its size – several feet in length, the **beef tapeworm** does not produce many symptoms. It thrives on carbohydrates consumed by its host, utilizing the tissue of its host for a source of protein. Thankfully, most beef tapeworms live a solitary life, but that life usually lasts twenty to twenty-five years. The common symptoms of this infection are diarrhoea, abdominal cramping, nervousness, nausea and loss of appetite.

The body is composed of successive segments (*proglottids*). The sum of the proglottids is called a strobila, which is thin, resembling a strip of tape, and is the source of the common name "tapeworm". The worm's *scolex* ("head") attaches to the intestine of the definitive host. In some species, the scolex is dominated by bothria, which are sometimes called "sucking grooves", and function like suction cups. Other species have hooks and suckers that aid in attachment.

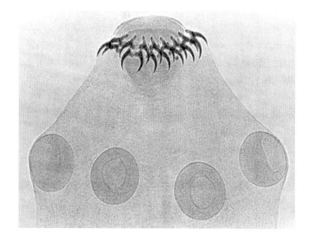

Taenia scolex with hooks

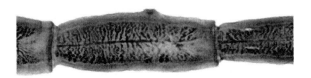

Taenia saginata proglottid

The **pork tapeworm** is similar to the beef tapeworm, but shorter in size. These worms are typically transmitted to their human host through undercooked pork, such as fresh or smoked ham or sausage. These parasites usually produce multiple worms living in the same host. Immature larvae can migrate into the muscles, heart, eyes and brain.

The **fish tapeworm** is the largest parasite found in humans. Commonly found in Scandinavia, Russia, Japan, Australia, the Great Lakes of North America, Canada and Alaska, this parasite can be contracted by eating raw or lightly cooked freshwater or migratory fish. The list of fish includes Alaskan salmon, perch, pike, pickerel and American turbot. The most common symptoms are pain and fullness of the abdomen, nausea and anorexia. The most debilitating effect of this infection is a B12 deficiency or pernicious anemia.

Hookworms (Ancylostoma species)

Hookworms[8,9] infect about 800,000.000 people as well as dogs and cats (domestic varieties). They live in the small intestine and produce 10,000 – 25,000 eggs per day. Their main source of food is their host's blood.

---

[8] Crompton, DW. Hookworm disease: Current status and new directions. Parasit Today 5:1-2, 1989.
[9] Schad, G., and Warren, K (eds). Hookworm disease: current status and new directions. Taylor and Francis, Philadephia, 1991.

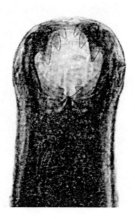

Hookworm

Guinea worms (fiery serpent – dracunculus medinensis)

This is not only a parasite of the undeveloped countries – it has been mentioned by the ancient Greek, Roman and Arabic scholars. It is found mostly in carnivores and omnivores and can grow to over one metre in length - female worms are found just under the skin (most often in the legs, ankles, feet). If it is not able to escape and find its way to the skin, it will become encapsulated in tissues and joints, causing serious complications.

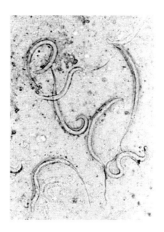

Guinea larvae from dog

Heartworms (Dirofilaria immitis)

Though usually found only in dogs, they can also occur in humans. The adult worm is quite large and lives in the arteries of the body – often causing inflammation and thickening of the heart – resulting in respiratory insufficiency, a chronic cough and vomiting. Many species of mosquitoes serve as vectors.[10]

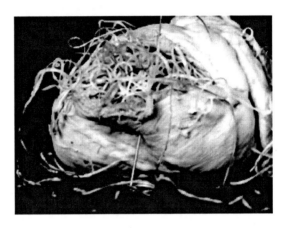

Heartworm in dog's heart

---

10 American Heartworm Society. Recommended procedures for the diagnosis and management of heartworm (Dirofilaria immitis) infection. *American Heartworm Society*, Batavia, Ill., 1992.

Warning signs of parasitic infestation

There are many different signs and symptoms of parasitic infestation – let us look at a few of the more common ones:

Itchy ears and nose	Men: sexual dysfunction
Forgetfulness	Slow reflexes
Gas, bloating	Unclear thinking
Loss of appetite	Yellowish face
Rapid heartbeat	Heart pain
Pain in the navel	Eating more than normal and still feeling hungry
Blurry or unclear vision	Pain in the back, thighs, shoulders
Lethargy	Numb hands
Burning sensation in the stomach	Women: problems with menstrual cycle
Dry lips during the day	Damp lips at night
Drooling while sleeping	Grinding teeth while asleep
Bed wetting	Anal itching

The signs of parasitic infection in humans

Constipation – some worms can physically obstruct certain organs. Blockage of the common bile duct in the gall bladder and the intestinal tract can make elimination infrequent and difficult.

Diarrhoea – some parasites, primarily protozoa, produce a prostaglandin that creates sodium and chloride loss that leads to frequent, watery stools.

Gas and bloating – some parasites live in the upper small intestine, where the inflammation they produce causes both gas and bloating. This problem worsens with the eating of hard-to-digest foods such as beans, raw fruits and raw vegetables. Persistent abdominal distension is a frequent sign of hidden invaders.

Irritable Bowel Syndrome (IBS) – parasites can irritate, inflame and coat the intestinal cell wall, leading to a variety of gastrointestinal symptoms and malabsorption of vital nutrients, particularly fatty substances. This malabsorption leads to bulky stools and excess fat in the faeces (steatorrhea).

Joint and muscle aches and pains – parasites can migrate and become enclosed in a sac (encysting) in joint fluids, and worms can encyst in the muscles. When this happens, pain becomes evident and is often assumed to be arthritis. Joint and muscle pain and inflammation are also the result of tissue damage caused by the body's ongoing immune response.

Anaemia – some intestinal worms attach themselves to the mucosal lining of the intestines and leach nutrients from the human host. If they are present in large enough numbers, they can create enough blood loss to cause a type of iron deficiency.

Allergy – parasites can irritate and sometimes perforate the intestinal lining, increasing bowel permeability to large undigested molecules. This can activate the body's immune response to produce increased levels of eosinophils. These eosinophils can inflame the body tissue, resulting in an allergic reaction.

Skin conditions – Intestinal worms can cause hives, rashes, eczema and other allergic-type skin reactions. Protozoa invasion can cause cutaneous ulcers, swelling and sores, papular lesions and dermatitis.

Granulomas – granulomas are tumour-like masses that encase destroyed larvae or parasitic eggs. They most often develop in the colon or rectal walls, but can also be found in the lungs, liver, peritoneum, and uterus.

Anxiety – metabolic waste and toxic substances from parasites can act as irritants to the central nervous system. Restlessness and anxiety are often the result of parasitic infestation.

Insomnia – awakening during the night, particularly between 2 and 4 a.m. are possibly caused by the body's attempts to eliminate toxic wastes via the liver.

Teeth grinding (Bruxism) – has been observed in cases of parasitic infection. Most notable in sleeping children, this is thought to be a nervous response to a foreign irritant.

Chronic fatigue – tiredness, flu-like complaints, apathy, depression, impaired concentration and faulty memory may all be symptomatic of malnutrition. In the presence of a parasitic infection, malnutrition results from malabsorption of proteins, carbohydrate, fats and especially vitamins A and B12.

Immune dysfunction – parasites depress immune system function by decreasing the secretion of IgA. IgA deficiency results from low levels, or complete absence of immune globulin A, which causes decreased immune function in the mucosal surfaces (e.g. the mouth, gastrointestinal tract, and lungs) and results in an increased risk of respiratory and gastrointestinal infections. It is associated with autoimmune diseases. The presence of parasites continuously stimulates the immune response and eventually can exhaust it, leaving the body vulnerable to bacterial and viral infections.

Other signs – such as blisters on the lower lip, constant wiping and scratching of the nose, restlessness and grinding of the teeth at night, dark circles under the eyes, hyperactivity, bed wetting, headaches, sensitivity to light, twitching eyelids and gums, rectum, or nose bleeds are signs that you may have parasites. These signs are also found in children.

Children

If you suspect that your child has parasites, simply answer the questions below – the more questions you answer positively, the higher the chances that your child is infested with parasites:

1. Does your child have dark circles under his eyes?
2. Is your child hyperactive?
3. Has you child been diagnosed with 'failure to thrive'?
4. Does your child grind or clench his teeth at night?
5. Does your child constantly pick his nose or scratch his behind?
6. Does your child have the habit of eating dirt?
7. Does your child wet the bed?
8. Is your child restless at night?
9. Does your child cry often for no reason?
10. Does your child tear his hair out?
11. Does your child have a limp that orthopedic treatment has not helped?
12. Does your child have a brassy, staccato-type cough?

13. Does your child have convulsions or an abnormal electroencephalogram (EEG)?
14. Does your child have recurring headaches?
15. Is your child unusually sensitive to light and prone to eyelid twitching, blinking frequently, or squinting?
16. Does your child have unusual tendencies to bleed in the gums, rectum, or nose?

Infants

1. Does your baby have severe intermittent colic?
2. Does your baby persistently bang his head against his crib?
3. Is your baby a chronic crier?
4. Does your baby have a blotchy rash around the perianal area?

Treatment: eliminating parasites

Due to the vast number of illnesses implicating parasites as the cause, a regular natural digestive detoxification program (including an anti-parasitic formula and colon cleanser to promote proper elimination), has been recommended by various naturopaths.

Ozone and parasites

One of the most effective treatments for the elimination of parasites in the large intestine is to cleanse the colon with ozonated water and hydrogen peroxide by colonic irrigation. This method is extremely lethal to all types of bad bacteria, food pathogens, parasites and viruses. As the colon becomes cleaner, the ozone and oxygen will reach other organs where parasites may be a problem.[11]

Why does ozone work so well? Healthy cells and friendly bacteria are aerobic, which means they need oxygen to survive. Unhealthy cells, parasites, pathogens and viruses are anaerobic – they can only survive in a non-oxygenated environment. It makes more sense to change the living environment of the parasite by making it richer in oxygen, and cleaner – conditions that are not so favourable to most parasites if you wish to eliminate them.

---

11 Please refer back to the section entitled Colon Hydrotherapy in Chapter 4 for a full description.

Dr. Hulda Clark's Herbal Parasite Cleanse

It would be impossible to get rid of the whole spectrum of parasites that we have in our bodies by taking vermicide drugs. Generally, these drugs target only one or two parasites at a time. Such medicines also tend to make you quite ill. Imagine taking a cocktail of such drugs to kill a dozen of your parasites! Good news, perhaps, for the drug makers but not for you.

The good news is that there are three herbs that can rid you of over one hundred types of parasites without provoking any side effects or interfering with any drug that you are already on. This is a herbal parasite cleansing programme that was put together by Dr. Hulda Regehr Clark, a biologist who studied biophysics and cell biology, as well as naturopathy. After many years of research she discovered that three herbs, when combined, have a strong synergy for eliminating many different types of parasites – here are the three herbs:

Black Walnut Hulls - (from the black walnut tree - *juglans nigra*) were used by the Indians of America as an anti-parasitic, anti-bacterial, anti-viral and anti-fungal remedy. Its active ingredients are juglone, tannin and iodine.

Wormwood (from the Artemisia shrub - *artemisia absinthum*) It is known for its vermicidal properties and helps those with a weak and under-active digestion. It also increases the acidity of the stomach and the production of bile. Wormwood contains sesquiterpene lactones (thujone and isothujone), which are thought to weaken parasite membranes. Wormwood also contains santonin, an effective remedy for parasitic diseases.

Common Cloves - (from the clove tree - *eugenia caryophyllata*) have anti-parasitic, anti-fungal, antiviral and anti-inflammatory properties. It also relieves pain/it is also a pain reliever/killer.

These three herbs must be used together as a single treatment. Black walnut hull and wormwood kill adult and developmental stages of at least one hundred parasites, while cloves kill the eggs. Only if you use them together will you rid yourself of parasites. If you only kill the adults, the eggs will soon incubate in your body and hatch into young adults. If you kill only the eggs, the million stages already at large in your body will soon grow into adults and make more eggs.

Flatworms, roundworms, protozoa, even bacteria and viruses are remarkably easy to kill using this herbal programme.

Supplements to take with the herbal parasite cleanse

Also beneficial to take concomitantly with Dr. Clark's Herbal Parasite Cleanse, **Ornithine** and **arginine** are two natural amino acids that detoxify ammonia as they help the body free itself from excessive nitrogen. They strengthen the immune defence by stimulating the production of more active and more effective White Blood Cells. They also protect the liver from damage caused by medications and chemicals, and stimulate the regeneration of the liver. Arginine is also involved with hormone secretion and reduces tumour growth.

What you need:

Black Walnut Hull Tincture

1. Wormwood capsules (200-300mg of wormwood per capsule)
2. Cloves capsules (500mg per capsule)
3. Arginine (500mg per capsule) – one capsule, twice daily
4. Ornithine (500mg per capsule) – one capsule, twice daily

Here is a summary of how to take the three herbs together over 14 days. Remember to drink plenty of water each day to flush the excreted toxins out of your system! The more water you drink, the more toxins your body will be able to expel as part of the parasite cleanse, and the better you will feel through the cleansing process:

	Black Walnut Hull Tincture	Wormwood Capsules	Clove Capsules
Day	Once a day, before a meal, in ½ a cup of water:	Capsules once a day, on an empty stomach, before a meal:	Capsules 3 times a day, with meals:
1	2 teaspoons	1	1,1,1
2	2 teaspoons	1	2,2,2
3	2 teaspoons	2	3,3,3
4	2 teaspoons	2	3,3,3
5	2 teaspoons	3	3,3,3
6	2 teaspoons	3	3,3,3
7	2 teaspoons	4	3,3,3
8	2 teaspoons	4	3,3,3
9	2 teaspoons	5	3,3,3
10	2 teaspoons	5	3,3,3
11	2 teaspoons	6	3,3,3
12	2 teaspoons	6	3,3,3
13	2 teaspoons	7	3,3,3
14	2 teaspoons	7	3,3,3

Dr. Clark's Herbal Parasite Cleanse

Homeopathics for parasitic infestation

These are certain homeopathic medicines that can be taken concomitantly with the herbal formulae – these have a more specific action depending on the parasite being targeted, such as:

ASCARIDES	TAPEWORM	HOOKWORM	PINWORM	THREADWORMS	OTHERS
Sabadilla – 30 C potency (3 x daily)	Cuprum metallicum – 3 C potency (3 x daily)	Thymol – 6 C potency (3 x daily)	Teucrium 30 C potency (3 x daily)	Santonium 30 C potency (3 x daily)	Cina 3 C potency (3x daily)
Spigelia – 30 C potency (3 x daily)				Felix mas – 3 C potency (3 x daily)	
Teucrium – 30 C potency (3 x daily)					
Santonium – 30 C potency (3 x daily)					

Additional remedies

Grapefruit Seed Extract is effective in destroying parasites and may be taken internally - two tabs, three times daily. The liquid can also used to wash raw fruits and vegetables before eating.

Cayenne, garlic, and turmeric all support proper immune system function and help destroy some worms. Garlic has a history of killing parasites including amoeba, hookworm, roundworm, pinworm and hookworm.

Barberry, Oregon grape and goldenseal have been used to eliminate giardia infections in the body.

Pumpkin seed, wormwood, sweet Annie, male fern root, tansy leaf, black walnut and clove are often recommended for the elimination of parasites.

Bromelain may help to destroy tapeworms.

To support your body with the nutrition the parasites may be robbing you of, take a high quality multivitamin and multimineral supplement.

Vitamin B complex may help prevent anaemia caused by parasites.

Supplement with a high quality probiotic such as acidophilus and bifidophilus (can be bought in capsule form) to rebuild intestinal flora – parasites thrive in an environment absent of proper intestinal flora.

Essential Fatty Acids may help protect the intestinal tract.

Aloe Vera Juice may be taken to soothe the system.

Witch Hazel may be used to reduce anal itching.

Shore up the defenses

A healthy immune system is the best defense against parasites and disease. Some of the things you can do to reduce the risk of parasitic infections are:

Drink pure water. Parasites are associated with many water-borne outbreaks and are highly resistant to conventional methods of disinfecting. Water that is properly purified with ozone is free of parasites.

Wash all fruits and vegetables. Scrape off the wax substance on the outer surface on any fruit or vegetable with a knife before washing. Anything with a nick or recess can harbour just about anything and should be cut out. Avoid eating grapes (or any other fruits) with open splits. Washing in ozonated water (you would need your own ozonator) mixed with hydrogen peroxide (one teaspoon per gallon of water) will kill parasites. Rinse well afterwards to remove peroxide residue. Some prefer to wash fruit and vegetables in chlorinated water, but chlorine and organic material do not mix well together as they are prone to produce carcinogenic compounds.

Thoroughly cook meats and fish. Do not eat raw or uncooked meats or fish. Check for worms, especially on fish. Spray with hydrogen peroxide or wash in ozonated water before cooking. Keep all work surfaces clean.

Use more cloves with every meal. Adding some cloves to food will help kill the parasite eggs in the intestinal tract. Cloves can be added to coffee or herbal teas as a flavouring agent.

Do not overuse antibiotics. Reducing the numbers of friendly bacteria in the colon through abusing antibiotics opens the door to the proliferation of parasites.

Practice good personal hygiene. Wash your hands before eating and after going to the bathroom, changing diapers, gardening or handling pets. Keep your fingernails short and clean. Parasites can live for two months under the fingernails.

Keep your living environment clean. Avoid breathing in the dust in your house as it can contain human skin, soil particles, or faecal material from dust mites and cockroaches. An easy test to determine if this is a problem is by looking across the room when the sunlight is shining through a window and checking for particles floating in the air. Then let the kids run around for a few minutes and recheck. The elimination of carpets reduces this problem considerably.

If pets are infested with parasites, de-worm and keep them outside. You are at a higher risk for contracting worms when pets are allowed indoors. Dogs and cats are host to many parasites that humans can contract. Garlic added to their food will help control some parasites. Animals can spread 240 diseases to humans, mainly through parasitic infestation.

Do not walk barefoot on warm, moist soil or while working in the garden. Parasites are abundant in soil and can be absorbed (penetrate) through skin cells. Fertilizers are added to garden soil and it is the pet's favourite place to go. Use gloves and shoes for protection.

Be vigilant when swimming in rivers, lakes, ponds, or public swimming pools. Avoid swallowing or drinking the water while swimming anywhere. Avoid swimming if cuts or open sores are present.

Global travel. There is a chance of picking up foreign parasites that are not indigenous to your home country – the risks are greater in countries where hygiene and food preparation standards are poor.

Specific Recommendations for Pregnant Women

If you are thinking of getting pregnant or are already so, then there are a few guidelines that you can follow to minimize the probability of getting infected – there is a chance that once you are infected, the parasites can travel into the baby's body too.

For minimizing risk against Toxoplasma, take the following measures:

❖ Exclude rare or undercooked meat and non-pasteurized dairy products from the diet.

❖ Have yourself tested for antibodies, preferably before becoming pregnant. A positive test would indicate past infection that will not be transmitted to the foetus. The presence of antibodies also lessens the likelihood that congenital transmission would occur should you be exposed again to the parasite during pregnancy. As an antibody-negative female you would thus be at greater risk of transmitting Toxoplasma to your foetus should you become infected during pregnancy.

❖ Test household cats for antibodies to Toxoplasma. Assuming that a cat is healthy, a positive antibody test indicates that the animal is most probably immune and not excreting oocysts (eggs) and thus would be an unlikely source of infection. A healthy antibody-negative cat is most probably susceptible to infection and would shed oocysts for one to two weeks after exposure to Toxoplasma. If possible, the cat should be tested before you become pregnant.

❖ Protect cats from infection (or re-infection) by preventing access to birds, rodents, uncooked meat and non-pasteurized dairy products.

❖ Avoid handling free-roaming cats because the fur or paws could be contaminated with oocysts, which might be transmitted by hand-to-mouth contact. Any cat allowed indoors should be kept off the bed, pillows, blankets, or other furnishings you use.

❖ Avoid handling any cat showing signs of illness.

❖ Avoid handling litter boxes. Even if a cat is antibody-positive and hence most likely immune, there exists a potential for re-shedding of oocysts (although in much smaller numbers than during the initial infection). For safety, litter boxes should be changed daily or every other day by another person, to eliminate any potential for accidental infection.

❖ Wear rubber gloves if working with garden soil. Uncooked vegetables, whether grown in a home garden or supplied commercially, should be washed thoroughly before ingestion, in case they have been contaminated by cat faeces.

❖ Make a habit of vigorously and thoroughly washing hands with soap and water after contact with soil, cats, non-pasteurized dairy products, uncooked meat or vegetables.

So, to recap:

Practice good hygiene. Wash your hands with soap and water before eating or preparing food, and especially after using the toilet.

When travelling to developing countries, avoid drinking the tap water, or eating ice, uncooked or undercooked foods and fruits that cannot be peeled.

Cook your fish, meat and poultry thoroughly. Undercooked meats can contain parasites.

When doing any kind of parasite cleanse, it is imperative to do it consistently for 14 days. This will allow the body to clear any active parasites as well as eliminate any newly hatched eggs or larvae.

Remember to drink plenty of water each day to flush the excreted toxins out of your system! The more water you drink, the more toxins your body will be able to expel as part of the parasite cleanse, and the better you will feel through the cleansing process.

Re-infestation will occur, so consider doing a parasite cleanse once or twice a year. Children are especially susceptible to parasites since they are always sticking things in their mouths.

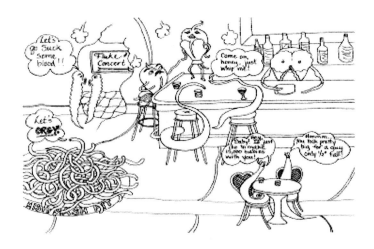

Chapter 7

Killing ourselves with toxic chemicals

In Chapter 4, we talked about general detoxification protocols for eliminating toxins from different organs and tissues of the body. This chapter has been written specifically to address the issue of heavy metal and xenobiotic[1] toxicity, as well as outlining natural ways in which these can be eliminated.

I became interested in heavy metals, particularly mercury, when I inadvertently discovered back in 1997 – after running a routine Hair Tissue Mineral Analysis (HTMA) on myself – that I had severely high mercury levels in my system (see column 'Hg' in the reports below – this is off the scale). In fact they were about 10 times higher than the acceptable levels, that's 1000 percent higher! This had occurred after removing about 10 amalgams with the help of a holistic dentist, here in Cyprus, who gave me chlorella as part of the detoxification protocol. I have since realised how misinformed the dentist was concerning toxic metal chelation protocols, as I learned many years later that chlorella is simply not enough to eliminate toxic metals from the body. There are many other dentists all over the world that are inadvertently poisoning people with mercury due to their ignorance. This chapter hopefully will highlight some of the adverse effects on health from mercury toxicity.

It was no surprise that I had many health problems in those days including hand tremors, memory loss, skin irritation, ataxia (poor balance), kidney pains and neurological disturbances. In fact, I was trying hard to keep some sort of balance to maintain my busy work schedule, not to mention bringing up a demanding family.

---

1 Xenobiotics are chemicals that are foreign to life that generally have detrimental effects on body systems.

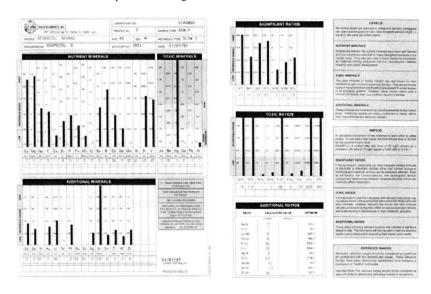

Dr. Georgiou's Hair Tissue Mineral Analysis results of 1997

It took me many years of study to discover how to remove this mercury from my body and regain my health. In the last few years, I have been actively involved in developing heavy metal detoxification protocols that have been scientifically proven to work and I will be discussing these, with case examples, towards the end of this chapter.

Xenobiotics

Toxic chemicals, otherwise known as 'xenobiotics' (*Greek:* 'foreign to life') which are scattered all over our planet from the North Pole to the South Pole, are being constantly researched, and the conclusion is that they are extremely toxic to humans as well as wildlife. Even though some chemicals have been taken off the market, those that remain are even more noxious than the ones already banned. Bioaccumulation in soils, water supplies and the tissues of animals and humans is a real problem, which results in these chemicals lingering for many, many years even after they have being banned. DDT, for example, has been banned for more than 25 years in the Western world, yet it is still being found in the tissues of wildlife in the arctic, as well as humans in many different countries.

A recent study noted that only five organochlorine compounds as well as mercury were found in marine mammals in the 1960's. Today over 265 organic pollutants and 50 inorganic chemicals have been found in these species.[2]

Other recent research has focused on how chemicals affect the thyroid and pituitary systems. Some chemicals have been identified as endocrine disrupters because they can interfere with the body's own hormones, which are secreted by the endocrine glands.

It is also emerging that endocrine disrupters can have many physiological effects not directly associated with the primary system. For example, the thyroid system is well known to regulate metabolism, but it is also a crucial component in foetal brain development in mammals, and too much or too little thyroid hormone at crucial points can do permanent damage.

The immune system is also vulnerable to hormone-mediated disruption. Chemicals can cause neurological problems, reproductive and developmental abnormalities as well as cancers. And researchers are only just beginning to disentangle the questions about the effects of chronic low-level exposure (as opposed to brief high doses of chemicals); combinations of chemicals and interactions between chemicals and other physiological and environmental factors.

Low dose exposure

Toxicologists studying chemical toxicity usually have a reference range of values which indicate the 'safe levels' of toxic chemicals. New research is showing, however, that even low-dose exposure[3] of mercury for example, is accumulative over time and can lead to children having decreased performance in areas of motor function and memory. Similarly, disruption of attention, fine motor function and verbal memory has also been found in adults on exposure to low mercury levels. It is an occupational hazard for dental staff, chloralkali factory workers, gold miners and those of similar

---

2 O'Shea, T.J., Tanabe, S., Persistent ocean contaminants and marine mammals: a retrospective overview. In: O'Shea, T.J. et al. (Eds.), 1999. Proceedings of the Marine Mammal Commission Workshop Marine Mammals and Persistent Ocean Contaminants, pp 87-92. Cited in Tanabe, S. Contamination and toxic effects of persistent endocrine disrupters in marine mammals and birds. *Mar Pollut Bull* 45:69-77, 2002.
3 Zahir, F., Rizwi, S.J., Haqb, S.K., Khanb, R.H. Low dose mercury toxicity and human health. *Environmental Toxicology and Pharmacology*, March 2005.
http://www.detoxmetals.com/images/newsletter/Low%20dose%20Hg%20exposure.pdf

professions. Mercury has been found to be a causative agent of various sorts for disorders, including neurological[4], nephrological, immunological, cardiac, motor, reproductive and even genetic disorders. Recently heavy metal mediated toxicity has been linked to diseases like Alzheimer's, Parkinson's, autism, Lupus, Amyotrophic lateral sclerosis, and even cancers. Besides this, it poses danger to wildlife. This low-dose toxicity and its effects on health will be the toxicologists' next goal for future research.

We are all toxic

Heavy metal poisoning is now so common that it is literally impossible to avoid it. There would not be many scientists knowledgeable in heavy metals and xenobiotics (foreign chemicals), who would disagree with the statement that 'We are all toxic.'

What is the proof? Even though I discussed this in Chapter 4, I will quickly recap for those that have not read this chapter – for those that have, there is a lot of new material mentioned here that is worth knowing. There are many studies that have found many of these heavy metals and xenobiotics in newborn babies. In September 2005, Greenpeace International, with the World Wildlife Fund, published a document entitled *Present for Life: Hazardous Chemicals in Umbilical Cord Blood.*[5] The research was a real eye-opener as it convincingly demonstrated that newborns tested for hundreds of different xenobiotics, showed high numbers and levels of these toxins. Specifically, the blood tests showed that these newborns had an average of 287 toxins in their bodies – 180 of these are known carcinogens.

Toxins in newborns

This study also quantifies the antibacterial agent triclosan in human blood, which was found in almost 50% of the samples. DDT, the notorious pesticide that is banned for

---

4 http://www.youtube.com/watch?v=VImCpWzXJ_w
5 Schuiling, J., van der Naald, W. (Greenpeace International, Greenpeace Netherland, World Wildlife Fund – UK), Present for Life: Hazardous Chemicals in Umbilical Cord Blood. Sept. 2005.
http://www.detoxmetals.com/images/newletter/Chemicals%20in%20newborns.pdf

agricultural use worldwide but which is still used in some places to control malaria, was still found in virtually all blood samples. Similarly, the organochlorine by-product and pesticide hexachlorobenzene – also subject to a global ban – was found in the samples. Perfluorinated compounds like PFOS and PFOA, used to make non-stick pans and water repelling coatings, were present in all but one maternal blood sample. PFOS was detected in all cord blood samples, and PFOA in half of them.

We could make the assumption that this study was conducted in America where the level of toxicity is probably higher, as compared with other countries. In order to address this

question let's examine a similar study conducted on pregnant women living in the North Pole, which most people feel is a clean part of the earth! The research was published in The Science of the Total Environment journal and was entitled, *Organochlorines and heavy metals in pregnant women from the Disko Bay area in Greenland.*[6]

Toxins in the North Pole

This study showed high concentrations of heavy metals – such as mercury – and organochlorines in the blood and fatty tissue of the Inuit people. This is attributed in particular to their high consumption of the meat and blubber of marine mammals.

In this present study, 180 pregnant women and 178 newborn babies were studied, amounting to 36% of the total number of births in the Disko Bay area during 1994-1996.

The pesticides found in the highest concentrations in maternal blood were DDE – 4.8 µg/l wet weight, trans-nonachlor – 1.6 µg/l.and hexachlorobenzene – 1.2 µg/l; while the total concentration of PCB (Aroclor 1260) was 19.1 µg/l. Calculated on a lipid basis, concentrations were slightly higher in maternal than in cord blood. The mercury concentrations were 16.8 µg/l in maternal blood and 35.6 µg/l in cord blood. In a linear regression analysis, the concentrations of

6 Bjerregaarda, P.U., Hansenb, J.C. Organochlorines and heavy metals in pregnant women from the Disko Bay area in Greenland, The Science of the Total Environment 245, 2000,195-202.
http://www.detoxmetals.com/images/newsletter/HMs%20in%20pregnant%20women%20in%20Greenland.pdf

organochlorines, mercury and selenium increased with maternal age. Concentrations of mercury and cadmium increased with the consumption of marine mammals, and cadmium was associated with smoking.

Toxins in wildlife

Similar studies have also shown that wildlife in the Arctic[7,8] is also being reduced/wiped out due to high levels of toxic chemicals in their environment, and that several Arctic mammal and bird species showing signs of chemical exposure are likely to have their health adversely affected. Some of the effects seen are potentially quite serious (e.g. immune suppression, hormone disturbances, as well as altered behaviour).

Toxic contamination through the generations

Another fascinating study conducted by the World Wildlife Fund set out to explore whether there was any relationship between the types and levels of contamination

found in 3 generations of families, and to examine possible links between contamination and a family's lifestyle, consumption patterns and everyday products. The report entitled, *Contamination: The Next Generation*[9] summarises the findings of the analysis of 104 different chemicals in the blood of 33 volunteers from 7 families living in England, Scotland and Wales.

The volunteers in each family spanned three generations, generally comprising the grandmother, mother and two children. The volunteers comprised 14 children, 13 adult parents and six grandmothers. The ages of the volunteers ranged from 9 to 88 years.

---

7 World Wildlife Fund. Killing Them Softly: Health Effects in Arctic Wildlife Linked to Chemical Exposures. 2006.
http://www.detoxmetals.com/images/newsletter/Chemicals%20in%20the%20arctic.pdf
8 Brown, V. (World Wildlife Fund). Causes for Concern: Chemicals and Wildlife – Toxic Chemicals, a Threat to Wildlife and Humans, Dec. 2003.
http://assets.panda.org/downloads/causesforconcern.pdf
9 WWF-UK. Contamination: the next generation. Results of the family chemical contamination survey, October 2004
http://www.detoxmetals.com/images/newsletter/Contamination%20-%20The%20next%20generation.pdf

All three generations tested, including the children, were contaminated by a cocktail of hazardous man-made chemicals. The results reveal that every child, from as young

as 9 years (none younger were tested), was contaminated by the same range of hazardous chemicals: organochlorine pesticides, PCBs, brominated flame-retardants, phthalates and perfluorinated ('non-stick') chemicals. Five chemicals found in each parent and grandparent was also found in every child.

While it might be expected that the chemical burden increases with age, the above study has shown that this conventional assumption is not always true: children can be more contaminated by higher numbers and levels of certain 'newer' chemicals than their parents or even their grandparents, despite being exposed to these chemicals for only a fraction of the time. These 'newer' chemicals include brominated flame retardants (used in sofas, textiles and electrical appliances) and perfluorinated chemicals (used in the manufacture of non-stick pans, coatings for takeaway food packaging and treatments for carpets, furniture, clothing and footwear).

The results also show that chemicals used daily were found in the families tested in the survey, including the children. For example, fifty seven per cent of the 7 people found to be contaminated by deca-BDE, a brominated flame retardant, were children. Of the volunteers tested, 82 per cent were contaminated by one or more perfluorinated chemicals. The perflourinated chemical, PFOA (perfluorooctanoic acid) was found in more than a third of the children tested. A related chemical PFOS (perfluorooctane sulphonate) was found in 5 of the family members tested.

There have been similar studies in the USA too – in July 2005, the Department of Health and Human Services, Centers for Disease Control and Prevention, published a 475-page document entitled, *Third National Report on Human Exposure to Environmental Chemicals*[10] which clearly indicates the growing number of chemical toxins present in all age-groups in the USA. The American Council on Science and Health published a document in May 2003 entitled, *Traces of Environmental Chemicals in the*

---

10 Department of Health and Human Services, Centers for Disease Control and Prevention. Third National Report on Human Exposure to Environmental Chemicals, July 2005. http://www.detoxmetals.com/images/newsletter/CDC%203rd%20Report%20on%20Chemical%20Exposure.pdf

Human Body: Are They a Risk to Health?[11] This research looked at the different types of xenobiotics found in US citizens, as well as their quantity. While chemicals that have been banned for many years are still being detected, generally there is a downward trend with up to 90% reduction in the last few decades of toxins such as DDT and lead.

Let's take a brief look at some of these more common xenobiotics chemicals that have detrimental effects on humans, as well as wildlife.

Perfluorochemicals (PFCs)

These compounds are chains of fully fluorinated carbon atoms of varying lengths, yielding chemicals that are extremely resistant to heat and chemical stress; and that repel both water and oil. Because of these properties PFCs, or chemicals that degrade into PFCs, have been widely used by industry since the 1950s as surfactants and emulsifiers; and in commercial products including stain or water protectors for carpets, textiles, auto interiors, camping gear and leather; food packaging; folding cartons and other paper containers; floor polishes, photographic film, shampoos, dental cleaners, inert pesticide ingredients as well as lubricants for bicycles, garden tools and zippers.

Their durability is extreme, particularly perfluorooctanoic acid (PFOA) – there is no evidence that they ever fully degrade, and they have been found in animals, humans and ecosystems worldwide.

The first public indication that PFOS and PFOA were problematic came on May 16, 2000 when '3M' (the primary global manufacturer of many perfluoroalkanesulfonates and PFOA) announced plans to phase out, by the end of 2001, the production of perfluorooctanyl chemistry – which underpinned their extremely successful Scotchgard™ and Scotchban™ product lines.[12]

A 2002 European study of PFCs has detected these compounds in bottlenose, common and striped dolphins, whales, bluefin tuna, swordfish

11 Kamrin, M. (The American Council on Science and Health). Traces of Environmental Chemicals in the Human Body: Are They a Risk to Health? May 2003 http://www.detoxmetals.com/images/newsletter/Environmental%20chemicals%20in%20human%20body.pdf
12 3M. (2000) 3M phasing out some of its specialty materials, May 16, 2000 press release.

and cormorants in the Mediterranean as well as ringed and grey seals, sea eagles and Atlantic salmon in the Baltic.[13]

Other research shows that these chemicals are now contaminating many wildlife species around the world, including polar bears in the Arctic, seals in Antarctica, dolphins in the river Ganges in India, albatrosses from Midway Atoll in the Pacific, turtles in the United States, gulls in Korea, cormorants in Canada and fish in Japan.[14]

Fluorinated telomers are used to keep grease from soaking through fast food containers such as pizza boxes, French fry holders, and food wrapping paper. The digestive system can break telomers down into PFOA and related chemicals. Newly revealed tests conducted by '3M' showed that a metabolite specific to the telomers was found in 85 per cent of the children tested.

Red Cross blood bank analyses, conducted by a team including scientists from the '3M' Company, estimated the average concentrations in humans to be 30-40 parts per billion (ppb), with males having higher levels.[15] By comparison, levels in wildlife have been measured at 940 ppb in common dolphin livers; 1100 ppb in ringed seals from the Bay of Bothnia and 270 ppb in long-finned pilot whale livers from the North Thyrrenian Sea.[16]

Harmful health effects of Perfluorochemicals (PFCs)

In 1979, '3M' administered four doses of PFOS to monkeys, and every monkey in all treatment groups died within weeks. Typically, when a study like this is conducted,

---

13 Kannan, K., Corsolini, S., Falandysz, J., Oehme, G., Focardi, S., Giesy, J.P. Perfluorooctanesulfonate and related fluorinated hydrocarbons in marine mammals, fishes and birds from coasts of the Baltic and Mediterranean Seas. *Environ Sci Technol* 1;36(15):3210-6, Aug 2000.

14 Geisy J.P. and Kannan K. Global Distribution of Perfluorooctane sulfonate in wildlife. *Env Sci Technol* 35:1339-42, 2001.

15 Taniyasu, S., Kannak, K., Horii,Y., Hanari, N.,Yamashita, N. A survey of perfluorooctane sulfonate and related perfluorinated organic compounds in water, fish, birds and humans from Japan. *Environ Sci & Technol* 37:2634-2639, 2003.

16 Olsen, G. W., Church, T.R., Miller, J.P., Burris, J.M., Hansen, K.J., Lundberg, J.K., Armitage, J.B., Herron, R.M., Medhdizadehkashi, Z., Nobiletti, J.B., O'Neill, E.M., Mandel, J.H., Zobel, L.R. Perfluorooctanesulfonate and other fluorochemicals in the serum of American Red Cross adult blood donors. *Environ Health Perspect* 111:1892-1901, 2003.

the researchers predict that the lowest dose will not cause any harmful health effects.[17]

In 1981 both DuPont and '3M' reassigned women of childbearing age working in their

production plants on learning that PFOA caused developmental abnormalities in laboratory animals. Within weeks of this discovery, DuPont found PFOA in the women's blood.

It was known as early as 1975 that fumes from hot pans coated with polytetrafluoroethylene can kill pet birds,[18] and battery chicks have died after exposure to polytetrafluoroethylene-coated light bulbs.[19] Laboratory experiments showed in 2003 that in rats, PFOS exposure can lead to loss of appetite, interrupted oestrus cycles and elevated stress hormone levels. PFOS was found to accumulate in brain tissue, particularly the hypothalamus, suggesting that PFOS crosses the blood-brain barrier and may interfere with reproductive hormones through the pituitary-hypothalamus process that stimulates their production.[20]

Recent laboratory studies with PFOA involving rats show low birth weight, small pituitary gland, altered maternal care behaviour, high pup mortality and significant changes in the brain, liver, spleen, thymus, adrenal gland, kidney, prostate, testes and epididymides.[21]

Several studies indicate PFOA increases oestrogens and leads to testosterone dysfunction in males. There is even more evidence that PFOA as well as chemicals that metabolize to PFOS and PFOA lead to an underactive thyroid, and thyroid dysfunction during pregnancy can lead to many developmental problems, including faulty brain development and

---

17 Kannan, et al., 2002.
18 Organization for Economic Cooperation and Development (OECD). (2002) Hazard Assessment of perfluorooctane sulfonate (PFOS) and its salts. November, 21 2002. Available online at: http://www.oecd.org/dataoecd/23/18/2382880.pdf
19 Environmental Working Group. PFC's: A Family of Chemicals that Contaminate the Planet, Part 6: PFC's in Animals Worldwide., 2003.
http://www.ewg.org/reports/pfcworld/part8.php
20 Ibid.
21 Austin, M.E., Kasturi, B.S., Barber, M., Kannan, K., MohanKumar, P.S., MohanKumar, S.M.J. Neuroendocrine effects of perfluorooctane sulfonate in rats. Environ Health Perspect 111:12:1485-1489, 2003.

neurological and behavioural problems that affect not only infants and young animals (or humans) but continue into adulthood. The Environmental Protection Agency (EPA) considers both PFOS and PFOA to be a carcinogen in animals, with testicular, pancreatic, mammary, thyroid and liver tumours most frequent in exposed rats.

All studies to date indicate perfluorinated compounds damage the immune system. In one experiment, a chemical very similar to PFOA called PFDA resulted in such atrophy of the thymus gland, (the source of T cells which attack bacteria, viruses and cancer cells) that the gland was undetectable upon clinical examination.

Phthalates

Phthalates are a group of chemicals used as softeners in a variety of plastic products, including the ubiquitous polyvinyl chloride (PVC). Products containing phthalates include medical devices (intravenous tubing, blood bags, masks for sleep apnea devices); building products (insulation of cables and wires, tubes and profiles, flooring, wallpapers, outdoor wall and roof covering, sealants); car products (car under-coating, car seats etc.) and children's products (teething rings, squeeze toys, clothing and rainwear). They are also used in some lacquers, paints, adhesives, fillers, inks and cosmetics.

The most common phthalate in the environment is di-(2-ethylhexyl)phthalate (DEHP), which comprises half of all phthalates produced in Western Europe, with 450,000 tonnes used per year. Concern about children's exposure to phthalates prompted the EU to ban six types of phthalate softeners in PVC toys designed to be mouthed by children under three years of age.

Both humans and wildlife may be exposed to various phthalates. Airborne phthalate esters are present at detectable levels across the surface of Earth. They were first identified in outdoor urban air and subsequently have been recognized as global pollutants and major constituents of indoor air, also present in household dust and Air Fresheners. Their presence in outdoor and indoor environments reflects their large emission rates coupled with moderate atmospheric lifetimes.

For example, a 2003 study of two groups of pregnant women, one in New York City and one in Krakow, Poland, compared the levels of four phthalates in the women's personal ambient air and measured the levels of the metabolites of these phthalates in the urine of the New York women.[22] All four phthalates were present in all the air samples, but air concentrations of di–isobutyl phthalate and DEHP were higher in Krakow than in New York. The study found that air was a significant source of exposure; that some women receive doses high enough to cause concern, and that there was a correlation between air and urine levels of some phthalates.

Other studies in the EU have also raised concerns with regard to current exposure levels. A recent study in Germany, for example, has concluded that exposure to DEHP may be far higher than previously thought. It reported that in 12 per cent of the Germans studied, phthalate levels exceeded the tolerable daily intake (TDI) used by the EU Scientific Committee for Toxicity, Ecotoxicity and the Environment. Exposure to DBP was also ubiquitous.[23]

Harmful health effects of phthalates

Some phthalates appear to exert endocrine disrupting effects, and can act against the male hormone androgen through pathways other than binding to androgen or oestrogen receptors. While there is little research on the effects of phthalates on wildlife per se, some studies suggest that there may be serious consequences for both wildlife and humans. Of particular concern is phthalate exposure in pregnant females: some researchers have proposed that the antiandrogenic properties of phthalates might be

linked to Testicular Dysgenesis Syndrome, the manifestations of which range from birth defects in males, including undescended testes, low sperm counts and testicular cancer.[24]

22 Adibi, J.J., Perera, F.P., Jedrychowski,W., Camann, D.E., Barr, D., Jacek, Ryszard, Whyatt, R.M. Prenatal exposures to phthalates among women in New York City and Krakow, Poland. *Environ Health Perspect* 111:14:1719-1722, 2003.
23 Kock et al,. An estimation of the daily intake of di(2-ethyl) phthalate (DEHP) and other phthalates in the general population. *International Journal Hygiene and Environmental Health*, 2003.
24 Sharpe R.M. The oestrogen hypothesis – where do we stand now? *International Journal of Andrology* 26:2-15, 2003; Skakkebaek, N.E. et al. Testicular dysgenesis syndrome: an

Numerous laboratory studies underpin the concern. For example, a study has shown that DEHP, BBP, and DINP administered to pregnant rats induced feminized breasts in the male offspring, as well as other reproductive malformations, including small testes in the cases of the DEHP and BBP exposed rats.[25]

There are also worries that exposure to manmade chemicals with hormone disrupting properties may be affecting the age of puberty. A study of Puerto Rican girls with premature breast development suggested a possible association with exposure to certain phthalates.[26]

US researchers recently reported the effects of DEHP on Leydig cells (testosterone-producing cells in the testes) in rats.[27] They found that prolonged exposure to DEHP caused the number of Leydig cells to increase by 40 – 60 per cent while simultaneously reducing testosterone production. At the same time, blood levels of both testosterone and oestrogens increased by 50 per cent. It is known that males with high levels of serum testosterone and luteinizing hormone (a hormone that triggers testosterone production) are at higher risk of early puberty and testicular tumours.

With regard to cancer, a recent study supported other research associating DEHP with liver cancer in rodents.[28] A 2003 Harvard study suggested another mechanism for the carcinogenic effect of phthalates. The researchers measured levels of eight phthalates in subjects and found an association between monoethyl phthalate (MEP) and increased damage to the DNA in the subjects' sperm.[29] This is the first study showing that

increasingly common developmental disorder with environmental aspects. Human Reproduction 16:5:972-978, 2001.

25 Gray, L.E. Jr., Ostby, J., Furr, J., Price, M., Veeramachaneni, D.N., Parks, L. Perinatal exposure to the phthalates DEPH, BBP, and DINP, but not DEP, DMP, or DOTP, alters sexual differentiation of the male rat. *Toxicological Sciences* 58:350-565, 2000.

26 Colón, I., et al., Identification of phthalate esters in the serum of young Puerto Rican girls with premature breast development. *Environmental Health Perspectives*, 108(9): p.895-900, 2000.

27 Akingbemi, BT., Ge, R., Klinefelter, GR., Zirkin, BR., Hardy, MP. Phthalate-induced Leydig cell hyperplasia is associated with multiple endocrine disturbances. *Proceedings of the National Academy of Sciences* 2004.

28 Seo, KW., Kim, KB., Kim,YJ., Choi, JY, Lee, KT., Choi, KS. Comparison of oxidative stress and changes of xenobiotic metabolizing enzymes induced by phthalates in rats. *Food Chem Toxicol.* 42(1):107-14, Jan 2004.

29 Duty, S.M., Singh, N.P., Silva, M.J., Barr, D.B., Brock, J.W., Ryan, L., Herrick, R.F., Christiani, D.C., Hauser, R. The relationship between environmental exposures to phthalates and DNA damage in human sperm using the neutral comet assay. *Environ.*

phthalates can induce such damage at levels presently found in the environment.

Other studies with phthalates show that accumulative effects can occur when there is exposure to more than one phthalate.[30] This underlines the growing concern with real life exposures to multiple pollutants, and the increasing realisation that current regulatory practices, based on testing chemicals in isolation, may not be protective.

Phenols, bisphenyl A and nonylphenol

Evidence for endocrine disruption by the widely used phenol compounds bisphenol A (BPA) and nonylphenol is mounting. BPA is mostly used to make polycarbonate plastic, which has a diverse range of application in making bottles, computer and electronics shells, CD's, crash helmets, and many other consumer products.

Certain compounds that can leach BPA are also used in the plastic linings of food cans

and in dental fillings, through which people can ingest small quantities. In December 2003, concerned about BPA in the plastic linings of food cans, the EU reduced the amount of BPA migration permitted by 80 percent to 0.6 milligrams per kilogram of food.[31] However, BPA remains widely distributed in consumer products.

Nonylphenolic compounds have been used in degreasing solutions and in leather and textile processing, as well as in de-icing fluid, paints, plastics, and pesticides. However, the EU has imposed restrictions on the marketing and use of nonylphenol and nonylphenol ethoxylates to a certain extent in cleaning products, textile and leather processing, agricultural teat dips,

---

Health Perspect 111:9:1164-1169, 2003.
http://ehp.niehs.nih.gov/members/2003/5756/5756.html
30 Foster, P M. Turner K J, Barlow N J. Anti-androgenic effects of a phthalate combination on in utero male reproductive development in the Sprague-Dawley rat: additivity of response. Toxicologist 66(1-S), 233, Mar 2000.
31 Environmental Data Services, Ends Daily 15th Dec 2003.

metal working, pulp and paper, cosmetics including shampoos and personal care products except spermicides.[32]

Harmful health effects of phenols

Fish have been shown to be susceptible to the endocrine disrupting effects of both nonylphenol[33] and BPA.[34] Exposure to either of these chemicals can cause male fish to make vitellogenin (an oestrogen-regulated protein produced by female egg-laying vertebrates and not normally produced by males or juveniles) and can also affect the formation of sperm. Before improved regulation, male fish in the river Aire in England were found to be feminised downstream of a wastewater treatment plant discharge containing alkylphenol ethoxylates from the textile industry. Many male fish were found with egg producing cells in their testes and reduced testis growth rate and size.[35,36]

Aquatic invertebrates seem particularly sensitive to these chemicals. For example, nonylphenol affects the freshwater algae Scenedesmus subspicatus, at levels of 3.3 micrograms per litre.[37] Molluscs in particular have shown effects at very low dose levels. For example, in the mollusc Potamopyrgus antipodarum, BPA and octylphenol, as well as a mixture of these and other chemicals in treated sewage effluent, stimulated egg and

---

32 Directive 2003/53/EC of the European Parliament and of the Council of 18 June 2003 amending for the 26th time Council Directive 76/769/EEC relating to restrictions on the marketing and use of certain dangerous substances and preparations (nonylphenol, nonylphenol ethoxylate and cement), *Official Journal* L 178 17-7-2003.
33 Jobling S., Sheahan D., Osborne J., Matthiessen P., Sumpter J. Inhibition of testicular growth in rainbow trout (Oncorhynchus mykiss) exposed to oestrogenic alkylphenolic chemicals. *Environ. Toxicol. Chem.*, 15, 194-202, 1996.
34 Sohoni et al, Reproductive effects of long term exposure to bisphenol A in the fathead minnow (Pimephales promelas), *Environ Sci Technol* 35: 2917-2925, 2001.
35 Environment Agency of England and Wales 1998; Endocrine Disrupting Substances in the Environment. What Should Be Done? The EA Bristol.
36 Commission of the European Communities. Proposal for a Directive of the European Parliament and of the Council relating to the restrictions on the marketing and use of nonylphenol, nonylphenol ethoxylate and cement. *COM* (2002) 459, 2002/0206 (COD).
37 Jobling, S., Casey, D. Rodgers-Gray, T., Oehlmann, J., Schult-Oehlmann, U., Pawlowski, S., Baunbeck, T., Turner, A.P., Tyler, C.R. comparative responses of molluscs and fish to environmental oestrogens and an oestrogenic effluent. *Aquat Toxicol* 29;65(2):205-20, Oct 2003.

embryo production at low doses and inhibited such production at high doses.[38]

This work supported a study in 2000 by some of the same researchers, showing that extremely low levels of BPA and octylphenol triggered malformed genitals of female ramshorn (freshwater) snail, Marisa cornuarietis, and the (saltwater) dogwhelk Nucella lapillus. In some of the freshwater snails, the excessive growth of the female glands and the egg masses ruptured the egg tube, and the snails died. This syndrome was referred to as superfeminisation. A number of other adverse changes were observed in both species. Another important finding was that in the freshwater snails, the medium doses of octylphenol produced more changes than either the highest or lowest doses.

Other researchers have shown that a single 48-hour exposure to 1 microgram per litre of nonylphenol, comparable to environmental levels, altered the sex ratio of oysters, reduced the survival of offspring and caused some oysters to become hermaphroditic.

A 2001 study exposing barnacles to concentrations of nonylphenol similar to those in the environment (0.01-10 micrograms per litre) disrupted the timing of larval development.[39] In addition to fish, other vertebrates also show effects when exposed to BPA. For example, in 2003, researchers reported that BPA at environmentally comparable doses, resulted in sex reversals and altered gonadal structures in the broad-snouted caiman, an alligator relative native to mid-latitude South America.[40] In another study, the offspring of pregnant mice exposed to BPA showed changes in ovarian and mammary gland tissues and disrupted fertility cycles as adults.[41] BPA was reported for the first time in 2001 to induce reproductive malformations in birds – specifically, in female quail embryos and male

---

38 Oehlmann, J., Schulte-Oehlmann, U., Tillmann, M., Markert, B. Effects of endocrine disruptors on Prosobranch snails (Mollusca: Gastropoda) in the laboratory. Part I: Bisphenol A and octylphenol as xenoestrogens. *Ecotoxicology* 9:383-397, 2000.
39 Billinghurst, Z., Clare, AS., Depledge M.H. Effects of 4-n-nonylphenol and 17beta-oestradiol on early development of the barnacle Elminius modestus. *J. Exper. Mar. Biol. Ecol.* 15;25(2);255-268, Mar 2001.
40 Stoker, C., Rey, F. Rodriguez, H., Ramos, JG., Sirosky, P., Larriera, A., Luque Munoz-de-Toro, M. Sex reversal effects on Caiman latirostris exposed to environmentally relevant doses of the xenoestrogen bisphenol A. *Gen Comp Endocrinol* 1;133(3)287-96, Oct 2003.
41 Markey, CM., Coombs, MA. Sonnenschein, C., Soto, AM. Mammalian development in a changing environment: exposure to endocrine disruptors reveals the developmental plasticity of steroid hormone target organs. *Evol Dev* 5(1):67-75, Jan-Feb 2003.

chicken embryos. The female embryos' oviducts developed abnormally and the males' testes were feminized.[42]

The exact mechanism by which BPA and nonylphenol exert their effects is not clear, but a recent in vitro study demonstrated a molecular mechanism by which BPA and nonylphenol interfere with both the activation and function of cellular androgen receptors.[43] In a 2002 study, nonylphenol tested on barnacle larvae induced DNA damage, possibly including mutations, and the authors speculate that this effect may be a mechanism by which higher level reproductive abnormalities are caused.[44]

Despite evidence from these and other studies, the low dose effects of BPA are still in dispute. Regulators in the EU have been reluctant to act, and further studies have been demanded.

Polybrominated flame retardants (BFRs)

Brominated flame retardants (BFRs) in furniture, building materials and clothing have become a serious concern as their levels are showing sharp increases in living organisms. The first BFRs were taken off the market in the early 1970s after a spill led to poisonings of livestock and farm families in Michigan. Three BFRs now dominate the market: TBBPA, the most widely used, primarily in printed circuit boards and in some plastics; HBCD and the deca-BDEs. The other commercial PBDEs (octa-BDE and penta-BDE) have been banned in the EU as of August 2004, and the state of California has taken similar action. However, because of their alarming spread and rate of accumulation in humans and animals, Europe's ban does not provide complete reassurance, particularly regarding the penta-BDE form used as a flame retardant in polyurethane foam elsewhere in the world.

---

42 Berg, C., Halldin, K., Brunstrom, B. Effects of bisphenol A and tetrabromobisphenol A on sex organ development in quail and chicken embryos. *Environ Toxicol Chem* 20(12):2836-40, Dec 2001.
43 Lee, HJ., Chattopadhyay, S., Gong, EY, Ahn, RS, Lee, K. Antiandrogenic effects of bisphenol A and nonylphenol on the function of androgen receptor. *Toxicological Sciences* 75:, 40-46, 2003.
44 Berg, C., Halldin, K., Brunstrom, B. Effects of bisphenol A and tetrabromobisphenol A on sex organ development in quail and chicken embryos. *Environ Toxicol Chem* 20(12):2836-40, Dec 2001.

Researchers recently reported levels of PBDEs in US breast milk.[45] Forty seven Texas women had an average level of 73.9 ng/g lipids. Such levels are sharply higher than those found in European studies. There are serious concerns about the transfer of BFRs to nursing infants, and some scientists are worried that BFRs might affect foetal development, including disruption of the thyroid system's role in foetal brain development.[46] In 2003 a WWFUK biomonitoring programme found deca-BDE in the blood of seven per cent of those tested.[47]

New research from Sweden has found high levels of several brominated flame retardants in the eggs of peregrine falcons from 1987-1999. The eggs of falcons living in the wild had significantly higher concentrations of the essentially unregulated deca-BDE than eggs of captive falcons. The fact that deca-BDE was found in eggs demonstrates that the chemical can cross cell membranes, contrary to what scientists had previously thought. The peregrine study represents the first time that the deca formulation has been found in wildlife.[48]

In 2002, one research team predicted that within 10 to 15 years, concentrations of BFRs in Great Lakes herring gulls may be higher than those of PCBs.[49] BFRs have also been found in sperm whales,[50] ringed seals from the Canadian Arctic,[51] mussels and several kinds of fish in Norwegian waters; and harbour seals in San Francisco Bay,[52] among other wildlife. Essentially, BFRs are being found wherever we look.

---

45 Schecter, A. Pavuk, M. Papke, O., Ryan, JJ., Birnbaum, L., Rosen, R. Polybrominated diphenyl ethers (PBDEs) in U.S. mothers' milk. *Environ Health Perspect* 111:14:1723-1724, 2003.

46 http://www.ourstolenfuture.org/NewScience/oncompounds/PBDE/2003/2003-0807schecteretal.htm Accessed 5 January 2004.

47 http://www.panda.org/about_wwf/where_we_work/europe/what_we_do/policy_and_events/epo/news.cfm?uNewsID=9941

48 Lindberg, P., Sellström, U., Häggberg, L., and de Wit, CA. Higher brominated diphenyl ethers and hexabromocyclododecane found in eggs of peregrine falcons (Falco peregrinus) breeding in Sweden. *Environ Sci Technol* 38;(1): 93-96, 2004.

49 Norstrom RJ, Simon M, Moisey J,Wakeford B,Weseloh DV. Geographical distribution (2000) and temporal trends (1981-2000) of brominated diphenyl ethers in Great Lakes herring gull eggs. *Environ Sci Technol.* 36(22): 4783-9, Nov 2002.

50 De Boer, J.,Wester, PG., Klamer, HJC., Lewis,WE., Boon, JP. Do flame retardants threaten ocean life? *Nature* 394:28-29, 1998.

51 Ikonomou et al., 2002a (cited in Birnbaum & Staskel, 2004).

52 Birnbaum & Staskal, 2004.

Harmful health effects of BFRs

Laboratory studies show that certain BFRs are highly toxic to aquatic animals (crustaceans),[53] and suggest effects on pubertal development, affecting the thyroid and liver in rats, as well as developmental neurotoxicity in mice.[54] A recent paper reported behavioural effects in mice pups at a relatively low dose.[55] In 1999 Swedish researchers reported that PBDEs and HBCD may have health effects similar to those of DDT and PCBs because of their ability to induce genetic recombination.[56]

While there are no published epidemiological studies on effects of BFRs on humans, the possible thyroid effects, based on tissue culture and animal studies, are a red flag. As with other chemicals, anything that affects foetal development merits particular study because of the profound, long-term, and often irreversible influence that early exposures have on the entire life of an organism.

Mercury: 'the big one'

Let us take a closer look at this toxic heavy metal – mercury – which I refer to as the 'Big One' as it is omnipotent and ubiquitous. There is probably not a living person on this planet, or living animal – whether domesticated or wild – that does not have their share of mercury toxicity. Mercury is a very toxic substance – more toxic than lead, cadmium, or arsenic.[57]

Mercury is listed as one of the top six most poisonous metals on Earth, with known human toxicity occurring at minimal doses – producing urine levels of 5 mcg/l – which is another way of saying 5 millionths of one gram.

---

53 Birnbaum & Staskal, 2004.
54 Birnbaum & Staskal, 2004.
55 Darnerud, P.O. Toxic effects of brominated flame retardants in man and in wildlife. *Environ Int* 29(6):841-53, Sept 2003.
56 Helleday, T., Tuominen, KL., Bergman, A., Jenssen, D. Brominated flame retardants induce intragenic recombination in mammalian cells. *Mutat Res* 19;439(2):137-47, Feb 1999.
57 Sharma, RP; Obersteiner, EJ., Metals and Neurotoxic Effects: Cytotoxicity of Selected Metallic Compounds on Chick Ganglia Cultures, *J Comp Pathol*, 91(2):235-44, 1981.

Basically, there are three forms of mercury:

1. Metallic Mercury (the metal) - used in oral thermometers, barometers, sphygmomanometers (devices used to test blood pressure), wall thermostats for heating and cooling, fluorescent light bulbs/tubes, some batteries, electric light switches – absorbed by breathing the vapour emitted.
2. Inorganic Mercury (like mercuric chloride or sulphate) - is created when emitted mercury vapour by natural sources, such as volcanoes, geothermal springs, geologic deposits, and the ocean combines with other elements to form salts (see Mercury Cycle). Human-related sources primarily include coal combustion, waste incineration, industrial uses, and mining.
3. Organic (such as methylmercury and ethylmercury) – in nature, this is produced by the methylation of inorganic mercury by bacteria. Man-made sources of methylmercury are from Thimerosal added to various vaccinations as well as the emissions from dental amalgam fillings.

The Mercury Cycle

The essence of the Mercury Cycle is the evaporation of inorganic Mercury from both natural and man-made sources into the atmosphere where it is then oxidized in the upper atmosphere and returned back to earth, most commonly in precipitation, in its inorganic mercury form. It is dispersed evenly throughout the environment and the inorganic mercury is biomethylized by bacteria into the more toxic formation, methyl mercury. Once converted, the methyl mercury then enters the food chain and biomagnifies up the food chain.

There are 6 universally recognized steps to the Mercury Cycle:

1. Degassing of Mercury from rock, soils, and surface waters, or emissions from volcanoes and from human activities.

2. Movement in gaseous form through the atmosphere.

3. Deposition of Mercury on land and surface waters.

4. Conversion of the element into insoluble Mercury sulphide.

5. Precipitation or biomethylation (adding a methyl group) into more volatile or soluble forms such as methyl mercury.

6. Re-entry into the atmosphere or biomagnify up the food chain.

Conceptual Biogeochemical Mercury Cycle

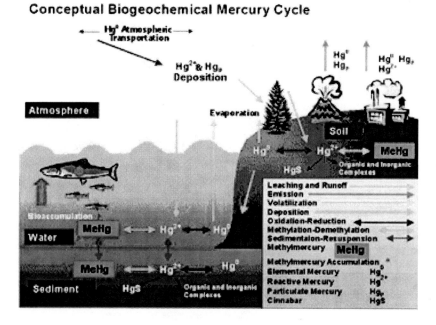

The Mercury Cycle[58]

There is considerable evidence suggesting that the inorganic form – also called 'ionic mercury' – is the most harmful. It is also the most difficult to remove from the brain and usually stays there permanently.

Many forms of mercury

Mercury's elemental symbol is *Hg*, which is derived from the Greek word *hydrargyrias*, meaning 'water silver.' As stated above, mercury is found in organic and inorganic forms. The inorganic form can be further divided into elemental mercury and mercuric salts. Organic mercury can be found in long and short alkyl and aryl compounds. Mercury in any form is toxic. The difference lies in how it is absorbed, the clinical signs and symptoms

---

58 Taken from http://www.ec.gc.ca/MERCURY/EH/EN/eh-b.cfm

and the response to treatment modalities. Mercury poisoning can result from vapour inhalation, ingestion, injection or absorption through the skin.

Elemental mercury is found in liquid form, which easily vaporizes at room temperature (the only metal to do so) and is well absorbed through inhalation. Its lipid (fat)-soluble property allows for easy passage through the alveoli into the bloodstream and red blood cells. Once inhaled, elemental mercury is mostly converted into an inorganic *divalent* or *mercuric* form, by *catalase* in the red blood cells. This inorganic form has similar properties to organic mercury. Small amounts of non-oxidized elemental mercury continue to persist and account for CNS toxicity.

Mercury is a multipotent cytotoxin that intervenes in the primary processes of the cell by bonding strongly with *sulfhydryl* and *selenohydryl* groups on albumen molecules in cell membranes, receptors and intracellular signal links, and by modifying the tertiary structure. The structure of albumen molecules is genetically determined, and this leaves ample scope for genetic *polymorphism* (taking many forms) to manifest itself in varying degrees of sensitivity and types of reaction to mercury exposure. Mercury is toxic because it induces production of free oxygen radicals and modifies the redox potential (oxidation reduction) of the cell (causing the cell to mutate).

Mercury in surprising places

The use of mercury in Medicine predates its use in dentistry by centuries. Mercury has been found in Egyptian tombs, indicating that it was used as early as 1500 BC. As far back as 500 BC there is evidence that India was using mercury as a drug. However, Arabic physicians first studied mercury as a drug and introduced the use of a mercurial ointment in the 10th century AD. It was towards the end of the 18th century that mercury found its way into medical practice in the US as a prescription item. In the late 18th century, antisyphlitic agents contained mercury. For centuries, mercury was an essential part of many different medicines such as diuretics, antibacterial agents, antiseptics and laxatives.

The Number One source of human contamination of inorganic mercury today is coal-burning plants, but the primary source of organic mercury contamination is right in your mouth – dental fillings composed of an amalgam of various metals, of which about 50% is the metallic form of mercury which can easily convert to the organic form of methylmercury. A small, tenth-of-a-gram mercury filling would release enough organic mercury lasting 27 years, which is pretty much a consistent chronic toxic exposure for the life of most fillings. At least seventeen separate studies have confirmed that dental patients absorb a daily dose of mercury derived from their mercury fillings.[59] We will look at this in more depth a little later. Mercury poisoning is usually misdiagnosed because of its insidious onset, nonspecific signs and symptoms and lack of knowledge within the medical profession. In Medicine today, mercury is used in various antiseptic agents as well as amalgams.

Mercury is found in many industries such as the manufacture of batteries, thermometers and barometers. It can also be found in fungicides used in the agricultural industry. Before 1990, paints contained mercury as an antimildew agent. On July 7, 1999, a joint statement by the American Academy of Pediatrics and the US Public Health Service was issued, alerting clinicians and the public to the dangers of *thimerosal*, an ethylmercury[60]-containing preservative used in vaccines. Although several sources contributing to the domestic mercury concentrations have been identified, human waste (faeces and urine) from individuals with dental amalgam fillings is believed to be the most significant source – greater than 80 percent.

It is in many of the foods we eat and it is also contained in a great many over-the-counter drugs and cosmetics; e.g. mascara, contact lens solution, haemorrhoid preparations, etc. The mercury ingredients used are *thimerosal, phenylmercuric acetate, phenylmercuric nitrate, mercuric acetate, mercuric nitrate, MB for merbromin* and *mercuric oxide yellow*. Thus, sensitization to mercury can come from a number of sources.

The chemistry of methyl mercury

As mentioned in chapter two, hair and blood are used as biological indicator media for methyl mercury in both the adult and foetal brains (in the latter case, maternal hair or cord blood). Methyl mercury accumulates copiously in growing scalp hair. Concentrations in the hair are a reflection of concentrations in the blood, but are about 250 times higher than in blood as they accumulate over time and are measured at much more

---

59 Richardson, GM. Inhalation of Mercury-Contaminated Particulate Matter by Dentists: An Overlooked Occupational Risk, Human and Ecological Risk Assessment, 9:1519-1531, 2003.
60 Ethylmercury – an organic form of mercury widely used as an antifungal agent.

concentrated levels. Hair levels are also proportional to concentrations in the target tissue – the brain. Longitudinal analysis of strands of scalp hair can reflect past blood and brain levels.[61]

Methyl mercury[62] is slowly metabolized into inorganic mercury mainly by microflora in the intestines, probably at a rate of about 1% of the body burden per day. Some demethylation also occurs in phagocytic cells. The biochemical mechanism is unknown. Although methyl mercury is the predominant form of mercury during exposure, inorganic mercury slowly accumulates and resides for long periods in the central nervous system. It is believed to be in an inert form – probably insoluble mercury selenide.[63]

Urinary excretion is negligible, to the order of 10% or less of the total elimination from the body. Methyl mercury undergoes extensive enterohepatic cycling - it is secreted into bile and is eliminated from the body by demethylation and excretion of the inorganic form in the faeces – about 90% of the methylmercury is eliminated from the body in the faeces.

The role of these two processes in suckling human infants is unknown. The high mobility of methyl mercury in the body is not due to lipid solubility, as claimed in some textbooks. It is present in the body as water-soluble complexes mainly, if not exclusively, attached to the sulphur atom of thiol ligands. It enters the endothelial cells of the blood–brain barrier as a complex with L-cysteine. The process is so specific that the complex with the optical isomer D-cysteine is not transported.

Structurally, the L-complex is similar to the large neutral amino acid L-methionine and is carried across the cell membrane on the large neutral amino acid carrier.[64] Methyl mercury is pumped out of mammalian cells as a complex with reduced glutathione. For example, it is secreted into bile as a glutathione complex. The glutathione moiety is degraded in the bile duct and gall bladder to a dipeptide and finally to the L-cysteine complex.

61 Amin-Zaki L, Elhassani S, Majeed MA, Clarkson TW, Doherty RA, Greenwood M. Intra-uterine methyl mercury poisoning in Iraq. *Pediatrics* 54(5):587–595, 1974.
62 Methyl mercury – an organic form of mercury made from the methylation of elemental mercury.
63 WHO. Environmental Health Criteria 101: Methylmercury. *International Program on Chemical Safety*. Geneva: World Health Organization, 1990.
64 Kerper LE, Ballatori N, Clarkson TW. Methylmercury transport across the blood-brain barrier by an amino acid carrier. *Am J Physiol* 267:R761–R765, 1992.

Presumably, in this form it is reabsorbed into the bloodstream to be returned to the liver, thereby completing the enterohepatic cycle[65].

The elimination of methyl mercury from the body varies from one tissue to another but generally fall in the range of 45–70 days. Thus, individuals with long-term regular exposure to methyl mercury attain a substantial body burden in about 1 year. Several thiol-containing complexing agents have been successfully used to remove methyl mercury from the body (e.g. in the Iraq outbreak: see Clarkson et al.[66]) An interesting example is a thiol-containing resin that, when given by mouth, traps the methyl mercury secreted in bile and carries it into the faeces. Perhaps the most promising complexing agent is N-acetylcysteine.[67] It enhances methyl mercury excretion when given orally, has a low toxicity, and is widely available in the clinical setting.

Mercury: crossing all barriers

Mercury is associated with 258 different symptoms, and copper – also found in amalgam – is associated with over 100. The severe toxicity of methylmercury is attributed to its ability to pierce any cell membrane in the body and cross all barriers, even the placental and blood-brain barriers. After crossing these barriers, methylmercury is converted back into the highly destructive ionic form and destroys all cell components in its path. The transportation mechanism into cells is its primary damaging component. Its conversion to ionic form then deposits the 'killer' form of mercury in areas it could never penetrate in the organic form. By this mechanism, methylmercury is credited with initiating degeneration and atrophy of the sensory cerebral cortex, paresthaesia, (numbness and tingling), autism, behavioural and emotional aberrations, as well as hearing and visual impairment.

In crossing the placenta, it can inhibit foetal brain development and bring on cerebral palsy or psychomotor retardation in the latter stages of development. Other symptoms of mercury toxicity include: anorexia,

---

65 Dutczak WJ, Ballatori N. Transport of the glutathionemethyl mercury complex across liver canalicular membranes on reduced glutathione carriers. *J Biol Chem* 269:9746–9751 1994.
66 Clarkson TW, Magos L, Cox C, Greenwood MR, Majeed MA, Damluji SF. Tests of efficacy of antidotes for removal of methylmercury in human poisoning during the Iraq outbreak. *J Pharmacol Exp Ther* 218:74–83, 1981.
67 Ballatori N, Lieberman NMW, Wang W. N-Acetylcysteine as an antidote in methylmercury poisoning. *Environ Health Perspect* 106:267–271, 1998.

depression, fatigue, insomnia, arthritis, multiple sclerosis, moodiness, irritability, memory loss, nausea, diarrhoea, gum disease, swollen glands, headaches and many others. Mercury amalgams have set us up for most of the health problems we see today.

Mercury and the central nervous system

The major poisonous effects of methyl mercury are on the central nervous system. Its toxic action on the developing brain differs in both mechanism and outcome from its action on the mature organ, so the two actions are treated separately here (for detailed reviews, see US EPA and ATSDR[68]). However, recent reports have raised the possibility that methyl mercury may have adverse effects on other targets in the body.

The action of methyl mercury on adults is characterized by a latent period between exposure and the onset of symptoms. This period can be several weeks or even months, depending of the dose and exposure period. Perhaps the most dramatic example of latency was in the case of the severe, ultimately fatal poisoning of a chemistry professor from exposure to dimethyl mercury.[69]

A single exposure from a spill of liquid dimethyl mercury took place in August. The professor continued her normal professional work without any apparent ill effects. In November she presented a paper at an overseas conference. It was not until late December that the first symptoms appeared. Within a few weeks the full syndrome of severe methyl mercury poisoning became manifest. Despite many decades of research on methyl mercury toxicology, the mechanism underlying this long latent period is still unknown.

Paresthesia – numbness, or a 'pins and needles' sensation, is the first symptom to appear at the lowest dose. This may progress to cerebellar ataxia, dysarthria, constriction of the visual fields and loss of hearing. These signs and symptoms are caused by the loss of neuronal cells in specific anatomical regions of the brain. For example, ataxia results from

---

68 U.S. EPA. Water Quality Criterion for the Protection of Human Health: Methyl Mercury. EPA 0823-R-01-001. Washington, DC: U.S. Environmental Protection Agency, 2001.
69 Nierenberg DW, Nordgren RE, Chang MB, Siegler W, Blayney MG, Hochberg F, Toribara TY, Cernichiari E, Clarkson T. Delayed cerebellar disease and death after accidental exposure to dimethyl mercury. *N Engl J Med* 338:1672–1675, 1998.

the loss of the granule cells in the cerebellum. The neighbouring Purkinje cells are relatively unaffected.

The transport of mercury vapour around the body

The escape of mercury vapour from amalgams is the primary source through which mercury gains access to the body. It is absorbed through the mucous membranes of the mouth and by direct inhalation into the lungs. The stomach and intestinal tract also absorb swallowed mercury, freshly formed from the highly reactive vapour in the mouth. All of these portals of entry allow mercury relatively direct access to the bloodstream, where binding to haemoglobin can take place. The majority of mercury in the blood is contained within the red blood cells.

Mercury is implicated in metal-induced autoimmunity with the emphasis on *multiple sclerosis* (MS), *rheumatoid arthritis* (RA) and *amyotrophic lateral sclerosis* (ALS). If everyone who had come down with MS, lupus, arthritis, epilepsy, leukaemia, ALS, diabetes, etc., could relate their disease to dental procedures, the ensuing legal battle would be for more money than exists. A dentist can't legally throw amalgam material or extracted amalgam filled teeth in the trash, bury them in the ground, or put them in a landfill, but the ADA and the EPA say it's okay to put it in people's mouths.

Exposure to mercury vapour causes accumulation of mercury in the brain and spinal cord. Mercury is often concentrated in neurons, especially motor neurons and astroglia cells. It has been suggested that mercury in low concentrations may affect phosphorylation and thereby intercellular signalling. Mercury inhibits the development of, and breaks down, cytoskeleton[70] structures in nerve cells. At approximately 0.35 $\mu g/g$ mercury in brain tissue, bonding of GTP (a binding protein) to tubulin is inhibited. This process is necessary for polymerization of *tubulin*, which in turn is a key component of the cytoskeleton. Concentrations of $HgCl_2$ below and close to 0.1 μM inhibit the growth of nerve germs and also cause retrograde degradation of the cytoskeleton in nerve cells.

---

70 Cytoskeleton - The internal framework of a cell, which plays an important role in cell movement, shape, growth, division, and differentiation, as well as in the movement of organelles within the cell.

Mercury and the autoimmune system

A recent study completed in 2003,[71] states that patients with certain autoimmune diseases such as lupus, multiple sclerosis, autoimmune thyroiditis and allergic disease 'often show increased lymphocyte stimulation by low doses of inorganic mercury in vitro.' In their study, they removed amalgams from a group of 35 patients with autoimmune diseases and replaced them with composites. When examined six months later, 71 percent had shown an improvement in health, with the greatest improvement in those with multiple sclerosis. Their conclusion: 'Mercury-containing amalgam may be an important risk factor for patients with autoimmune diseases.'

Pendergrass and Haley[72] in 1997 performed a study published in the journal *Neurotoxicology*. In their study, they showed concentrations of mercury vapour, known to be released by dental amalgams in people, increased mercury concentrations in rat brains from 11- to 47-fold higher than controls. At this level, the mercury produced the identical lesions seen in Alzheimer's disease (*neurofibrillary tangles*) by interfering with normal tubulin maintenance.

The effects of mercury on glutamate

A second mechanism producing neurodegenerative diseases is even more impressive, called *excitotoxicity*.[73] This is a mechanism by which excess glutamate accumulates outside the neuron, thereby leading to the death of the cell by an excitation process, which has been linked to mercury neurotoxicity since as early as 1993. More recent studies have confirmed this mechanism and clearly demonstrate – even in concentrations below that known to cause cell injury – that mercury can paralyze the glutamate removal mechanism, leading to significant damage to synapses, dendrites and neurons themselves.

---

71 Charles S. Via, Phuong Nguyen, Florin Niculescu, John Papadimitriou, Dennis Hoover, and Ellen K. Silbergeld, Low-Dose Exposure to Inorganic Mercury Accelerates Disease and Mortality in Acquired Murine Lupus Environmental Health Perspectives • Vol 111, No. 10, August, 2003.
72 J. C. Pendergrass, B. E. Haley, M. J. Vimy, S. A. Winfield and F. L. Lorscheider, Mercury Vapor Inhalation Inhibits Binding of GTP to Tubulin in Rat Brain: Similarity to a Molecular Lesion in Alzheimer's Disease Brain, *Neurotoxicology*, 18(2), 315-324, 1997.
73 Blaylock, R.L. Excitotoxins: The Taste that Kills. Health Press, New Mexico, 1997.

This glutamate removal mechanism is critical to brain protection. Additionally, mercury in very low concentrations increases glutamate release, primarily by stimulating the brain's immune cell, the *microglia*. Chronic microglial activation, as seen with mercury exposure, has been solidly linked to all of the neurodegenerative diseases.

At least two studies have shown that mercury increases the toxicity of glutamate. Interestingly, excess glutamate can also produce the same neurofibrillary tangles seen with mercury exposure. In essence, we have the mechanism by which these diseases are produced by mercury vapour and know that it can occur in concentrations commonly found in people having dental amalgam fillings.

According to Dr Boyd Haley, Professor of Medicinal Biochemistry at the University of Kentucky:

'If you have something that's been put in your mouth that you can't dispose of in a waste basket without breaking environmental protection laws, there's no point in keeping it around, there's no point in taking that type of risk – there's no point in exposing people to any level of mercury toxicity if you don't have to......

' .....there is no doubt in my mind that low levels of mercury present in the brain could cause normal cell death, and this could lead to dementia which would be similar to Alzheimer's disease....

'We can't go inside a living human being and look at their brain, so we have to work outside, and do scientific experiments such as we've done. And to the best that we can determine with these experiments, mercury is a time-bomb in the brain, waiting to have an effect. If it's not bothering someone when they're young, when they age it can turn into something quite disastrous.'

Mercury and yeast infections

Toxic metals interfere with the normal energy patterns in acupuncture channels by setting up interference patterns in the meridians. The body, in trying to protect itself against mercury, creates a problem of yeast infection.

One of the natural absorbers of heavy metals is the yeast: *candida albicans* (refer back to chapter 5 for more details on Candida) – the body attracts yeast into the intestines to act as a natural sponge for the mercury. Heavy metals such as mercury act as free radicals, which are highly reactive, charged particles that damage body tissues. Free radicals prevent nutrients from entering the cells and wastes from leaving, and block enzymes necessary for the body's detoxification processes. Mercury can bind to the DNA of cells, as well as to the cell membranes, distorting them and interfering with normal cell functions. The immune system no longer recognizes the target as part of the body and will attack it.

The mechanisms of mercury toxicity in the central nervous system

Nerve endings in the peripheral nervous system constantly scan their environment, engulfing foreign particles and bringing them across the cell membrane for inspection. These substances may then travel all the way up from the foot to the spinal cord to be presented to the nerve cells there. As it travels up the axon, mercury destroys a substance called *tubulin*, used as insulation for *neurofibrils* in the *microtubules*, effectively destroying the nerves.[74]

Within 24 hours of injecting a minute dose of mercury into a muscle anywhere in the body of test animals, it is detectable in the spinal cord and brain. The mercury is also found in the kidneys, lungs, bloodstream, connective tissue, adrenals and other endocrine glands. In the brain, it tends to congregate in the hypothalamus, which regulates the autonomic nervous system, and in the limbic system, believed to be the seat of the emotions.

As stated above, the most devastating effect of mercury in the nervous system is that it interferes with energy production inside each cell. Nerve cells are impaired in their ability to detoxify and nurture themselves. The cell becomes toxic and dies, or lives in a state of chronic malnutrition. It is common for heavy metals to migrate to and accumulate in nerve *ganglia* (nerve relay stations). As a heavy metal (which means heavier than water), mercury tends to accumulate in the lowest parts of the body, such as the floor of the mouth, the pelvic floor, and the feet.

---

74 See www.detoxmetals.com/Hg-Destroys.html for a video demonstrating this.

Mercury attacking the tissues

Once mercury reaches its destination tissue, it has many ways in which it may express its toxicity:

- ❖ Altered cell membrane permeability
- ❖ Alteration of tertiary structure
- ❖ Alteration of enzyme function
- ❖ Interference in nerve impulses
- ❖ Alteration of the genetic code
- ❖ Inhibition of DNA repair
- ❖ Interference with endocrine function
- ❖ Contribution to autoimmune disease
- ❖ Digestion and absorption alteration
- ❖ Contribution to the development of antibiotic resistance
- ❖ Damaging the heart muscle
- ❖ Inhibiting the CNS.

A number of studies have shown that the heart is sensitive to mercury toxicity – one study with idiopathic cardiomyopathy found that in some cases their heart muscle contained a dose of mercury that was 22,000 times higher than that seen in the hearts of other people of similar age. With heart failure rates rising exponentially, no one is really looking at the possibility that vaccines, dental amalgams and other sources of mercury are the cause.

Methyl mercury and the foetal brain

Methyl mercury crosses the placental barrier. Levels in cord blood are proportional to, but slightly higher than levels in maternal blood. Levels in the foetal brain are about 5-7 times that in maternal blood.[75] Brain-to-blood ratios in adult humans and other primates are approximately within the same range.

Health effects of primary concern include damage to babies' developing brains when pregnant women are exposed to methylmercury, with effects

---

75 Cernichiari E, Brewer R, Myers GJ, Marsh DO, Lapham LW, Cox C, Shamlaye CF, Berlin M, Davidson PW, Clarkson TW. Monitoring methylmercury during pregnancy: maternal hair predicts fetal brain exposure. *Neurotoxicology* 16(4):705–710, 1995.

on intelligence, learning ability and behaviour.[76] Adults and children exposed to excessive doses of methylmercury can also suffer from effects on memory, cognitive and sensory functions, and motor coordination.[77]

Most methylmercury in the embryo comes from the mother eating fish which is contaminated. The EPA's safe exposure estimate for methylmercury has dropped twice in the past 16 years, as new science has identified adverse effects in children exposed in the womb at lower and lower doses.

Emerging evidence indicates that the safe dose may drop even lower in the future. Just how long a foetus can tolerate a dose of methylmercury above a 'safe level' with no observable adverse effects is a matter of ongoing debate.

Compounding this uncertainty is the lack of effective education and outreach to pregnant women about methylmercury risks and the near total absence of information for pregnant women on the levels of mercury in the fish they buy. New data from the US Centers for Disease Control and Prevention (CDC) show that about 10 percent of all women of childbearing age have blood methylmercury levels above the dose that may put their foetus at risk from adverse neurological effects.

If these women were to increase their consumption of certain fish species in hopes of benefiting their babies during pregnancy, they could expose their foetuses to potentially hazardous levels of methylmercury.

Mercury toxicity in fish

About 95% of methyl mercury ingested in fish is absorbed into the gastro-intestinal tract, although the exact site of absorption is not known. It is distributed to all tissues in a process completed in about 30 hours. About 5% is found in the blood components and about 10% in the brain. The concentration in red blood cells is about 20 times the concentration in plasma.

---

76 National Research Council. Toxicological Effects of Methylmercury. Washington, D.C: National Academy Press, 2000.
77 Clarkson, TM., Magos, L and Myers, GJ. The Toxicology of Mercury – Current Exposures and Clinical Manifestations. N. Engl J Med 349 (18): 1731-1737, 2003.

Fish and shellfish are an important part of a healthy diet. Fish and shellfish contain high-quality protein and other essential nutrients, are low in saturated fat, and contain omega-3 fatty acids. A well-balanced diet that includes a variety of fish and shellfish can contribute to heart health and children's proper growth and development. So, women and young children in particular should include fish or shellfish in their diets due to the many nutritional benefits.

However, as I mentioned in chapter 4, nearly all fish and shellfish contain traces of mercury. For most people, the risk from mercury by eating fish and shellfish is not a health concern. Yet, some fish and shellfish contain higher levels of mercury that may harm an unborn baby or young child's developing nervous system. The risks from mercury in fish and shellfish depend on the amount of fish and shellfish eaten and the levels of mercury in the fish and shellfish. Therefore, the US Food and Drug Administration (FDA) and the Environmental Protection Agency (EPA) are advising women who may become pregnant; pregnant women, nursing mothers and young children to avoid certain types of fish and eat fish and shellfish that are lower in mercury.

Guidelines for minimizing mercury exposure from fish and shellfish

By following these 3 recommendations for selecting and eating fish or shellfish, women and young children will receive the benefits of eating fish and shellfish and be confident that they have reduced their exposure to the harmful effects of mercury.

1. Do not eat shark, swordfish, king mackerel, or tilefish because they contain high levels of mercury.
2. Eat up to 12 ounces (2 average meals) a week of a variety of fish and shellfish that are lower in mercury.
3. Five of the most commonly eaten fish that are low in mercury are shrimp, canned light tuna, salmon, pollock and catfish.

Another commonly eaten fish – albacore ('white') tuna has more mercury than canned light tuna. So, when choosing your two meals of fish and shellfish, you may eat up to 6 ounces (one average meal) of albacore tuna per week.

Check local advisories about the safety of fish caught by family and friends in your local lakes, rivers, and coastal areas. If no advice is available, eat up to 6 ounces (one average meal) per week of fish you catch from local waters, but don't consume any other fish during that week.

Follow these same recommendations when feeding fish and shellfish to your young child, but serve smaller portions.

On January 12, 2001, government health officials issued new advisories warning women to limit fish consumption during pregnancy to avoid exposing their unborn children to unsafe levels of methylmercury.

In February 2009, the Zero-Mercury Working Group[78] published a report entitled "Mercury in Fish is a Global Health concern.[79]" "Mercury contamination of fish and mammals is a global public health concern," said Michael Bender, report co-author and member of the Zero Mercury Working Group. "Our study of fish tested in different locations around the world shows that internationally accepted exposure levels for methylmercury are exceeded, often by wide margins, in each country and area covered."

The Food and Drug Administration (FDA), which regulates commercially sold fish, recommends that pregnant and nursing women and young children not eat any shark, swordfish, tilefish, or king mackerel, but then recommends 12 ounces per week of any other fish.

The Environmental Protection Agency (EPA), which makes recommendations to states about safe mercury levels in sport fish, allows up to 8 ounces of any fish per week for pregnant women with no prohibitions on consumption of any individual fish caught recreationally.

These restrictions are steps in the right direction, but they need to be tightened significantly to adequately protect women and their unborn children from the toxic effects of methylmercury.

---

78 The Zero Mercury Working Group is an international coalition of more than 75 public-interest non-governmental organizations from around the world, formed in 2005 by the European Environmental Bureau and the Mercury Policy Project/Ban Mercury Working Group. The aim of the group is to continually reduce emissions, demand and supply of mercury from all sources we can control, with the goal of eliminating mercury in the environment at EU level and globally. See www.zeromercury.org
79 http://www.zeromercury.org/press/090210-MercuryFishRelease.pdf

The nutritional benefits of fish complicate the task faced by health officials when protecting the public from methylmercury. Protein, omega-3 fatty acids, Vitamin D, and other nutrients make fish an otherwise exceptionally good food for pregnant mothers and their developing babies.

Some research suggests that the risk of cardiovascular disease increases with methylmercury exposure.[80] In extreme cases, methylmercury poisoning can lead to paralysis, coma and even death.

A new Mercury Policy Project (MPP) report recently published entitled, *Mercury in Fish: An Urgent Global Health Concern,*[81] explains that the mercury risk is greatest for populations whose per capita fish consumption is high, and in areas where pollution has elevated the average mercury content of fish. But methylmercury hazards also exist where per capita fish consumption and average mercury levels in fish are comparatively low – in cultures where fish-eating marine mammals are part of the traditional diet, mercury in these animals can add substantially to total dietary exposure.

Widespread health problems from mercury exposure

There seems to be a schizophrenic policy regarding the control of toxins in the World at large – on the one hand there are concerted efforts by authorities to clean up mercury from the atmosphere, while also banning mercury thermometers, barometers and the like, but on the other hand the US Food and Drug Administration (FDA) and the Public Health Services seem to be covering up the dangers of mercury in amalgams, fish and vaccinations. This policy can be summed up in a few words: 'The love of money is the root of all evil.' Peer-reviewed studies have established that adverse health affects have been associated with mercury vapour derived from amalgam fillings.[82]

Dr. Boyd Haley, Chair and Professor of the Chemistry Department at the University of Kentucky and a proponent and researcher of the dangers of mercury, believes that the US Centers for Disease Control (CDC) and the FDA are strongly influenced by the pharmaceutical and vaccine industries

---

80 Konig, A., et al. A Quantitative Analysis of Fish Consumption and Coronary Heart Disease Mortality. *Am J Prev Med* 29 (4): 355-346, 2005.
81 Mercury in Fish: A Global Health Hazard, Zero Mercury Working Group, Mercury Policy Project, Feb. 2009.
82 Lorscheider, FL; et al., Mercury Exposure from Silver Tooth Fillings: Emerging Evidence Questions a Traditional Dental Paradigm. *FASEBJ.* 9:504-8, 1995.

and that they have been derelict in their duty to safeguard the health of the American People. As a result of their delinquency, we have been systematically poisoned by mercury derived from silver amalgam fillings in our teeth, and also our children who have been severely damaged by vaccines containing *thimerosal* (a mercury-based preservative used in vaccines – see below for more details on this).

Toxicity caused by excessive mercury exposure is now becoming recognized as a widespread environmental problem and is continuing to attract a great deal of public attention. A National Academy of Sciences study [83] published in July 2001 estimates that up to 60, 000 children born in the US each year may be affected by mercury toxicity, and in March of 2002 an environmental group charged the FDA with failing to warn the public of the dangers of mercury contamination from eating tuna, which contains high levels of mercury.

The World Health Organization reports that the amount of mercury absorbed daily by the average human body is 0.3 micrograms (mcg) from water and air, 2.61 mcg from fish and 17 mcg from dental amalgams (silver fillings). Uptake of up to 100 µg daily has been observed in extreme cases. Research points out that mercury vapour is 80% absorbed into the blood, and that in animal studies, mercury vapour goes directly from the nose to the brain, following nasal nerve pathways. Amalgam fillings release mercury for as long as 70 years. Someone with 8 amalgams could release 120 mcg into the saliva per day.

The maximum mercury exposure allowable by the US Environmental Protection Agency (EPA) is less than 0.1mcg per kilogram of body weight per day, to be absorbed into the human body.

Mercury causes adverse health effects in dentists and dental personnel[84,85,86,87]. Dentists have 4 times as much of a body burden of

---

83 NAS. National Academy of Sciences Report: Toxicological Effects of Methylmercury. C. R.A. Goyer, *National Academy Press*: pp. 344, 2000.

84 Ngim, CH; et al., Chronic Neurobehavioral Effects of Elemental Mercury in Dentists, *Brit J Indust Med*, 49:782-90, 1992.

85 Echeverria, D; et al., Behavioral Effects of Low-Level Exposure to HgE Among Dentists. *Neurotoxicol Teratol*, 17(2):161-8, 1995.

86 Shapiro, IM., et al., Neurophysiological and neuropsychological function in mercury-exposed dentists. *The Lancet* 1, 1147-1150, 1982.

87 Uzzell, BP., et al., Chronic low-level mercury exposure and neuropsychological functioning. *J of Clin and Exper Neuropsych*. 8, 581-593.

mercury as an average non-dentist. Dental workers show 50-300% more mercury in hair and fingernails than the average population.

Dental amalgams – a closer look

> *'The mercury uptake from amalgam is the dominating source for inorganic mercury in the central nervous system and is the major source of total mercury uptake in the population.'*
> Maths Berlin, a leading Swedish toxicologist

So, what is an amalgam? It was dentists who, over 150 years ago discovered a new, less expensive way to fill cavities in teeth, rather than using gold and silver alone. This was a mixture of an assortment of metals such as mercury (45% - 52%),[88] silver (30%) and small amounts of copper, zinc and tin.

Denying the truth about the dangers of amalgam toxicity

Initially, back in those early days, the American Society of Dental Surgeons opposed its use as they knew that mercury was so toxic. However, so many dentists were using it that the original society collapsed and the rogue dentists replaced it with a new one – the American Dental Association (ADA), which is still in existence. This has now grown to be a powerful lobby in Washington and other states. After 150 years, the ADA is still allowing over 180 million mercury-containing amalgam fillings to be placed in people's mouths, including young children!

The ADA has been covering up the danger by saying that the mercury is 'locked in' to the tooth and is not released from the filling itself. The scientific evidence is now so overwhelmingly against this lie that the ADA had to eventually admit that mercury is released from amalgam fillings (as a vapour) and that over 80% of this is absorbed into the body. Amalgams release mercury even quicker when a person chews or drinks hot liquids. This is a shocking realisation given that everyone alive today will chew and drink hot liquids on occasions![89]

---

88 Sandra Denton MD: Proceedings of the First International Conference on Biocompatibility 1988.
89 http://www.iaomt.org/videos

Consumers aren't being told the truth: that amalgam fillings contain 50% mercury – a known neurotoxin. Worse, they are deceived: the ADA still uses the deceptive word 'silver' to describe a product that is mainly mercury, thus hiding the product's main ingredient.

In previous years the ADA has managed to de-license various dentists who proclaimed amalgams to be dangerous, and strictly enforced a Gag Rule[90] In response, these dentists have taken the issue to court, protecting their right, among others, to Free Speech. And yet today, member dentists of the ADA who talk against mercury, or even mention that mercury 'might' be toxic, run a high risk of being expelled as well as having their licenses revoked. The ADA even calls it 'unethical and unprofessional conduct' to inform patients of the potential dangers of the most hazardous metal known to mankind. Yet European countries like Sweden[91] have legislated a total ban on all amalgams and other products containing mercury, after spending years reviewing the scientific research.

Yielding to scientific pressures, the ADA now admits that mercury is indeed released from amalgam fillings even after placement, but state that it is perfectly safe and still support the use of amalgam fillings. They claim their use is safe, based on over 150 years of use, and that no scientific evidence shows mercury exposure from dental fillings causes any known disease. Yet the American Dental Association ADA does admit there is a potential hazard for dental office personnel with the handling of dental amalgam and recommend that dentists use a 'no-touch' technique, because dentists and their staff might become contaminated. They admit that the 'scrap' amalgam – the excess amalgam left over after filling a tooth – also constitutes a hazardous threat because of continuous vapour release.

There is no scientific evidence showing amalgam's safety, and mixed dental amalgam has never had US Food and Drug Administration (FDA) research or approval. If it were to be classified as a *class II* medical device and made to undergo the rigorous testing needed to prove safety, it would never pass.

After filing petitions, testifying at Congressional hearings, providing state fact sheet laws, testifying at Scientific Advisory Committee hearings, and

---

90 The Gag Rule is a pillar of the ADA's agenda to block consumers from learning that the major component of amalgam is Mercury. The Gag Rule instructs dentists to abandon their allegiance to patient health care - to remain silent or face disciplinary action.
91 http://www.sweden.gov.se/sb/d/11459/a/118550

writing hundreds of letters, the Consumers for Dental Choice (CDC)[92] eventually won their ten-year battle to get the FDA to comply with the law and recently (2008) classify mercury amalgam. The FDA website[93] now states:

'Dental amalgams contain mercury, which may have neurotoxic effects on the nervous systems of developing children and foetuses.[94] ... Pregnant women and people who may have a health condition that makes them more sensitive to mercury exposure, including individuals with existing high levels of mercury bio burden, should not avoid seeking dental care, but should discuss options with their health practitioner.'

Each amalgam filling has as much mercury as a thermometer, and its poisonous vapours are constantly emitted from the teeth to the brain, a particular risk, according to the US government, to the developing brain of the child. As mentioned earlier, the foetus is at the greatest risk of all if the pregnant woman has dental fillings drilled out or implanted, because of the proven transport of mercury through the placenta. So too is the nursing infant of a woman with amalgam dental fillings, because of the transport of mercury into the breast milk.

Confirmation of the escape of mercury vapour and ions from amalgam dental fillings is provided by The World Health Organization (WHO) Environmental Health Criteria 118 document (EHC 118) on inorganic mercury. It clearly states that the largest estimated average daily intake and retention of mercury and mercury compounds in the general population, is from dental amalgams, not from food or air.

The nuts and bolts of mercury vapour inhalation from amalgams

Mercury vapour inhaled into the lungs is absorbed almost 100 percent and immediately passes into the bloodstream. It takes approximately four minutes before mercury is converted or oxidized into an ionic state from its elemental vapour state. While in its elemental form, mercury vapour is

---

92 www.toxicteeth.org
93 www.fda.gov
94 Mercury has been removed from thermometers and vaccines, controls have been tightened on mercury emissions from coal power plants, and pregnant women have been warned about consuming fish tainted by mercury.

lipid (fat) soluble and readily passes through the blood-brain barrier or the placental membrane.

> *'Worldwide there are over 4,000 research papers indicating that mercury is a highly toxic substance. How can dentists be so thoughtless as to place one of the deadliest toxins in existence two inches from our brains?'*
> Tom Warren

It can also accumulate in other organs and tissues of the body. The estimated average daily intake of mercury from dental amalgams is 3.8 - 21 micrograms per day. Two-thirds of the body burden of mercury is derived from the mercury vapour released from amalgams. The static release of mercury vapour from amalgam fillings that are not being stimulated, which goes on 24 hours a day, 365 days a year, is a major contributor to total mercury body burden. Large amounts of mercury vapour are released during chewing. After only ten minutes of gum chewing, there is an average increase in mercury release of 15.6 times more than during the resting state in test subjects. That converts to a 1,560% increase in mercury release.

Mercury levels in autopsy tissue samples, including the brain, have been shown to correlate with the total number of surfaces of amalgam restorations. The estimate for the

rate of release in people with amalgam restoration is 2-17 µg Hg/day[95]. The most recent estimate based on applying pharmacokinetic parameters to steady-state plasma levels in people with amalgam suggests an average intake of between 5 and 9 µg Hg/day.[96] Kingman et al, in a study [97] correlating urinary excretion of mercury with amalgam surfaces, estimated that 10 amalgam surfaces would raise urinary levels by 1 µg Hg/L. As discussed below, these are far below toxic levels. However, excessive chewing, such as occurs when smokers try to stop smoking by using nicotine-containing chewing gum, may lead to urine levels in excess of 20

---

95 WHO. Environmental Health Criteria 101: Methylmercury. International Program on Chemical Safety. Geneva: World Health Organization, 1990.

96 Sandborgh-Englund G, Elinder C-G, Johanson G, Lind B, Skare I, Ekstrand J. The absorption, blood levels and excretion of mercury after a single dose of mercury vapour in humans. *Toxicol Appl Pharmacol* 150:46–153, 1998.

97 Kingman A, Albertini T, Brown LJ. Mercury concentrations in urine and whole blood associated with amalgam exposure in a US military population. *J Dent Res* 77:461–467 1998.

µg Hg/g creatinine, thereby approaching occupational health safety limits.[98]

Increased amounts of mercury are excreted in the faeces of individuals with amalgam fillings. Engqvist et al.[99] found that only 25% of the total mercury in faecal samples was in the form of amalgam particles in samples taken from six adults with a moderate load of amalgam fillings. About 80% of an oral dose of amalgam particles or mercuric mercury attached to sulfhydryl groups was excreted in the faeces. Interestingly, 60% of an oral dose of vapour dissolved in water was retained. Previously it had been assumed that intake of vapour was due solely to inhalation.

> *The World Health Organization has calculated that the average human daily dose of mercury from various sources are: Dental amalgam = 3.0 - 17.0 mg/day (Hg vapour) Fish and Seafood = 2.3 mg/day (methylmercury); Other food = 0.3 mg/day (inorganic Hg) Air & Water = Negligible traces (NOTE mg = Micrograms).*

Mercury readily mixes with food and is swallowed with it. The body uptake from inorganic mercury, swallowed with saliva, can be as much as hundreds of micrograms per day for individuals with a large number of amalgam fillings. Urinary excretion is a common indicator of mercury toxicity, even though faecal excretion of mercury is twenty times greater than the corresponding urinary excretion.

There is a statistical correlation between the mercury concentration in saliva and the number of amalgam fillings. The United States government has determined and ruled that the continual exposure to mercury from amalgam fillings is not without risk to patients.

> *'You wouldn't take a leaky thermometer, put it in your mouth, and leave it there 24 hours a day, 365 days a year. Yet that's exactly what happens when an amalgam filling is installed in your mouth.' – Dr Michael Ziff*

---

98 Sallsten G, Thoren J, Barregard L, Schutz A, Skarping G. Long-term use of nicotine chewing gum and mercury exposure from dental amalgam fillings. *J Dent Res* 75:594–598, 1996.
99 Engqvist A, Colmsjo A, Skare I. Speciation of mercury in faeces from individuals with amalgam fillings. *Arch Environ Health* 53:205–213, 1998.

Mercury vapour is released when you chew or grind your teeth. Additionally, minute rusted particles of the amalgam are being abraded and taken up by your food or saliva and swallowed. Intestinal enzymes and bacteria both produce *methylmercury*, an even more toxic form than elemental mercury, which may act upon these minute particles of mercury filling. Over time the amalgam fillings corrode and 'rust' which releases molecules of mercury into the oral cavity.

Conventional amalgam was routinely placed until 1976, when the new state-of-the-art amalgams (50% mercury and 30% copper) were introduced. These emit up to 50 times more mercury than the earlier, conventional amalgam fillings. That means that every new high-copper amalgam filling placed today has the effective toxic equivalent of fifty of the older amalgam fillings.

If other dental work is also present in the mouth, such as gold crowns, nickel crowns and removable bridges or braces, the mercury emission further increases from the amalgam. This is due to the electrical current generated by the presence of dissimilar metals in an electrolyte medium such as saliva. Heat will reliably increase the rate of escape of mercury vapour from amalgam fillings. Vapour detectors, held above amalgams, have revealed an increase from 3 micrograms to over 500 micrograms ten seconds after a hot drink was swallowed.

Chronic inhalation of mercury vapour from amalgam fillings for twenty years or more can result in the accumulation of pathologic quantities of mercury in the brain and other critical organs and tissues. Human autopsy studies of accident victims have shown a positive correlation between the numbers of mercury amalgam dental fillings and the concentration of mercury in the brain. The onset of clinically observable signs or symptoms of mercury toxicity may take as long as 20-30 years to appear, depending on a person's biochemical individuality.

Several recent reviews have discussed in detail the uptake, distribution, excretion, metabolism, and kinetics of inhaled mercury vapour.[100,101,102] A

100 U.S. EPA. Mercury Report to Congress Office of Air Quality and Standards. Washington, DC: U.S. Environmental Protection Agency, 1997.
101 ATSDR. Toxicological Profile for Mercury. Atlanta, GA:Agency for Toxic Substances and Disease Registry, 1999.
102 WHO. Environmental Health Criteria 118. Inorganic Mecury. International Program on Chemical Safety. Geneva: World Health Organization, 1991.

brief summary is presented here with an update from recent reports. About 80% of inhaled mercury vapour is retained in the body. However, approximately 7-14% is exhaled within a week after exposure. The half-time of the process is about 2 days.

The dissolved vapour accumulates in red blood cells and is carried to all tissues in the body. It crosses the blood–brain and placental barriers. The half-time of distribution to the plasma compartment is approximately 5 hours.[103]

In a trial with nine adult subjects, the amount of time to reach a peak value was 9 hours, within a range of 7-24 hours. The amount of mercury in plasma at the time of the peak concentration was 4% of the inhaled dose (95% confidence limit: 3-5%).

Approximately 7% of mercury is deposited in the cranial region after a single exposure to nontoxic levels of the vapour. The kidney is the main depository. Once the vapour has entered the cell, it is subject to oxidation to divalent inorganic mercury. The oxidation step is catalyzed specifically by the enzyme catalase, with endogenously produced hydrogen peroxide as the other substrate. The process is inhibited by ethanol. As a result, workers who drink a moderate amount of alcohol tend to retain less of the inhaled vapour, therefore become less toxic.

The finding that the half-time for exhalation from the lung is about 2 days, suggests that the halftime for the oxidation in body tissues is about the same. Studies with radioactive tracers indicate that the rate of overall excretion of mercury from the body can be described by a single half-time of about 58 days, corresponding to an excretion rate of slightly more than 1% of the body burden per day.

The effects of mercury on reproductive health

The uterus is a collection centre for mercury. Dr. Hal Huggins, a pioneer dentist in the USA who has written much on the effects of mercury, reported that more than 90% of the imbalances created by sex hormone disturbances were corrected within a few weeks of amalgam removal. His

---

103 Sandborgh-Englund G, Elinder C-G, Johanson G, Lind B, Skare I, Ekstrand J. The absorption, blood levels and excretion of mercury after a single dose of mercury vapour in humans. *Toxicol Appl Pharmacol* 150:46–153, 1998.

patients noted differences in fertility, less pain during periods, relief from endometriosis and a trend toward optimization of the days of menstrual flow.

PMS is one of the most common symptoms to change after amalgam removal. Amenorrhea, or the complete absence of a menstrual flow, also responds to amalgam removal. This is usually in women in their twenties or thirties. Even in women who have gone through a sort of premature menopause in their early forties, the periods may start up again for a couple of years. This has resulted in surprise pregnancies. Women should avoid pregnancy for at least six months after amalgam removal.

Lubricated condoms and birth control creams or gels have mercury as the primary spermicidal. It is not required that the word 'mercury' appear on the label, as it is assumed that everyone knows that mercury is in there.

Pelvic symptoms, in both men and women, are very commonly caused by metal toxicity of the *Frankenhauser's ganglion*. This can account for premature ejaculation and an enlarged prostate in men, and endometriosis, pelvic pain, and hormonal dysfunction in women. Neural therapy cleans up this area through the painless injection of the Frankenhauser's ganglion (just above the pubic bone) with a local anaesthetic. This opens up most of the ionic channels in the cell wall. The cell is then able to excrete much of its toxic components. This spurs the body to dump large amounts of mercury into the urine.

A unisex society!

I was recently interviewed by a journalist here in Cyprus and towards the end of the interview she casually commented that there was a shortage of 'real men' as they all seem to be feminized! I have heard similar comments on a number of occasions and it is true that men have lost a lot of their masculinity and women their femininity. Can chemicals be playing a role in the development of a unisex society?

The simple answer is 'yes' and science seems to support this. Dioxins and PCBs have been found to be tampering with the male and female behaviour patterns of children. Such effects might be due to the ability of

PCBs and dioxins to disrupt the sex hormones, as both these chemicals are known to have sex hormone-disrupting properties.[104]

The sex hormones not only influence reproduction, but also non-reproductive behaviour that manifests sex differences.[105] In Europe, researchers studying Dutch children exposed to background levels of pollution found that the effects of prenatal exposure to PCBs were different for boys and girls. In boys, higher prenatal PCB levels were related to less masculine play, whereas in girls, higher exposure was linked with more masculinized play. On the other hand, higher prenatal dioxin exposure was associated with more feminized play in boys as well as girls. While this work is controversial, these effects are alarming and warrant more research to verify and understand the full implications.

Phthalates and bisphenol A are also known to have oestrogen (female sex hormone) mimicking properties, and as such are hormone-disrupting chemicals. In addition to effects on the uterus in animals, they are reported to cause reduced nursing behaviour; more masculine play behaviour in females and increased aggression in males. They are also known to eliminate the sex differences in open-field behaviour.

Obesity and toxicity

There is now mounting evidence showing that obesity, which is reaching pandemic proportions, has a direct relationship to toxicity. This role has received additional support from a recent review[106] which presents a provocative hypothesis to explain the global obesity epidemic: chemical toxins. This article presents data showing that the current epidemic in obesity cannot be explained solely by alterations in food intake and/or decrease in exercise. There is a genetic predisposition component of obesity; however genetics could not have changed much over the past few decades. This suggests that environmental changes might be responsible for at least part of the current obesity epidemic.

---

104 Damstra T, Barlow S, Bergman A, Kavlock R, Van Der Kraak G, eds. Global assessment of the state-of-the-science of endocrine disruptors. International Programme on Chemical Safety, 2002. http://ehp.niehs.nih.gov/who
105 Mylchreest E, Sar M, Cattley R, Foster PMD. Disruption of androgen-regulated male reproductive development by di(n-butyl) phthalate during late gestation in rats is different from flutamide. *Toxicol Appl Pharmacol* 156: 81-95, 1999.
106 Baillie-Hamilton, PF. Chemical Toxins: A hypothesis to explain the global obesity epidemic. *J. Alt. and Comp Med.* 8, 185–192, 2002.

Indeed, the level of chemicals in the environment is purported to coincide with the incidence of obesity, and examples of chemicals that appear to cause weight gain by interfering with elements of the human weight control system - such as alterations in weight-controlling hormones, altered sensitivity to neurotransmitters, or altered activity of the sympathetic nervous system - are noted.

Indeed, many synthetic chemicals are actually used to increase weight in animals. This article/chapter provides fascinating examples of chemicals that have been tested for toxicity by standard tests, which resulted in weight gain in the animals at lower doses than those that caused any obvious toxicity. These chemicals included heavy metals, solvents, polychlorinated biphenols, organophosphates, phthalates and bisphenol A. This is an aspect of the data which has generally been overlooked.

Diagnosis of heavy metal toxicity

The diagnosis of heavy metal toxicity must take into account the exposure history, clinical signs and symptoms and laboratory tests. While the US Centers for Disease Control has steadily dropped the 'allowable level' of lead in the blood over the last fifteen years, there remains a problem with using blood levels to evaluate toxicity in the first place. Blood levels may not accurately reflect the total body burden of toxic metals. High blood levels are usually only found in acute toxic metal exposure, or in people exposed to high levels of toxins over a long period of time. In chronic low level exposure however, the blood levels may actually be low, due to redistribution of the toxins throughout the body, while bone and other tissue levels remain high.

Hair tissue mineral analysis (HTMA)

Hair analysis is a method of determining toxin exposure which is popular with many clinicians. The amount of mercury in the hair is determined by first digesting the hair in acids and then using a spectrometer such as ICP-MS to measure accurately, to parts per billion, the levels of mercury.

What are we measuring from hair, and why? When the body has toxic metals circulating in the blood, the first thing that it tries to do is remove them from circulation. This is because the toxic metals are prone to do a lot of damage to different cells of the body through their vicious free radical activity. The first place that the body stores these metals is in the

266

inert tissues such as the hair and nails, which are situated outside the body and therefore would do the least harm. When these storage sites are full then the body will start distributing and storing the metals in other less inert tissues and organs such as fat, liver, kidneys, thyroid, brain and other organs.

The hair sample taken represents about a two month 'history' of what has been circulating in the blood – the typical sample of hair is about 1 inch long and this takes about two months to grow. Therefore, the levels of metals in the hair correlate quite well with the levels in the circulating blood – if there are no metals circulating in the blood during the last two months, then there is a good probability that none will appear in the hair either.

This is a far more clinically significant test that facilitates the practitioner's clinical decision-making as it is showing a timeline or history of progress, not simply a snapshot. There are also many advantages to using this over the urine pre-post provocation test using chemical provocation agents because:

It is a 'gentle' way to proceed as there is no aggressive mobilization and release of large quantities of metals – as with the chemical chelators[107] – which can greatly exacerbate symptoms of neurological problems such as MS, cancer, autism, cardiovascular diseases and others.

The history of progress can be mapped over time as the decline in toxic metals shown on the HTMA is an indication that the storage sites in the body are also diminishing. If the levels are still high on the HTMA, then this is an indication that the storage sites are still loaded and that HMD® chelation should be continued for longer. HMD® is a natural, heavy metal chelator that we will talk about more below.

It is not the 'snap-shot' picture provided by urine tests, which are difficult to interpret over time (see below).

---

107 The word 'chelation' comes from the Greek word 'chelos' which stands for 'claw' – these are chemical or natural substances that attach to toxic metals and help in their removal from the body.

The HTMA is **far more cost effective** than the urine tests – costing the patient about $85 every two months.[108]

The HTMA is very quick, and easily implemented by an assistant in any clinical setting. It also negates the compliance problems often faced by practitioners when they ask the patient to collect urine over a 24-hour period.

Urine and faeces testing

Urine and faeces testing can also be used, but as we have already mentioned these are really only 'snapshots' of metabolic activity in the body at the time of collection, which usually runs over a 24-hour period. The differences between the baseline sample and the post-provocation sample when a provocation agent such as EDTA or DMSA is used are not really comparable as they are arbitrary figures. These tests are fine for research purposes but do not really help the practitioner to make clinical judgements for the best interest of the patient.

What can we do to protect ourselves?

The answer to this question is two-fold. Firstly we can push for legislation to ban a lot of the harmful chemicals which have been researched, and are known to be detrimental to animals and humans. Secondly, we need to be able to detoxify our bodies in order to eliminate many of these chemicals. Given that we are exposed to these literally daily, this process must be an ongoing one.

Treating heavy metal toxicity using conventional chelators

Many health practitioners use synthetic chelating agents such as DMPS, DMSA, EDTA and others to mobilise and eliminate heavy metals from the body. There are advantages

and disadvantages to using these. One advantage is the power of their mobilising activity – they are quick to mobilise and eliminate certain metals in the body, but this may place a huge burden on the body's detoxification systems. Further, symptoms have been reported by natural medical physicians throughout the US, such as intractable seizures in

---

108 www.detoxmetals.com/Hair-Testing.html

paediatric patients and multiple sclerosis in adult patients, due to taking high doses of DMSA, (also known as Succimer), over extended periods of time. [109,110,111]

The above are valid reasons to at least be cautious in the use of DMSA for the treatment of mercury-toxic paediatric patients. The fragile brains and nervous systems of children, and particularly those with autism, PDD and seizure disorders, should be handled with considerable care so as not to increase the damage. As of March 2009, as I write, the Federal Drug Administration (FDA) in the USA is considering removing DMSA from the market, but the motives for this move remain unclear.

DMSA and DMPS can certainly be life-saving drugs in cases of ACUTE metal poisoning. Toxicologists have noted that synthetic chelators should only be used in cases of ACUTE metal poisoning, or as a last resort for intractable chronic poisoning. Natural methods are preferable and should be exhausted first.

Natural heavy metal chelators – do they work?

It is not safe to use chemical chelators on an ongoing basis, but natural ones can be used instead, much like a supplement, on a daily basis. There are a number of purported natural heavy metal chelators on the market, but literally none of these have been investigated in depth using double blind, placebo controlled trials, except one. Do natural heavy metal chelators actually work?

The natural product called HMD®, [112,113,114] mentioned in chapter 4, has undergone a 'gold standard' double blind, placebo-controlled study using 350 people, at a cost of over one million US Dollars.

---

109 Smith, DR., et al, Succimer and the urinary excretion of essential elements in a primate model of childhood lead exposure, *Toxicological Sciences*, 54 [2] 473-80, Apr 2000.
110 Mann, KV. and Travers, JD., Succimer, an oral lead chelator, *Clinical Pharmacology*, 10 [12] 914-22, 1991.
111 Jorgensen, FM., Succimer: the first approved oral lead chelator, *American Family Physician*, 48 [8] 1495-1502, 1993.
112 Georgiou, G.J. The Discovery of a Unique Natural Heavy Metal Chelator. *Explore!* Volume 14, Number 4, 2005.
113 Georgiou, G.J. Natural Heavy Metal Chelators: Do They Work? *Explore!* Volume 16, Number 6, 2007.

It can be used safely over long periods of time with no side effects and is presently being tested to see its efficacy in eliminating some of the xenobiotics mentioned in this chapter.

HMD® is a Patent-Pending, proprietary synergistic blend of three natural ingredients:

1. Chlorella Growth Factor (CGF)
2. Organic Coriandrum sativum leaf tincture
3. Homaccord of cell-decimated, energized Chlorella

Research on HMD®

The research initially began as a health impact study to determine the levels of heavy metals in 374 metal foundry workers in Russia. These were randomly chosen from a workforce of 2,000 people and screened using Hair Tissue Mineral Analysis (HTMA) in a reputable US laboratory specializing in this type of analysis, using Inductively Coupled Plasma – Mass Spectrometers (ICP-MS) technology. There were four major heavy metals identified in this sample that were present at very high levels and were common to the entire workforce as they were by-products of the production process – these were lead, antimony, cadmium and arsenic.

The research design was a double blind, placebo-controlled study. Neither the participants, researchers, nor the analytical chemists doing the spectrometry analysis knew which treatment protocol each participant belonged to. The coding was stored in the co-ordinator's safe until it was time to interpret the statistical data. All participants signed an Informed Consent Form after discussion of the research protocols. There was a medical team on 24-hour standby to deal with any potential side-effects.

Each participant had to acquire a baseline sample of urine (24-hour collection) and faeces before taking HMD®. Both urine and faeces samples were taken in order to determine the excretory route used by the various substances tested. These samples were returned to the research team and circumspectly recorded in preparation for spectrometry, using the foundry's in-house instrument. Further ICP-MS analyses were conducted using two independent laboratories in Russia and the USA.

---

114 Georgiou, G.J. A Natural Heavy Metal Chelator Is Born: It's Use With Paediatric Cases. *British Naturopathic Journal* Volume 24, Number 1, 2007.

Table 1 below shows the summarized results of a number of different trials over a 3-year period. In order to make sense of the data, there was a group of people who were in the placebo group – these people took an initial urine and faeces sample, then they began taking a weak solution of chlorella (the same dosage as used for the experimental group mentioned below). The chlorella solution had been shown in previous trials not to mobilize metals in any way.

After a 24-hours period another urine sample was taken, and after 48-hours another faeces sample was taken. The difference between the baseline sample and the final sample is expressed in Table 1 below as the mean percentage increase of toxic metals after provocation – this is given for both the placebo group that took the inert chlorella as well as the experimental group that took the HMD®. 'U' denotes the Urine samples and 'F' the Faeces samples. The Mercury results are from a recent independent trial which is discussed in more detail below.

The experimental group followed exactly the same protocol as the chlorella group, as mentioned above, but they took the HMD® - 40 drops in the morning, 50 drops at lunch and 60 drops in the evening; all taken in a little water before food for both groups. Further research showed that similar results were achieved when taking 50 drops x 3 daily which is the present dosage recommended.

The mean percentage increase of heavy metals after provocation with HMD® is compared with the elimination while using a placebo (a mild chlorella tincture).

METALS	Mean % increase after provocation (Experimental group)	Mean % increase after provocation (Placebo group)	Number in sample	t-test results	Degrees of Freedom	Significance (p =)
ARSENIC-U	7,409.00	11.16	84	-	-	p<0.0005
ARSENIC-F	59.83	61.13	84	-	-	p<0.05
LEAD-U	466.47	-16.95	84	-	-	p<0.005
LEAD-F	142.16	-6.012	84	-	-	p<0.05
CADMIUM-U	67	-27.91	84	-	-	p<0.05
CADMIUM-F	43.13	22.62	84	-	-	p<0.05
ANTIMONY-U	59.16	14.91	84	-	-	p<0.05
ANTIMONY-F	50	6.61	84	-	-	p<0.05
NICKEL-U	80	5.52	77	t = 1.425	76	p<0.158
BISMUTH-U	564	7.95	19	t = 2.109	18	p<0.04
URANIUM-U	707	18.23	76	t = 1.015	75	p<0.03
MERCURY-U *	448	0.799	56	t = 5.395	55	p<0.0005

Table 1: HMD® data over a number of trials conducted over a 3-year period

* Mercury trial was conducted separately and the results of this are discussed below.

There were no serious side effects during the trials. Two people complained of a minor, transitory headache. Kidney, heart, liver and electrolyte blood tests showed that there were no pathological parameters in the post urine and faeces samples in all people tested, suggesting that HMD® is a 'gentle' chelator that does not place undue stress on the kidneys and liver.

Moreover, Heart Rate Variability Testing (HRV), a measure of the functioning of all the physiological systems of the body, showed a significant increase in 40% of the people tested in only 48 hours after provocation with the HMD®. It is predicted that HRV scores would be greatly improved if the HMD® were taken for much longer periods of time.

Independent Mercury trial using HMD®

Over the last year a voluntary group of clinical patients from the DaVinci Natural Health Centre in Cyprus, were used to test the efficacy of HMD® on mercury. All urine analyses were conducted on a mercury-dedicated PSA Atomic Fluorescence Spectrometer, measuring at levels of parts per billion. This involved a total of 56 patients who participated in a 24-hour provocation trial using HMD® at dosages of 40, then 50 and 60 drops throughout the day. Initial 6-hour baseline pre-urine samples were collected, along with a 24-hour collection for the post-urine sample.

There appears to be a 448% increase in eliminated mercury in the post-test after 24 hour provocation with HMD® in the 56 people tested, as compared with the pre-test baseline sample. Moreover, there was a negligible increase in mercury in the control group that was given only powdered chlorella in a little alcohol as a placebo. There was a statistically significant difference between the percentage increase of mercury in the post-sample as compared with the controls (t = 5.395, df = 55, p<.0005).

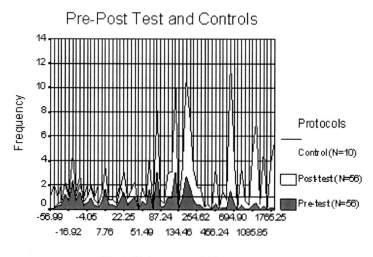

Percentage Increase of Mercury in Pre-Post Test and Controls

Liver and kidney serum test results during the HMD® pre-post provocation trials

During the HMD® research trials, blood samples were taken from a small group of people (N=16) to determine the effects of the HMD® provocation on liver and kidney function tests. The average percentage increase was calculated from the pre-and post sample figures of these biochemical tests.

Table 2 below shows the percentage increase of these biochemical parameters in the post-serum samples (during the taking of HMD®, as compared with the baseline serum sample before HMD® was taken. Overall, there are small average increases in creatinine, bilirubin, urea, ALT and AST, but nothing that surpassed pathological parameters. The minimum and maximum levels are also shown, but generally the higher levels were present in one individual only.

LEVELS OF LIVER & KIDNEY FUNCTION TESTS DURING HMD® PROVOCATION					
	CREATININE	BILIRUBIN	UREA	ALT	AST
% INCREASE	11.95	3.15	25.35	16.74	5.25
MINIMUM	0	0	0	0	0
MAXIMUM	42.80	20.19	53.73	75.00	38.46
N=	16	16	16	16	16

Table 2: Details of the liver and kidney function tests

It can be concluded from these tests that HMD® is a gentle chelator that does not adversely affect liver and kidney function tests and is tolerated by most people of all ages. However, based on clinical use of HMD® over the last 5 years, it would be advisable for the practitioner to use a universal drainage remedy that can work concomitantly on all detoxification systems including the liver, kidney, skin, lymph and blood – I have formulated such a natural herbal drainage remedy called Organic Lavage.[115]

---

115 See www.detoxmetals.com for more details

Natural heavy metal chelation protocol

I have been working on a natural, heavy metal chelating protocol based on scientific and clinical evidence for over five years now. This is what I suggest can be used for most cases of heavy metal toxicity – I have called it the HMD ULTIMATE DETOX PROTOCOL and it consists of the following:

HMD® – 50 drops x 3 daily for adults[116] – sensitive adults who have chronic diseases or compensated detoxification organs, as well as people with neurological diseases such as multiple sclerosis and the like, as well as autistic people should begin with half this dose, or less, and increase by one drop x 3 daily, every day until they reach a comfortable level.

ORGANIC LAVAGE – this is a herbal formula of wild-crafted and organic herbs such as Silybum marianum (Milk Thistle Seed), Taraxacum officinale (Dandelion Root), Arctium lappa (Burdock Root), Trifolium pratense (Red Clover Tops), Curcuma longa (Turmeric Root), Hydrangea arborescens (Hydrangea Root) and Arctostaphylos uva ursi (Bearberry Leaf). This herbal formula is designed to facilitate detoxification of the liver, kidneys, lymphatics and skin, as well as cleanse the blood and act as a natural anti-inflammatory. Adult dosage: 25 drops x 3 daily for adults, or more as directed by a practitioner.

ORGANIC CHLORELLA – there are many concerns about finding good quality, clean Chlorella that is void of heavy metals and xenobiotics. We have searched and travelled far and wide, and found an excellent source that is provided with a Certificates of Analysis with each pot. This chlorella comes from the western coast of Hai-Nan Island, China's southernmost island. Hai-Nan Island is a tropical island with an excellent climate and lies on the same latitude as Hawaii. The non-industrialized, pollution-free, tropical island offers favourable growth conditions for chlorella, including intense sunlight, pure water, and clean air. Available in 500mg tabs, adult dosage should be 2 tabs x 3 daily.

LIPOIC ACID – I believe that when metals and other xenobiotics are mobilized in the body, there should be some protection against free radical damage. Lipoic acid is that extraordinary antioxidant which is both water

---

116 See www.detoxmetals.com/dosages for full details

and fat soluble, able to penetrate the brain and other nervous tissues, and is therefore able to protect all parts of the body against free radical damage.

MINERALS – flushing the body with high levels of most of the minerals and trace elements will prevent the metals from re-entering the cell, as well as providing the raw materials for enzyme systems to reactivate, including detoxification systems. The easiest way is to take a colloidal multi-mineral formula in solution, otherwise a good-quality, high-potency, multi-mineral capsule will suffice.

I will often fine-tune this protocol depending on the needs of the patient, but generally this works well for most cases as a basic protocol.

Further Research

During the 5 years of experience with HMD® we have had many reports from women of all ages who have suffered from chronic endocrine problems, of coming back into balance while using HMD® for 2-3 months. Many of these women suffered from irregular periods, heavy bleeding, PMS and other hormonal imbalances.

Based on this anecdotal evidence we believe that HMD® is eliminating other chemicals (xenobiotics) such as Bisphenyl A and Phthalates which are known endocrine-disrupting chemicals, as described above. Preliminary trials have already been done which have shown that indeed this is the case – HMD® is eliminating the xenobiotics through the urine. However, the sample of people tested is small so further trials need to be conducted in this area before any scientific papers can be written.

The next chapter will deal with a topic that is related to heavy metal toxicity, 'The Dangers of Modern Dentistry.' I will not be discussing the dental amalgam issue in depth as this has already been covered in this chapter, but I will be touching on topics such as the safe removal of amalgams, as well as the problems with root canal fillings and dental foci.

Chapter 8

The dangers of modern dentistry

In the last chapter I discussed the dangers of mercury amalgam fillings, but this is only one of the dangers that people face when going to a dentist.

It is estimated that 70% of all medical illnesses are directly or indirectly caused by human intervention in the dental structures (teeth and jawbones). This includes: Impacted teeth, infected root canalled teeth, new and recurrent decay around old fillings, cysts, bone infections in areas of previously extracted teeth, granulomas and areas of bone condensation to osteitis represent some of the more common factors.

Dental mercury poisoning in focus

In Chapter 7 I have described in detail the effects of mercury on health in general, as well as discussing the health issues related to dental amalgam fillings. Here is a brief summary of some of the findings:

The World Health Organization has found the average individual can absorb as much as 120 micrograms of mercury per day from his or her amalgam fillings, a level which is considered a toxic dose.

Further research has shown a positive correlation between the concentration of mercury in mothers' breast milk and the number of dental amalgams in these women's mouths. The mean level of mercury in the milk of amalgam-free mothers was less than 0.2mcg/litre, while milk from mothers with one to four amalgam fillings contained 0.50 mcg/litre, with five to seven fillings at 0.57mcg/litre and more than seven fillings at 2.11 mcg/litre.

Dr Murray Vimy, clinical associate professor of the Department of Medicine, as well as several other medical researchers from the Departments of Radiology, Medicine and Medical Physiology at the University of Calgary in Canada, have spent more than a decade examining the effects of amalgam fillings on sheep, monkeys and humans. Their published evidence conclusively proves that mercury from amalgam fillings migrates to tissues in the oral cavity, the lungs and the gastrointestinal (GI) tract, causing a 'time-released poisoning'. Vimy's animal studies, which were met by ridicule within the dental community, have been vindicated by the work of Professor Vasken Aposhian, Head of the Molecular and Cellular Biology Department of the University of Arizona in Tucson. Aposhian and his team graded the amalgam filling content of human volunteers, from which they were given an amalgam score.

New evidence on human health shows that mercury fillings in pregnant women may also affect the growing foetus. In 1989, the University of Calgary Medical School published evidence that showed that within three days of placing amalgam fillings in pregnant sheep, mercury showed up in the blood, pituitary glands, liver and kidneys of their lambs. By 33 days (around the time of birth), most foetal tissue had higher levels of mercury than that of the parent animals. During nursing, the mother sheep were found to have eight times more mercury in their milk as in their blood.

More recently, Professor Gustav Drasch, a forensic toxicologist and his colleagues at the Institut fur Rechtsmedicine in Munich, examined the brain, liver, and kidneys of dead human babies and foetuses that had been aborted for medical reasons. They found these levels the mercury levels correlated significantly with the number of amalgam fillings in their mothers. Meanwhile, children were found to have accumulated mercury in their kidneys apparently from the mothers' amalgams, to a similar extent that adults do from their own fillings. As most of the children weren't breastfed, or only for a short period, the researchers concluded that mercury must have passed through the placenta.

Current research suggests that mercury vapour from fillings may be a predominant underlying cause of a broad spectrum of conditions, ranging from gum disease, migraine, headaches, poor memory, depression, anxiety, mental lethargy, chronic fatigue, allergies such as eczema and asthma, sensitivity reactions to food and inhalants, rheumatism, arthritis, backache, kidney disease, Alzheimer's disease, Parkinson's disease, multiple sclerosis and other neurological disorders.

In light of the evidence for such wide-ranging mercury poisoning effects, many patients and dentists then began replacing amalgams with alternative materials, without realizing the risks involved in the amalgam removal process. The removal of toxic materials calls for specially-prepared, expert handling and many dentists are simply not trained or equipped for the job.

Dental amalgam fillings slowly leak mercury, tin, silver, copper and sometimes nickel. All of these metals have various degrees of toxicity. A fairly large mercury filling contains enough mercury to kill a child if given as a single dose!

Mercury and tin are prime neuro-toxic substances. Mercury has the ability to destroy and or damage the transport fibres inside each nerve. The latest research from one of the top German toxicologists, Max Daunderer, MD, reveals that the entire jawbone (upper and lower) has become a toxic waste dump for the following substances:

❖ Pesticides
❖ Solvents (mostly present in lower jaw)
❖ Formaldehyde (mostly lower jaw)
❖ Amalgam (mercury, tin, copper and silver) – jawbone and maxillary sinus
❖ Palladium (from gold/palladium alloys) – mostly upper jawbone

Through biopsies, Daunderer found that virtually all inhaled toxins are stored in the jawbone in the areas adjacent to the root tips. Also of great interest is Daunderer's serial biopsies on malignant tumours in patients that had amalgam fillings and found, predictably, mercury in the tumour. The concentration is highest in the centre of the tumour (malignant melanoma, brain cancer, bladder, stomach, colon and tongue cancer).

The most common symptoms caused by amalgam fillings are:

❖ Chronic fatigue
❖ Tendency to chronic inflammatory changes – rheumatoid arthritis, phlebitis fibromyalgia, irritable bowel syndrome
❖ Chronic neurologic illnesses, especially when numbness is one of the primary symptoms
❖ Lowering of pain threshold.

Removing amalgams can seriously damage your health! TAKE PRECAUTIONS BEFORE REMOVAL!

I have already mentioned in the previous chapter the dreadful health consequences that I had as a result of mercury amalgam removal, without taking safety precautions and being on a proper chelation protocol. Therefore, I must issue a strong warning here for all those who are

279

thinking of removing their amalgams without the proper preparation – DO NOT DO IT! Do not go to any dentist and begin to remove amalgam fillings without understanding the safety precautions that you need to take. I will outline some of these below so there will be no excuse for ignorance.

Removing amalgams safely

A dental mercury detoxification protocol is a demanding task. If you intend to remove any metal fillings from your mouth, the following steps can help prevent plenty of grief and suffering. There are a few safety issues that you should have in mind:

1. The mercury in the filling is in the elemental form. It easily penetrates the rubber dam[1] and all mucous membranes (the oral cavity, GI tract and lungs).
2. Mercury is highly volatile when heated. The dental drill operating at 100,000 rpms will generate much mercury vapour during the removal procedure.
3. It is estimated that 80% of the mercury vapour inhaled enters the body through the lungs and is distributed to various bodily tissues and organs, with the potential for causing severe illness.

Despite the fact that the very best precautions are taken to prevent mercury exposure during dental removal, some exposure still occurs. Therefore, the patient needs to take detoxification agents to chelate any mercury and prevent inadvertent absorption.

Patient protection protocol

Here are some guidelines for removing amalgams – most of these follow Dr. Huggins' protocol[2] but has been somewhat adapted based on my experience and research with mercury detoxification– he is one of the leading research dentists in this field of Holistic Dentistry and has written much based on his empirical knowledge.

---

1 A rubber dam is used in the mouth to cover the back of throat so that less mercury vapour and debris from the amalgam removal is swallowed.
2 http://www.hugginsappliedhealing.com

Always prepare your body as best as you can before, during and after amalgam removal. It is always prudent to observe the heavy metal detoxification protocols in Chapter 7 before removing any amalgams. It may take three to six months to prepare your body to withstand the potential mercury intoxication from the removal process. Otherwise, you risk ending up with more health problems than when you started. The good health of the human organism must be built up and maintained so it can withstand the risks of amalgam removal. Even if the removal is done at a modern dentistry office with a biological setup, accidents with hazardous materials can happen anywhere! I have seen too many patients who developed very serious chronic disease after mercury amalgam removal – heart disease, cancer, MS and other degenerative diseases.

While the detoxification protocols are crucial, there are other preparations to help optimize health, too, such as proper nutritional support. Chapter 6 regarding nutrition provides another line of defense to strengthen your body. The stronger your body is, the more capable it will be to handle an accidental mercury overdose.

It is imperative to be on a safe chelation protocol using HMD®, Organic Lavage, Chlorella[3] and a potent nutritional supplementation program before, during and after the amalgam removal. A rule of thumb is to use the chelation and the supplements protocols long BEFORE you start the amalgam removal – at least 3 months – to remove some of the toxic metal burden that you already have. You should also continue the chelation protocol throughout the removal procedures, and for at least six months to a year thereafter. Only after all symptoms have subsided and hair testing[4] has shown that you are low on toxins can you relax the protocol, but always be on guard regarding this issue. Observe and listen to your body. Tell your practitioner about your symptoms. He or she should correlate them with further testing to guide you.

Only once you are in good shape should you dare to have the mercury amalgams removed by a qualified, experienced, capable and fully-equipped biological dentist. While nearly any dentist is technically qualified to replace your amalgam fillings, less than 1 per cent of dentists have any clue on how to do it properly, so that your risk of mercury

---

3 See www.detoxmetals.com for more details of these protocols.
4 http://www.detoxmetals.com/THMA.html

poisoning is minimized. Do it right the first time and you will save yourself the grief and expense associated with severe mercury poisoning-derived diseases.

Do not extract more than one amalgam every month. This will buy you time to detoxify your body slowly. Better safe than sorry. If you are not in a desperate hurry, allow even longer spacing between amalgam removals.

It is best if the dentist measures the electrical potential of each amalgam filling in order to determine the sequential order in which the restorations should be carried out. The most negatively charged tooth is the one that is removed first, followed by the next negatively charged and so on. Never work on both sides of the head in any one sitting.

Do not take Vitamin C the day of dental procedures. Vitamin C by mouth will shorten the effect of the dental anaesthetic to literally around 10 minutes – after that it gets painful! The IV form of Vitamin C does not do this for reasons unknown, but even 500 milligrams in the tablet form will detoxify the anaesthetic adequately to let you feel the pain of drilling or surgery.

It is wise to get a practitioner like myself who can perform a VEGA or ART test, to determine whether the composite materials that will be used to fill the tooth after the amalgam is removed, is immune-compatible with you.

At the Davinci Natural Health Centre we take a sample of the patient's hair from the nape of the neck and this is sent to a lab in the USA for mineral and toxic metal testing. This Hair Tissue Mineral Analysis provides a baseline of metals and minerals present in the blood over the previous two months and can then be compared with another hair test a couple of months later.

Observe the Patient Protection Protocol as closely as is possible during removal procedures. Complete protection includes the use of the rubber dam during amalgam removal and the use of a face flannel soaked in charcoal or chlorella powder placed over the face of the patient, to absorb any stray mercury. Moreover, the mouth can also be painted with a slurry mix of chlorella powder and water – the rubber dam can also be coated with this chlorella slurry. A cotton roll can also be coated with chlorella and placed as a reservoir around the teeth to catch escaping mercury vapour. It is best for the holistic dentist to remove the filling in as large chunks as possible to minimize vapourization of mercury during drilling. A copious amount of water should be used to cool the drill and contain the amalgam dust, and reduce vapour formation. There should be a large high-power suction hose at the side of the patient's mouth leading to a special mercury filter outside the clinic premises.

It is best to use nasal oxygen during the whole procedure as this allows the patient's face to be covered with a flannel coated with chlorella or charcoal while they are still able to breathe in through the nose. The presence of a negative ion generator in the dental office will also facilitate the removal of mercury vapour. If your dentist does not have all these safety protocols in their office then you need to assess what you could do without. A dentist that takes none of these precautions will only worsen your health, so it is best to search for another dentist rather than risk your health further.

If surgery is done during the procedure, use ice packs immediately after the procedures are finished, as well as magnets if desired, to help the inflammation. Minimal travel after surgery is advisable (i.e. one or two miles) as the vibration in a car can release a blood clot, resulting in the famous painful 'dry socket.' Smoking after surgery will almost guarantee the formation of a painful dry socket. Be forewarned.

If your dentist is using vitamin B12 in an IV then tell them not to – Vitamin B12 in any form is a methylator, and methyl mercury is extremely damaging to your nervous system.

The International Academy of Oral Medicine and Toxicology (IAOMT)[5] posts correct and incorrect protocols for amalgam removal for dentists. Read every word and discuss the issues raised with your dentist, as well as your holistic medicine practitioner. I would not necessarily adopt all their guidelines, like the possibility of removing two amalgams in one visit, but their overall recommendations are a good starting point. Bear in mind that judgment and discretion in dealing with individual cases is crucial. The IAOMT website also contains images of how a biological dentist goes about removing amalgams.

---

5 See http://www.iaomt.org

What to expect following the safe removal of amalgams

There is no doubt that the safe removal of amalgams can greatly facilitate the healing of many health issues that are related to mercury toxicity. However, the key words are 'safe removal.' The following published scientific references have been compiled by Bernie Windham, a chemical engineer who has spent years researching the hazardous health effects of mercury amalgam poisoning:

For a period of one week following amalgam removal the levels of mercury increase approximately 30%. Within 2 weeks levels reduce significantly.[6,7] (Symptoms may initially increase before improving).

Removal of amalgam fillings results in significant reduction in body burden and mercury in body waste.[8,9]

Total reduction of mercury in blood and urine levels is often reduced by 80% within a few months following removal.[10]

In a German study of Multiple Sclerosis patients whose amalgam dental fillings were removed, 85% recovered from illnesses.[11,12]

In interviews of a large population of Swedish patients who had amalgams removed it was found that virtually all reported significant permanent health.[13]

---

6 Begerow, J et al, Long-term mercury excretion in urine after removal of amalgam fillings, *Int Arch Occup Health* 66:209-212, 1994.

7 Molin, M et al, Kinetics of mercury in blood and urine after amalgam removal, *J Dent Res* 74:420, IADR Abstract 159, 1995.

8 Katsunuma et al, Anaphylaxis improvement after removal of amalgam fillings, Annals of Allergy, 1990, 64(5):472-75 & Drouet, M et al, Is mercury a respiratory tract allergen?, *Allerg Immunol Paris*: 22(3):81, 1990.

9 Begerow, J et al, Long-term mercury excretion in urine after removal of amalgam fillings, *Int Arch Occup Health* 66:209-212, 1994.

10 Barregard, L et al, People with high mercury uptake from their own dental amalgam fillings, *Occup Envir Med* 52: 124-128, 1995.

11 Klinghardt, D. IAOMT Conference & tape, 1998; large study by M.Daunderer (Germany) of MS patients after amalgam removal. (over 200 cases)

12 Daunderer, M. Handbuch der Amalgamvergiftung, Ecomed Verlag, Landsberg, 1998.

A 17-year study of an even larger population had similar results [14,15] (i.e. 89% of those reporting allergies had significant improvement or total elimination. Extrapolated to the U.S. population, this would represent over 17 million people with allergies who would benefit).

Body mercury burden was found to play a role in resistant viral infections such as Chlamydia trachomatis and herpes. Many cases can be effectively treated by antibiotics only after removal of mercury. [16,17]

Thousands of documented cases are available supporting improved health and/or cure of serious chronic illnesses after removal of mercury amalgam fillings coupled with nutritional, antioxidant and detoxification treatment (see list and references below):

---

13 Langworth, S et al, Amalgamnews and Amalgamkadefonden, 1997. (www.tf.nu) & Berglund, F, Bjerner/Helm, Klock, Ripa, Lindforss, Mornstad, Ostlin, Improved Health after Removal of dental amalgam fillings, *Swedish Assoc. Of Dental Mercury Patients*, 1998. (www.tf.nu) (over 1000 cases)

14 Foundation For Toxic-Free Dentistry. Compilation of health consequences resulting from amalgam removal of 1569 patients, (compiled by type of health problem and consequences after removal for 31 major types of health problems), *Bio-Probe* Home Page, 1997.

15 Press Release, Swedish Council for Planning and Coordinating Research (FRN), Stockholm, 19 February, 1998.

16 Omura Y et al, Heart Disease Research Foundation, NY, Role of mercury in resistant infections and recovery after Hg detox with cilantro. *Acupuncture & Electro-Theraputics Research*, 20(3):195-229, 1995.

17 Eriksen, SE. et al, Effect of mercuric chloride on macrophage- mediated resistance mechanisms against infection, *Toxicology*, 93:269- 297, 1994.

Allergies,[18] ALS,[19] Alzheimer's,[20] anxiety & mental confusion,[21,22] arthritis,[23] asthma,[24] Chronic Fatigue Syndrome,[25,26,27] Crohn's disease,[28] depression,[29] dizziness, endometriosis,[30] epilepsy,[31] eczema,[32] gastro intestinal problems,[33] infertility,[34] leukemia,[35] (lupus, migraines, multiple

---

18 Ziff, MF. Documented clinical side effects to dental amalgams, ADV. Dent. Res. 1(6):131-134, 1992; & Ziff, S., Dentistry without Mercury, 8th Edition, 1996, Bio-Probe, Inc., & Dental Mercury Detox, Bio-Probe, Inc. http://www.bioprobe.com. (cases: FDA Patient Adverse Reaction Reports - 762, Dr. Hanson, M - Swedish patients - 519, Dr. Lichtenberg, H - 100 Danish patients, Dr. Larose, P - 80 Canadian patients, Dr. Siblerud, R - 86 Colorado patients, Dr. Zamm, AV - 22 patients) (& over 1000 additional cases of significant improvement reported to FDA).

19 Merritt's Textbook of Neurology, 9th Ed., Williams and Wilkins, Baltimore, p668, 1995; & Redhe, O et al, Recovery from ALS after removal of dental amalgam fillings, Int J Risk & Safety in Med 4:229-236, 1994; & Vanacore, N et al, Dirparimento di Scienze Neurologiche, Univer. La Sapienza, Roma, Med Lav (Italy), 86(6): 522-533, Nov 1995.

20 Tom Warren, Beating Alzheimer's, Avery Publishing Group, 1991.

21 Davis, M (ed), Defense Against Mystery Syndromes, Chek Printing Co., March, 1994 (case histories documented).

22 Malt, UF et al, Physical and mental problems attributed to dental amalgam fillings, Psychosomatic medicine, 59:32-41, 1997 (100 cases).

23 Tanchyk, AP. Amalgam Removal for Treatment of Arthritis, Gen Dent, v42,n4, p354, July 1994.

24 Seidler, A et al, Possible environmental factors for Parkinson's disease, Neurology 46(5):1275-1284, 1996; & Vroom, FO et al, Mercury vapour intoxication, 95: 305-318, 1972; Ohlson et all, Parkinsons Disease and Occupational Exposure to Mercury, Scand J. Of Work Environment Health, Vol 7, No.4: 252-256, 1981.

25 Huggins, H & Editors of Alternative Medicine Digest, Chronic Fatigue, Fibromyalgia & Environmental Illness, Future Medicine Publishing, Inc, p197, 1998.

26 Adolph Coors Foundation, Coors Amalgam Study: Effects of Placement and Removal of Amalgam fillings, 1995. Internations DAMS Newsletter, p17, Vol VII, Issue 2, Spring 1997, (31 cases).

27 Malt UF et al, Physical and mental problems attributed to dental amalgam fillings, Psychosomatic medicine, 59:32-41, 1997, (100 cases).

28 Davis, M (ed), Defense Against Mystery Syndromes, Chek Printing Co., March, 1994 (case histories documented).

29 Do amalgam fillings influence manic depression? Journal of Orthomol. Medicine, 1998, http://www.depression.com/news/news_981116.htm

30 Ziff S. and Ziff M. Infertility and Birth Defects: Is Mercury from Dental Fillings a Hidden Cause? Bio-Probe, Inc., 1987.

31 Klinghardt, D, Migraines, Seizures and Mercury Toxicity, Future Medicine Publishing, 1997.

32 Dr. Kohdera, Faculty of Dentistry, Osaka Univ, International Congress of Allergology and Clinical Immunology, EAACI, Stockholm, June 1994; & Heavy Metal Bulletin, Vol 1, Issue 2, Oct 1994, (160 cases cured).

33 Langworth, S et al, Amalgam news and Amalgamkadefonden, 1997. (www.tf.nu) & Berglund, F, Bjerner/Helm, Klock, Ripa, Lindforss, Mornstad, Ostlin), Improved Health

chemical sensitivities, multiple sclerosis,[36] neuropathy/paresthesia, Parkinson's), oral keratosis,[37] rages and anger,[38] schizophrenia,[39] tachycardia and heart conditions.[40]

Let us now move on and examine another danger of dentistry that is overlooked by many practitioners, dentists and their patients, but which can be a potential 'time-bomb' too.

Root canals and dental foci

In recent years there has been a reawakening of the dangers of oral infections and their potential disastrous effects on systemic health. Dead and infected teeth are often treated 'conservatively' in modern dentistry by performing a treatment called Root Canal Therapy. The aim is to 'save' a tooth which has become infected or dead, in an attempt to make it functional and pain free.

---

after Removal of dental amalgam fillings, Swedish Assoc. Of Dental Mercury Patients, 1998, (www.tf.nu) (over 1000 cases).

34 Dr. Gerhard, I and Dr. Roller, E et al, Tubingen Univ. Gynecological Clinic, Heidelberg, 1996; & Gerhard, I et al, Heavy Metals and Fertility, *J of Toxicology and Environmental Health*, Part A, 54:593-611, 1998.

35 Ziff S. and Ziff M. Infertility and Birth Defects: Is Mercury from Dental Fillings a Hidden Cause? Bio-Probe, Inc, 1987.

36 Davis, M. (ed), Defense Against Mystery Syndromes', Chek Printing Co., March, 1994 (case histories documented).

37 Skoglund, A. *Scand J Dent Res* 102(4): 216-222, 1994; and 99(4):320-9,1991; Ostman, PO et al, Clinical and histologic changes after removal of amalgam, *Oral Surgery, Oral Medicine, & Endodontics*, 81(4):459-465, 1996, (77 cases).

38 Malt, UF et al, Physical and mental problems attributed to dental amalgam fillings, *Psychosomatic medicine*, 59:32-41, 1997, (100 cases).

39 Huggins, H. It's All in Your Head: Diseases Caused by silver-mercury fillings, USA: Life Sciences Press, 1990; & Observations From The Metabolic Fringe, ICBM conf. Collarado,1988; & Center for Progressive Medicine, 1999, http://www.hugnet.com (Over 1000 cases).

40 Ziff, MF et al, A Persuasive New Look at Heart Disease As It Relates to Mercury, Bio-Probe, Inc., & J. of American College of Cardiology V33,#6, pp1578-1583, 1999.

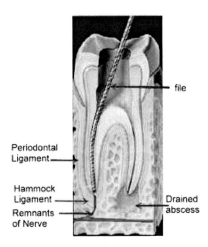

Cleaning a root-canal with a round burr

So how is a root canal performed? First, the nerve in the large pulp chamber at the top of the tooth is cleaned out using a round bur on a slow speed drill. Then the canals are cleaned with a series of tiny files which look like flexible pins with serrations along their lengths (see image above). The dentist will begin with a very thin burr followed by progressively thicker files until the entire mass of the nerve is removed and the sides of the root canals are made smooth and clean.

As the filing progresses, the tooth is washed or irrigated with a dilute solution of laundry bleach (Clorox) or a 2% solution of chlorhexidine in order to wash out the debris, and to sterilize and chemically neutralize any dead tissue that may be missed by the files.

When the root canal is completely clean, it is dried out with tiny paper points, and each canal is fitted with the appropriate diameter rubber cone that will entirely fill and block that canal. Each file is numbered to denote its diameter, and there is a corresponding rubber cone size to be used in canals finished to that size file. The rubber is a special form called gutta percha. It is less refined than regular rubber and is somewhat gummy, sticking to the walls of the canal and thoroughly waterproofing them.

After scraping out the inside of the tooth the dentist will attempt to disinfect the tooth and the canals to eliminate any source of infection. The canal is then filled with a combination of cement and Gutta Percha in an attempt to completely occlude these canals. This is supposedly to prevent any microorganisms from entering the tooth either through the crown or the root.

If you consider pain control, mechanical function and aesthetics to be the limit of good dental treatment, then you will have 'SAVED' the tooth.

If systemic effects are included in your concept of dentistry, than you must understand that all that has happened, is that you have kept dead, infected tissue, buried in the bone, within a couple of inches from your brain.

For some obscure reason we are all conditioned to think that teeth are not a part of the body, but that they are inert calcified material; and that they are sort of dead anyway. Dentistry is the only one of all the medical & para-medical professions that thinks it is a good idea to keep dead, gangrenous tissue in the body. The way to do this is to perform a root canal treatment.

One eminent Endodontist says:[41]

'It is wrong to speak of "Root Canal Therapy" - it as a dead tooth; it is more correct to describe such a tooth as non-vital or, better, pulpless. Even though the central blood supply to the tooth has been lost, the tooth itself still retains its connection to the body via the periodontal membrane and the cementum.'

This is like saying that even though the blood supply to your leg may be completely cut off, it would be wrong to suggest that the leg is dead, because it is still connected to your body by your hip joint! The Oxford dictionary defines 'non-vital' as 'Fatal to Life.' It defines 'dead' as 'No longer alive.'

The bacteria, yeasts and other organisms which enter the tooth do not die when the oxygen supply is reduced (as happens inside the root canal system). They undergo what is called a pleomorphic change and become 'anaerobic' bacteria. They literally change form and become bacteria that do not need oxygen to live. With the establishment of infection, the microbial flora changes from an initially predominant facultative gram

---

[41] Meinig, GE. Root Canal Coverup. *Price-Pottenger Nutrition Foundation Journal*, vol. 18, No. 3, pp.6, Nov. 1994.

positive flora to a completely anaerobic gram negative bacteria when the canals have been infected for 3 months or more.[42]

> **'80% of patients' health problems can be partially traced to the mouth.'**
>
> - Dietrich Klinghardt MD, Ph.D. (www.neuraltherapy.com)

It is now known that dead teeth are usually heavily infected with gram negative anaerobic bacteria. Sundqvist[43] isolated 88 species of bacteria out of 32 root canals with periapical[44] disease.' Only 5 of those bacteria could grow in air.

Other organisms such as yeasts, fungi and 'cell-wall-deficient forms' (Lida Mattman[45]) also inhabit this tissue. The dead teeth thus become a focus of infection which can cause numerous disease states throughout the body. Anaerobic bacteria produce incredibly potent neurologic and haemolytic toxins. A true 'toxin factory.'

Boyd Haley, Ph.D., a researcher at the University of Kentucky has estimated that 75% of root canalled teeth are infected. Another researcher, Hal Huggins, DDS,[46] has shown that the toxins liberated by infected root canalled teeth are almost 1000 times more toxic than botulism. Botulism is the most toxic substance known.

Austrian researchers have exhaustively studied the finer details of the entire dental structure. They have established that there is a lively metabolic interchange between the interior and exterior milieu of the tooth, and that this two-way process takes place along many thousands of

---

42 Fabricius L, Dahlen G, Ohman AE, Moller AJR. Predominant indigenous oral bacteria isolated from infected root canals after varied times of closure. *Scand J Dent Res* 90: 134–144, 1982.
43 Sundqvist G. Taxonomy, ecology, and pathogenicity of the root canal flora. *Oral Surg Oral Med Oral Pathol* 78(4):522–530, Oct 1994.
44 The tissues around the apex of a tooth root, including the periodontal membrane and the alveolar bone.
45 Mattman, LH. Cell Wall Deficient Forms: Stealth Pathogens. 3rd edition, USA: BioMed Publishing Group, 1997.
46 Huggins, HA and Levy, TE. Uninformed Consent: The hidden dangers in dental care. USA: Hampton Roads Publishing Co., 1999.

hyperfine capillary canals, joining the pulp cavity to the exterior surface of the tooth.

Very careful conservative measures may possibly seal off the vertical central dentinal canal, but they will never reach the lateral 'twigs' branching off from this tube. Nor can they ever close off the innumerable capillary canals. Some protein will always remain in these secondary spaces. If this protein becomes infected, toxic catabolic products, such as thio-ethers, thio-ethanols and mercaptans[47] will be produced, and conveyed into the organism.

In 1960, it was established by W. Meyer (Goettingen) that within devitalized teeth the dentinal canals and dental capillaries contain large microbial colonies. The toxins produced by these microbes in a tooth with a root filling can no longer be evacuated into the mouth, but must be drained away through the cross-connections and unsealed branches of the dentinal and capillary canals into the marrow of the jawbone. From there, they are conveyed to the tonsils, and thus the flow systems of the body. In fact, the conservative treatment may literally convert a tooth into a toxin producing 'factory' as described above.

Bartelstone (USA) and Djerassi (Bulgaria) have reported that endodental exchange may also take place in the opposite direction. If radio-iodine, I-131, is deposited in an evacuated pulp cavity which is then sealed off with a filling, the iodine will appear in the thyroid some twenty hours later, as can be demonstrated by taking a scintograph of the thyroid region. Similarly, dyes can be washed out of a sealed pulp cavity. Any substance produced by any of the structures in the oral cavity, teeth, gums or tonsils, will be drained by the lymphatic system and carried directly to the thyroid gland.

The close interlacing of the lymphatic and endocrine systems in the head, make it unavoidable that brain cells are more intensively toxic by the circulating focogenous agents and may suffer particularly heavy damage. The lymph ducts of the head region join Waldeyer's tonsillar ring[48], and if there is such congestion, waste fluids will be pressed through the porous base of the skull into the lymphatic spaces of the brain. Toxogenous

---

47 See below for a full description of thio-ethers and mercaptans, and their role in triggering cancer
48 A ring of lymphatic tissue in the nasopharynx joining the tonsils and adenoids

changes, especially within autonomic nuclei, are regularly found in cancer patients, as verified in the 1930's by Muehlmann (USSR); and they may be a consequence of a life-long inhibition of cerebral aerobiosis due to focogenous intoxication.

All these findings prove conclusively that within solid dental structures, there may proceed an unimpeded substantial interchange in either direction through the dental tubules (see image below). Dentinal tubules are microscopic channels which radiate outward through the dentin from the pulp to the exterior cementum or enamel border.[49] These tubules contain fluid and cellular structures. Consequently, odontogenic toxins, wherever they may have been produced, are able to diffuse and circulate within these tubules into the body tissues.

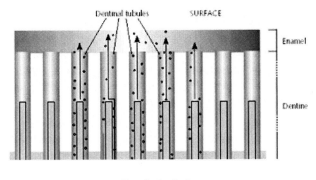

Dentinal tubules

The German study group of Eger-Miehlke has investigated the pathogenic significance of these 'endotoxins,' They examined the changes in healthy experimental animals following the injection of accurately defined, minimal quantities of the endotoxins from an odontogenous granuloma.

A single injection of a minimal dose seemed to develop a defence-activation effect. But after repeated injections, there was severe liver damage, and the animals died within weeks. Apart from the fatal liver damage, inflammatory and degenerative changes were found in all other organs, especially in the joints, muscles and blood vessels. These results brought clear experimental proof for the first time that focogenic toxins act

---

49 Ross, MH., Kaye, GI and Wojciech, P, Histology: a text and atlas. 4th edition, pp 450, 2003.

as causal agents for severe diseases in animals, corresponding to similar chronic conditions in man.

The most dangerous of all odontogenous toxins are undoubtedly the thio-ethers, (which I mention above), for instance dimethylsulfide. Other severe toxins from root-canal bacteria include thio-ethanols and mercaptans, which have been found in the tumours of women who have breast cancer. These toxins drain through the lymphatic system down the cervical chain of lymph nodes and ultimately in to the breast tissue.

In a series of tests performed at Dr. Issel's[50] clinic it was observed that patients with odontogenous and tonsillar foci had a heightened level of dimethylsulfide in their blood. After intensive treatment of the foci, this level returned to normal in just a few days.

Thio-ethers are closely related, both in their structure and their effect, to mustard gas and other poison gases used in the First World War. To give you an idea of its poisonous effects the following is a list of the major symptoms:

- ❖ Blistering of the skin
- ❖ Eye soreness
- ❖ Vomiting
- ❖ Internal and external bleeding
- ❖ Bronchial tube damage with stripping of the mucous membrane
- ❖ Throat feels like it is closing with sensations of choking.

Thio-ethers are 'partial' antigens: haptens,[51] and thus they also tend to combine with the normal proteins in the body, 'denaturizing' them. Such denatured proteins become 'non-self' or foreign agents, which the body must deal with. The production of antibodies adapted to the situation will be provoked, and they will home in on the target antigens wherever they are. The process of 'auto-aggression' will be set in motion: self-destruction of agents alien to the organism. Extensive structural cellular damage will result and help create the environment for cancer.

---

50 http://www.issels.com
51 A substance capable of reacting with a specific antibody but cannot induce the formation of antibodies unless bound to a carrier protein or other molecule.

Druckrey Heidelberg[52] found, among other things, that transformation of a normal cell into a malignant cell requires a certain quantity of a carcinogen – the carcinogenic minimum dose. It does not matter whether this quantity is supplied in a single dose or in a number of smaller doses, because the toxic effects of each dose are stored, and accumulate without loss.

The carcinogens held primarily responsible for the development of spontaneous cancer in man are those which inhibit the aerobiosis even in minimal quantities without at the same time immediately destroying the cell; and which are constantly present in the organism in this minimal concentration of either endogenous or exogenous origin. They can therefore accumulate during the normal life expectancy.

With recent advances in molecular biological methods, the endodontic microflora is being continually reclassified. Molecular biological methods like PCR (Polymerase Chain Reaction) have enabled amplification of small amounts of nucleic acids and allowed for identification of bacteria that would be detectable by culturing techniques. A recent such study using PCR techniques revealed a number of bacterial species.[53]

The predominantly isolated bacteria in the root canal, namely Fusobacterium nucleatum, comprises three subspecies – nucleatum, polymorphum and vincentii. The majority of the Streptococcus species include S. anginosus and S. mitis. Peptostreptococcus micros and P. anaerobius comprised of 1/3 of the samples in the study by Sundqvist, while 34 % of the root canals comprised of black-pigmented anaerobic rods, mainly Prevotella intermedia; and 6 % constituted P.loescheii and P. denticola. Porphyromonas endodontalis was more predominant than P. gingivalis among the black-pigmented asaccharolytic species. Eubacterium alactolyticum and E. lentum were isolated in a third of the root canals.

Actinomyces species comprised 15 % of the microflora and the dominant species was A. israelii (11%). Actinomyces israelii has been found to be commonly associated with root canal failures. Gram negative asaccaharolytic rods were identified as Fusobacterium and Bacteroides

---

52 To Hermann Druckrey on the occasion of his 80th birthday. *Journal of Cancer Research and Clinical Oncology*. Volume 108, Number 1, July 1984.
53 George, M., Ivančaková, R. Root Canal Microflora, Acta Medica, (Hradec Králové) 50(1):7–15, 2007.

when butyric acid and acetic acid, or succinic acid, respectively, was formed during fermentation.

Table 1 below summarizes the types of bacteria found in root canals of teeth.

GRAM POSITIVE COCCI	GRAM NEGATIVE COCCI
Streptococcus anginosus	Capnocytophaga ochracea
S. gordonii	C. sputigena
S. oralis	C. curvus
S. mitis	
S. sanguinis	Veillonella parvula
Enterococcus faecalis	Campylobacter rectus
Peptostreptococcus micros	
Peptostreptococcus anaerobius	
GRAM POSITIVE RODS	**GRAM NEGATIVE RODS**
Actinomyces israelii	Fusobacterium nucleatum
A. naeslundii	Prevotella intermedia
Eubacterium alactolyticum	Prevotella melaninogenica
Eubacterium lentum	Prevotella denticola
Eubacterium timidum	Prevotella buccae
Eubacterium brachy	Prevotella oralis
Eubacterium nodatum	Prevotella loescheii
Propionibact. propionicum	Porphyromonas gingivalis
P. granulosum	Bacteroides gracilis
Porphyromonas endodontalis	
Lactobacillus	

Table 1 – Bacteria Isolated from Root Canal of Teeth

Adapted from Sundqvist, 1992 a, b, 1994; Le Goff et al, 1997, R. M. Love, H. F. Jenkinson, 2002

What can be done?

So, what happens when we have a dead tooth in our mouths? Unfortunately there are no good alternatives for this situation. The only treatment for dead tissue in the body is to remove it. It is impossible to sterilize the canals. The medicaments and antibiotics used do not penetrate the dentine tubules. Dr. Weston Price,[54,55] a famous dental researcher who wrote prolifically (two-volume work totalling 1,174 pages), was even able to culture bacteria from teeth which had fuming formaldehyde poured over them. Even the recent dental literature reflects this:

'It is now known that complete sterilization of an infected root canal is very difficult to achieve and complete removal of all pulp tissue remnants frequently is not possible.'[56]

Therefore the treatment of choice is to extract a dead tooth rather than root-fill it. It is also important to remove any infected tissue from around the tooth. This usually requires a very easy surgical approach to access the end of the socket. Although this does not sound attractive, the results generally are, and the actual surgery is usually very easy.

Dentists are usually taught to extract teeth with forceps, and that any infected tissue left in the bony socket will be dealt with by the cells of the immune system. This does sometimes happen. Often, though, the bone will heal around the infected tissue, which remains indefinitely as an infected hole in the bone. These areas are usually colonized by gram negative bacteria. They are called areas of osteitis or NICO Lesions (Neuralgia Inducing Cavitational Osteonecrosis). NICO lesions can act as foci of infection and also neural foci, just as the root treated teeth can. This is the main reason that a surgical approach is used for most extractions.

Dr. Bouquot[57] in 1992 reported 1,995 cases of neuralgia osteonecrosis (dead bone neuralgia) and relates these with facial neuralgia or trigeminal neuralgia. In 70% of these cases the facial neuralgia disappeared completely after the necrotic bone was surgically removed. NICO's are very difficult to spot on X-rays or MRI scans – one of the best ways of detecting a NICO is with Autonomic Response Testing (ART). IF you

---

54 Price, WA. Dental Infections: Oral and Systemic, being a contribution to the pathology of dental infections, focal infections and the degenerative diseases (Volume 1). USA: The Penton Publishing Company, 1923.
55 Price, WA. Dental Infections and the Degenerative Diseases: Being a contribution to the pathology of functional and degenerative organ and tissue lesions (Volume 2). USA: The Penton Publishing Company, 1923.
56 Phillip Delivanis Oral Surgery Vol 52 No 4, 1981.
57 Bouquot, JE. Brief review of NICO (Neuralgia-Inducing Cavitational Osteonecrosis). *Journal of Oral Surgery, Oral Medicine and Oral Pathology*, March 1992.

touch the fingertip on the gum opposite the root of the extracted tooth while muscle testing, if there is a NICO the muscle will become weak.

Neural therapy using procaine can help to unblock the NICO and the muscle will test strong. The messages of the autonomic nervous system, travelling over the acupuncture meridians from that tooth area to the disabled or painful site have been blocked and neural therapy help to repolarise the cell membranes and release the blockage.[58]

Dr Dietrich Klinghardt, in a study entitled, 'The Tonsils and Their Role in Health and Chronic Illness,'[59] provides compelling literature and his own insights about how a root canal can damage overall health systemically. He mentions various ways:

1.   By acting on the neural mechanism (by affecting the autonomic nervous system)

2.   By having a toxic effect (release toxins altering the patient's biochemistry). Toxins freed from root canal-filled or dead teeth contain very deleterious thio-ethers related to the deadly gas 'LOST' used in WWI as mentioned above.

3.   By having an allergic effect: if proteins are released from dying or dead teeth ('necrotoxins') the immune system may become sensitized and overreact. Once the patient is sensitized there may be cross-reactivity with regular foods, amino acids and a whole host of chemicals and bio-chemicals. The patient's symptoms may be multiple chemical sensitivity or food allergies.

Dr Dietrich Klinghardt is a medical doctor, a neurologist and an expert in his field. He also cites many respectable researchers who have contributed to unraveling the mystery behind how root canals cause cancer, heart disease, allergies, multiple chemical sensitivities and any other known or unknown disease – just like mercury. It is crucial, therefore, that all dental foci are treated because they could be the causative factor of your severe chronic disease – from your weak immune system to your heart disease, to your cancer.

---

58 Meinig, GE. Root Canal Cover-Up. USA: Bion Publishing, 2000.
59 Available at http://www.neuraltherapy.com/a_tonsils.asp

Recent research by Ralph Turk and Fritz Kronner in Germany has shown that even the act of drilling a tooth causes severe energy disturbance.60 Turk describes the modern dental turbine rotor as a sort of time bomb and that its damaging intensity has been completely missed by the vast majority of dentists. There are many likely reasons, not least being the fact that, despite water cooling, the temperature of the dentine rises by as much as 10 degrees after just a few seconds of drilling. This is akin to cooking the tooth.

This denaturation destroys the viability of the tooth and its ability to resist bacterial invasion. From over 6,000 cases studied, it was uniformly seen that, as soon as a tooth was visited by a high-speed drill, focal osteitis trouble began in connection with that tooth within 2 years. It is possible to reduce the damage by taking sensible detoxification protocols before, during and after a dental programme. Such elementary measures would include vitamin C, charcoal (to absorb toxins), homeopathic support and immune drainage remedies, such as HEEL's lymphomyosot or Pascoe's Pascotox.[61]

Focal infection theory

A 'focus of infection' has been defined as 'a circumscribed area infected with microorganisms which may or may not give rise to clinical manifestations. A 'focal infection' has been defined as 'sepsis arising from a focus of infection that initiates a secondary infection in a nearby or distant tissue or organs.'

Curtis, an eminent dentist said many years ago that, "…a focal infection is a localized or generalized infection caused by the dissemination of organisms or toxic products from a focus of infection. It probably would be better defined as a metastatic infection."[62]

It has been known for over 150 years, that focal infections in dead, root-canal treated teeth can in fact release organisms and their toxins into the

---

60 Turk, R. Iatrogenic damage due to high speed drilling, paper presented at the Scientific Session at the dedication of the Princeton Bio Center, New Jersey, 13th June, 1981.
61 Mumby, S. Virtual medicine: A new dimension in energy healing. Thorsons, London 1999.
62 Curtis, A.C.: Focal infection. American Textbook of Operative Dentistry.
7th ed. M.L. Ward, ed. Lea & Febiger, Philadelphia, 1840.

body. These can then initiate disease states in other parts of the body. Stortebecker has even demonstrated that these organisms and their toxins can be transported directly back to the brain via the blood, and also by transport along the nerve fibres. Other researchers have demonstrated that parts of the brain can be directly infected from dead teeth.[63,64,65,66]

There is also research which demonstrates the presence of Tumour Necrotising Factor[67] at the end in the apical area of infected roots.[68,69,70,71] Tumour Necrosis Factor is capable of causing diseases and syndromes such as chronic wasting syndrome, anorexia and excessive weight loss; bone resorption through the activation of osteoclasts, as well as other inflammatory disease states.

Mechanisms of focal infection

The origin of many toxic or metastatic diseases may be traced to primary local or focal areas of infection. Two mechanisms can produce focal infection:[72]

1. An actual metastasis of organisms from a focus
2. The spread of endotoxins or toxic products from a remote focus to other tissues by the blood stream.

---

63 Black R., Laboratory model for Trigeminal Neuralgia. *Adv. Neuro.* 4:651-8, 1974.
64 Westrum LE., Canfield RC., Black R., Transganglionic degeneration in the spinal trigeminal nucleus following the removal of tooth pulps in adult cats. *Brain Res* 6:100:137-40, 1976.
65 Westrum LE., Canfield RC., Electron microscopy of degenerating axons and terminals in the spinal trigeminal nucleus after tooth pulp exterpation. *Am J Anat.* 149:591-6, 1977.
66 Gobel S., Bink J., Degenerative changes in primary trigeminal axons and in neurons in nucleus caudalis following tooth pulp extirpation in the cat., *Brain Res.* 132:347-54, 1977.
67 A member of a family of proteins, which induce necrosis (death) of tumour cells and possess a wide range of proinflammatory actions.
68 K.E Safvi *J. Endo.* vol 17 No 1, Jan 1991.
69 Bando Y, Henderson B, Meghji S, Poole S, Harris M. Immunocytochemical localization of inflammatory cytokines and vascular adhesion receptors in radicular cysts. *J Oral Pathol Med* 22(5):221-7, May 1993.
70 Wang CY, Stashenko P. Characterization of bone-resorbing activity in human periapical lesions. *J Endod* 19(3):107-11, March 1993.
71 Iwu C, MacFarlane TW, MacKenzie D, Stenhouse D. The microbiology of periapical granulomas. Oral Surg Oral Med Oral Pathol 69(4):502-5, April 1990.
72 Mechanism of Focal Infection J Am Dent Assoc Vol 42:619-633, June 1951.

Also in the same Journal of the American Dental Association we read:

"If the bacteria pass the barrier (of the abscess wall) a number of things may happen:

1. The bacteria may travel to another free surface where they begin to grow.

2. The bacteria can travel to distant parts of the body by way of the lymphatics or the blood. Some bacteria will be eradicated by the lymph nodes while others can greatly stress the lymph nodes causing lymphadonitis, which may convert to an abscess. If the bacteria get through the lymph nodes, they may:

(a) multiply in the blood, setting up an acute or chronic septicemia.

(b) be carried live to a suitable nidus where they infect the surrounding tissue.

(c) produce a slow but progressive atrophy with replacement fibrosis in various organs of the body.

3. The byproducts of bacteria such as endotoxins may reach remote parts of the body.

4. The bacteria at the focus may undergo autolysis or dissolution and again some of these endotoxins may cause allergic reactions in various tissues of the body."

The pathogenic significance of these endotoxins has been investigated by the German study group of Eger-Miehlke. They examined the changes in healthy experimental animals after injection of accurately defined, minimal quantities of the endotoxins from an odontogenous granuloma.

A single injection of a minimal dose seemed to develop a defence-activation effect. But after repeated injections, there was severe liver damage, and the animals died within weeks. Apart from the fatal liver damage, inflammatory and degenerative changes were found in all other organs, especially in the joints, muscles, and blood vessels.

These results brought clear experimental proof for the first time that focogenic toxins act as causal agents for severe diseases in animals corresponding to similar chronic conditions in man.

The most dangerous of all odontogenous toxins are undoubtedly the thio-ethers, for instance dimethylsulfide. Thio-ethers are closely related, both in their structure and their effect, to mustard gas and other poison gases used in the First World War.

The extreme toxicity of the poison gases and thio-eithers can be attributed to the following properties:

❖ They are weakly alkaline and 'electro-negative,' and have a natural affinity for 'electro-positive' cells such as those of the transit tissues as well as those of the defensive tissues.
❖ They are fat-soluble and therefore have a natural affinity for fat-soluble structures such as the mitochondria of the cells.

The action of thio-ethers is effected in three main ways:

1. Since thio-ethers tend to combine with electro-positive metal ions and many co-factors of enzyme systems, the body will be led into a downward spiral of nutritional deficiencies.
2. Thio-ethers are 'partial' antigens and haptens[73], and can set up auto-immune responses leading to extensive cellular and tissue damage over time.
3. Thio-ethers can disrupt the aerobic mechanisms of the cell and trigger the cell into an anaerobic respiratory cycle – this is the beginning phase of the development of the cancer cell, as postulated by the famous biologist, Prof. Otto Warburg,[74] twice winner of the Nobel Prize.

After root canal treatment when the pulp is removed, slowly over time the thio-ethers will be released into the circulation and paralyze the critical aerobic respiration of the cell.

---

73 A hapten is a small molecule which can elicit an immune response only when attached to a large carrier such as a protein; the carrier may be one which also does not elicit an immune response by itself.
74 Warburg O. On the origin of cancer cells. *Science* 23:309-14, 1956.

In 1931 Freeman reported, "There is no question that bacteria or their toxins are not limited by the fibrous capsule."

The dental literature basically talks about the susceptible patient (regarding thio-ethers and other endotoxins) as being:[75]

- ❖ Those that are immune-compromised or have defective lymphatic drainage.
- ❖ Patients with heart disease, heart valve prosthesis and other chronic diseases.
- ❖ Patients that may be taking prolonged antibiotic, corticosteroid and immunosuppressive drugs.

The late Patrick Stortebecker, Professor of Neurology at the Karolinska Institute in Stockholm, Sweden, carried out a series of experiments in the 1960s which were very interesting. He injected tooth bone margins under pressure with radio-opaque dyes and then took X-rays of the skull. What he showed was that most head veins do not have valve control and therefore blood could travel backwards into the cranium – his radio-opaque dye appeared all over the head, far away from the tooth which was injected[76].

> *'If I had to choose between Medical or Dental for our patients, I would eliminate the Medical side, for in our experience no one can overcome chronic health problems without Biological Dentistry.'*
>
> Thomas Rau MD, Paracelsus Clinic (www.paracelsus.ch)

If the tooth in question should happen to be infected, the results could be very adverse indeed. Bacterial toxic matter could be propelled into the cranium and there set up an unwanted focus of infection right inside the skull. Stortebecker himself mentioned the obvious risk of cavernous sinus thrombosis and suppuration. This was once a killer condition.

---

75 Baumgartner, J. and Harrison, H. The incidence of bacteremias relate to endodontic procedures. *Nonsurgical endodontics J of Endodontics* Vol 3, No 5, May 1976.
76 Stortebecker P. Dental Caries as a Cause of Nervous Disorders. Bio-Probe Inc, Orlando, USA, 1986.

The cavernous sinus is a large vein reservoir at the base of the brain and if it should clot and become filled with purulent matter, widespread meningitis and brain abscesses would almost inevitably result.

Stortebecker also had another disease model for multiple sclerosis, which is very persuasive. Through extensive research he was able to show that most plaques of nerve de-myelination (the unmistakable sign of MS) were located around blood vessels.[77] No-one else has noticed this important fact before.

He speculated that the back-pressure on veins had shunted toxic matter into the brain tissues, where foci of inflammation and myelin loss are instigated. What was particularly convincing was that MS cases with optic neuritis (leading to blindness) generally had bad teeth and inflammation plaques in the brain, whereas those who had leg weakness or paralysis, with de-myelination plaques in the spinal cord, had pelvic or other lower-body disease foci.

Even in the light of all this evidence, the dental profession generally still continue to suggest that focal theory is old fashioned and that root canal treated teeth do not act as foci of infection.[78,79] Yet one study cites at least 150 different species of bacteria at the end of the root of dead teeth stating: "These infections are predominantly anaerobic."[80] These bacteremias can be extremely dangerous for people with defective heart valves, rheumatic fever and vascular diseases. The authors of this study add: 'Other forms of systemic diseases such as brain abscesses, haematological infection and implant infections have also been related to oral micro-organisms.'

---

77 Ibid.
78 Heimdahl A., Hall G, Hedberg M, Sandberg, H. Detection and Quantitation of Lysis-Filtration of bacteremia after different oral surgical procedures. *J Clin Microbiol* 28(1): 2205-9, 1990.
79 Debelian GJ., Olsen I., Tronstad L. Profiling of Propionibacterium Acnes recovered from root canal and blood during and after endodontic treatment. *Endod Dent Traumatol*, 8(6):248-54, 1992.
80 Debelian GJ., Olsen I., Tronstad L. Systemic diseases caused by oral microorganisms., *Endod Dent Traumatol*, 10(2):57-65 1994.

Another study has shown the same anaerobic organisms in both the blood as well as the dead tooth – indicating the same organism migrated from the dead tooth into the blood, where it does not belong.[81]

Neural focal interference

So far we have talked about root canal treatments and the microorganisms they contain causing various disease states in the body – this is one form of focus. There is another focus which was developed by two German doctors called the Heuneke brothers. What they found was that areas of dead tissue, scar tissue, foreign bodies, cystic tissue and infected tissue could interfere with the body's regulatory systems. They called these areas 'Foci of Neural Interference.'

The 'focus' is defined by Pichinger and Kellner as a 'Chronic devious localised alteration in the connective tissue, which can cause the most diversive reactions out of its immediate environment, and consequently is located in a permanent active relationship with the localised and general immune system.'

Any chronic inflammation, any scar, any degenerative or other alteration can obviously satisfy this condition. The focus is embedded in the mesenchymal[82] base tissue and in that way has direct contact with the capillary system of the blood and lymphatic vessels and the neuro-vegetative nerve fibre. This produces the connection to the whole organism. Through any of these conduction systems, it will be able to cause distant actions in other organs. The focal nerve impulse will be first projected into the vegetative centres, where it can cause a vegetative dysregulation, which likewise can become retroactive to the whole organism again. On the other hand, focal toxins and bacteria will be infiltrated by the vessel systems where they are able to spread their infectious, toxic and allergenic properties everywhere.[83]

---

81 Debelian GJ., Olsen I., Tronstad L. Bacteremia associated with endodontic therapy *Endod Dent Traumatol*, 11(3):142-9, 1995.
82 The part of the embryonic mesoderm that consists of loosely packed, unspecialized cells that are set in a gelatinous ground substance, from which connective tissue, bone, cartilage, and the circulatory and lymphatic systems develop.
83 More Cures for Cancer Translation from the German by Dr. Josef Issels, Helfer Publishing E. -Schwabe, Bad Homburg FRG.

A neural interference field will create an imbalance in the body's regulatory mechanisms, which include the tissue fluid around all of the cells of the body. Dead and infected teeth fulfil all the criteria to become Primary Foci of Neural Interference. The imbalance in the regulatory system will then either create or potentiate disease states in other parts of the body, which are remote from the original focus. These disease states will often coincide with areas of the body that are on the same acupuncture meridians as the primary focus. This has been verified by the work of Voll who was a German physician and electro-acupuncturist. For example we often see disease states in the areas of the reproductive system, kidney and knees in relation to non-vital front teeth.

The mouth and teeth are a primary source of focal infection and neural interference fields. No other parts of the body have dead tissue routinely left in place. The only thing which seems to separate individual reactions is the state of that person's immune system, and genetic factors. Consequently other factors which may reduce immune function will allow a greater reaction to the non-vital teeth. (e.g. mercury from dental amalgam fillings will have a direct and deleterious effect on the immune system).

So, how can this be redressed?

The next obvious question is 'How do you fill the space?' The solution depends on the location of the space and the condition of the adjacent teeth and or lack of teeth in the area. It will usually involve the creation of some sort of bridge or partial denture. Each person must be assessed individually.

Some dentists prefer to recommend the fitting of titanium implants – I do not believe that this is a good solution as electric currents generated by these devices may also act as a neural interference field. Zirconium implants are the new ones being touted as 'safer,' but the evidence has not yet been established that this is the case. There are of course very large profits to be made from each implant, which costs about $1,500 per tooth.

Very recently I was suffering from low back pain without understanding its cause – I had adjusted my spine using osteopathy and chiropractic manpulations by skilled practitioners a number of times, as well as my Primus Metatarsus Supinatus (PMS) using Prof. Rothbart's proprioreceptive insoles – but to no avail. I was taking glucosamine for over 6 months, along with other supplements.

There was a molar in the lower right quadrant of my mouth that was giving me pain – the X-ray showed that there was an infection in the bone that needed to be seen to immediately, and the only way of dealing with this was to have the tooth extracted. This took place under the supervision of a holistic (or biological) dentist who carefully injected Sanum isopathic remedies84 into the bone to help any anaerobic bacteria undergo pleomorphic changes into less pathogenic forms. I also used combinations of silver liquid protein 500ppm, grapefruit seed extract; echinacea and goldenseal, oregano oil and large doses of buffered vitamin C.

A little while after the extraction, my low back pain literally disappeared completely. I was absolutely convinced that it was the tooth extraction and clearing of the infection that was responsible for this dramatic turn in my health as discovered/described by H. Kolb[85] and summed up/confirmed by Tom Warren when he wrote/said:

"I have been told about a woman who had a breast tumour. Oncologists (cancer specialists) do not like to operate if there are signs of other infection. Her physician asked the woman to have an abscessed tooth taken care of before surgery. Immediately after the dental appointment, while lidocaine was present in her system, the woman had a Thermography X-ray that revealed a thin white line extending from her tooth, down her neck, through the tumour in her breast and on down into her stomach. In light of the discovery, her physicians decided not to operate. Four months later the tumour disappeared. That was the first time direct connection to disease following an acupuncture meridian was clinically observed and was an immeasurably important observation for western medicine. Every tooth has a separate acupuncture meridian running though major organs in the body.."

---

84 The Sanum remedies I recommend in chapter 5 to normalize pathogenic Candida
85 Kolb H. Spontanous remission of severe backache following oral rehabilitation. *Quintessenz*, 27(4):35-6), April 1976.

Teeth and acupuncture medians

Just as described by Warren and Kolb above, the acupuncture meridians are 12 in total and some of these pass through each tooth – over the years there have been maps of these teeth that have been modified and adapted by researchers familiar with testing the acupuncture meridians.

Below is a typical map of the teeth indicating the acupuncture meridians running through each tooth.

Acumeridian Tooth-Organ Relationships from various sources including Gleditsch and Klinghardt (www.NeuralTherapy.com).
Compiled by Dr. Ralph Wilson (www.naturalworldhealing.com)

As an example, if we take the right upper (tooth 1) and lower (tooth 32) molars, the heart and small intestine meridian run through these two teeth. A focus in these teeth will likely lead to the following symptoms: Right shoulder, elbow, hand (ulnar), sacroiliac, foot, toes and middle ear. Right heart, right duodenum, terminal ileum. CNS. Anterior pituitary.

One thing I have alluded to above is the relationship between teeth and the acupuncture meridians, which are 'energy lines' that run through the body and 'energetically feed' organ systems. A tooth focus can directly block one of these meridians, causing energy blockages in various organ systems.

One example is of a 50-year old man who was athletic, conscious of his nutrition, affluent and generally enjoyed life to the full. On a routine medical examination for insurance purposes he found that his PSA levels were high – further examination of the prostate, including a biopsy, led to the diagnosis of stage II adenocarcinoma of the prostate. When he came to the DaVinci Centre for the IDEL Diagnostic programme, one of the major issues that we discovered was an incisor on the right bottom quadrant (tooth 25) that is connected to the bladder and kidney meridian and runs through the prostate.

In fact, this tooth was capped after a riding accident four years previously, and the patient remembers quite specifically how a few months later he was getting prostate problems, including partial erectile failure and nocturnal micturition that he never suffered from before. When an X-ray of this incisor was taken it was clear that there was a large abscess at the root of the tooth – when the tooth was extracted a small sac of pus with a vile smell came out with it. If this tooth focus had not been identified and removed, then the chances are that this man would not be alive now, let alone completely cured and leading a full life again.

I have also seen a number of women with breast cancer who had tooth foci on the stomach meridian – this has been validated by other practitioners such as Dr. Thomas Rau from the Paracelsus Clinic in Switzerland,[86] who found that of 150 women with breast cancer, 98% had a disturbance on the stomach meridian – the breast belongs to the stomach meridian. Of these 150 women, there were only 3 patients who did not have a root canal in a tooth linked to the stomach meridian. These women were further compared with women in the same age range who did not have breast cancer – only 30% of these had root canals, which is a statistically significant difference.

---

86 Dr. Rau, Paracelsus Clinic, Switzerland – www.Paracelsus.ch

Symptoms of dead teeth

The types of disease states which relate to dead teeth are so numerous that it is impossible in an article of this size to discuss them all. They range from head and neck pain all the way through to rheumatism and cancer.[87]

The most common symptom is in the form of head and neck pain. This may range from mild headaches to migraines to Trigeminal Neuralgia. Sinusitis is very often associated with non-vital and root canal treated teeth, especially if they are in the upper arch.

Dr. Weston Price found that most patients with non-vital teeth had some thyroid dysfunction. A number of other researchers and physicians are finding a relationship between cancer and non-vital teeth. Reduced immune function is common. Eye and ear problems are common with root treated teeth.

Rheumatic and arthritic changes are almost the norm amongst people with dead teeth in their mouths. Many heart problems[88,89] and nervous disorders are associated with dead teeth. Multiple Sclerosis has also been linked to the toxins and organisms from dead teeth.[90,91]

The location of the tooth, the types of organisms inside it and the nature of the person's genetic make up will determine the areas of disease found clinically. The one thing that is certain is that if you are sick you should look very carefully at all non-vital teeth, whether root treated or not.

At the Davinci Natural Health Centre all patients undergoing the IDEL Diagnostic Programme[92] will have their teeth checked using ART, VEGA

---

87 Genco R. Current View of Risk Factors for Periodontal Disease; *J. Periodontol* Oct 1996.
88 Beck J, Garcia R, Heiss G, Vokonas PS, Offenbacher S. Periodontal disease and cardiovascular disease. *J Periodontol* 67 (10 Suppl):1123-1137, Oct 1996.
89 Herzberg MC, Meyer MW. Effects of oral flora on platelets: possible consequences in cardiovascular disease. *J Periodontol* 67 (10 Suppl):1138-1142, Oct 1996.
90 Stortebecker P. Chronic dental infections in the etiology of Glioblastomas. 8th int congress Neuropathy. Washington D.C. Sept 1978 *J Neuropth. Exp. Neurology* 37(s) 1978
91 Dental Caries as a cause of nervous disorders, 1981.
92 The IDEL Diagnostic Programme is a comprehensive diagnostic protocol involving many different testing protocols, including testing tooth foci with VEGA and ART – see www.docgeorge.com/IDEL-Diagnostic-Programme.html

testing, panoramic X-rays and other methods to determine whether there are tooth foci present.

Allergy to dental materials used to restore teeth

There are many types of dental materials that are used by dental professionals today ranging from gold alloys (containing palladium, silver, platinum and iridium), mercury fillings, acrylic denture material which contains methyl methacrylate, chrome cobalt partial denture framework, nickel based crowns and composite resin crowns containing polyurethane. It is possible that these dental materials can cause allergic responses resulting in intractable pain, chronic fatigue, food allergies, chronic sinusitis and headaches.

The dental liners or bases used under permanent restorative filling materials can also be the causative agent for an allergic response and body toxicity. A new toxicity disorder discovered by Dr. Omar M. Amin, Ph.D.,[93] Neurocutaneous syndrome (NCS), linked components (ethyltoluene sulfonamide and zinc oxide) in the calcium hydroxide dental bases (Dycal, Life and Sealapex) as sources for the observed symptoms of NCS.

The neurological aspects of NCS are characterized by pinprick and/or creeping, painful and irritating movement sensations – often interpreted as parasite movements – subcutaneously or in various body tissues or cavities including the head. In no case was the movement sensation related to parasites, which were always proved to be absent. Additional neurological symptoms include memory loss, brain fog and lack of concentration and control of voluntary movements; pain, depleted energy and a depressed immune system, all of which may invite various opportunistic infections. In many cases, lesions are associated with swellings in the arms and legs. Blood vessels may also become enlarged and elevated, the head may become hot and turn red; and the gums and teeth may turn gray.

---

93 For those interested in reading the full text of Dr. Amin's article, Toxicity from dental sealants causing neurocutaneous syndrome (NCS), a dermatological and neurological disorder, it is available on the following web site: www.holisticdental.org

Amin's study concluded that the toxicity of the dental sealants (Dycal, Life and Sealapex) was well demonstrated in studies conducted in patients under controlled laboratory conditions, by many workers.

Electrogalvanism

It is well known and can easily be measured using a simple voltmeter and ammeter, that when two dissimilar metals are present in the mouth with the presence of saliva, an electric current will flow. Saliva acts as an electrolyte when it mixes with amalgam fillings, to create a measurable electric current of 900 millivolts (enough power to light a small torch bulb). This current overpowers the body's normal 450 millivolts, interferes with energy flow to the brain and is suspected to be a catalyst in many illnesses.

Other alloys, such as nickel in the metal base of bridges and under porcelain crowns, have been documented to lower the T-4 and T-8 lymphocyte levels.[94] In predisposed patients, exposure to nickel can be a contributory factor in the development of cancer of the lungs, nasal passages and larynx.

Any metal materials in the mouth such as gold crowns, chrome cobalt partial dentures, mercury fillings and titanium implants, will set the stage for galvanic currents. In 1985, a research team (Knappworst, Gura, Fuhrmann and Enginalev) revealed that when mercury fillings were in close proximity to gold crowns, the mercury release was ten times greater when compared to mercury fillings alone.[95] Electro galvanism is frequently the cause for the following symptoms:

❖ Lack of concentration and memory
❖ Insomnia
❖ Psychological problems
❖ Tinnitus
❖ Vertigo
❖ Epilepsy
❖ Hearing loss

---

94 Eggleston, D. Effect of Dental Amalgam and Nickel Alloys on T-Lymphocytes: Preliminary Report, *J. Prosthetic Dent*, 51(5);617-623, 1984.
95 Stortebecker, P. Mercury Poisoning from Dental Amalgam - a Hazard to Human Brain. USA: Bio Probe.

❖ Eye problems
❖ Mouth pain

Removing the mercury and other metals and replacing them with biocompatible non-metal restorations will resolve the galvanic issue.

Dental implants – bone graft and metallic incompatibility

When teeth are lost due to poor nutrition, then you have a choice of fitting brand new metallic implants – these have now become very fashionable – with a price tag of around $1,500 per tooth.

Are these metallic implants a good choice? Before these were available people would either fit permanent or removal bridges.

Dr. Douglas Swartzendruber, a professor at the University of Colorado and later Dean, was asked: "How safe are dental implants?" He had supervised the development of a blood test that determined whether dental materials were safe or not according to immune reactivity in the blood. The question was specifically regarding metals that showed non-reactivity to the immune system such as zirconium, presuming that as implants they would be acceptable. His answer was surprising: "Anything implanted into bone will create an autoimmune response. The only difference is the length of time it takes," he replied.

"Are you talking about autoimmune diseases?" he was asked.

"That's what an autoimmune response is," he replied.

"But don't the serum immunology compatibility tests show them to be safe?"

"To use them in the mouth as crowns or bridges is okay – they are outside the body, so to speak, but the moment you implant anything into bone, you create a non-self-reaction in which the immune system says: ('you are not registered as bone, therefore you are a foreign body, and must be removed.')."

When the blood chemistry from people having their implants removed was measured, researchers from TERF96 found that the red blood cell readings stayed on the low side – or dropped. This lack of recovery in the haemocrit or blood cell count led to the suspicion that anaerobic bacteria might be living adjacent to the implants. Other offenders, like mercury, nickel and aluminium, create changes in chemistry – but so can these particular bacteria. With DNA sampling available, researchers looked at the bone and unusual looking tissue around implants.

Many implants were hard to remove as they were encased in a 'shield' that the body had created in its wisdom, to limit the amount of toxins that it would endure. Ironically, this hard bone (a blending of artificial with natural bone) was thought by many scientists to represent the implant success. So, utilizing DNA identification, both implanted bone and implanted metals were looked at for the presence or absence of anaerobic bacteria.

Anaerobes live in the absence of oxygen, and are usually more pathogenic than aerobic bacteria – a couple of common ones being botulism and tetanus, which can be lethal.

Below are the results of DNA testing utilizing checkerboard analytical techniques to determine the presence of some basic anaerobes. There are probably more, because these tests were limited to 85 of the most common anaerobes. Just the activity of one microbe, like Streptococcus pneumonia, or Clostridium botulinum (botulism), or Corynebacterium diphtheria, can be adequate to reduce a recipient's quality of life.

The disease conditions that are commonly associated with the presence of certain bacteria found in metallic implants and bone grafts are also included below:

❖ Cemella morbillorum – meningitis – acute invasive infections of the inner lining of blood vessels.

---

96 TERF (Toxic Element Research Foundation), a non-profit research foundation, is dedicated to stimulating interest in the research community as well as informing the public to become aware of potential problems associated with dental materials and procedures – www.terftalks.com.

❖ Porphyromonas gingivalis – alters integrity of the endothelinal lining of vessels; enhances athrogenesis.

❖ Prevotella intermedia – contributes to heart disease – penetrates cells therefore, hiding from the immune system and antibodies.

❖ Staphlococcus anginosus – induces platelet clumping in heart valves, causing infective endocavolitis.

❖ Veillonella parvula – pathogen related to infection in sinuses, heart, bone and central nervous system.

❖ Strep constellatus – reported with myocardial abscess, narrowing of the ventricular system and severe brain swelling.

❖ Prevotells melaninogenica – can cause infections like abscesses and bacteraemia at wound sites (post surgical), genital tract and periodontal disease.

These bacteria are primarily located in the tissue and blood immediately surrounding the implants, or within the bone proper of the implanted 'sterile' cadaver bone. Implanted bone was not found to dissolve and turn into normal bone, as suggested, but sometimes was the consistency of a piece of coral, but mostly it was just mushy goo laden with anaerobic bacteria. There was no attachment to surrounding bone.

The other relatively consistent result was in the level of porphyrins, which increased. Normally when dental toxins are removed the level of urinary porphyrins decrease as the level of heme and ATP increase in the cell. When the implants were removed, the porphyrin levels increased, as more was being excreted by the incubating toxic bacteria entering the blood system around the putrefying bone of the implant. Porphyrins will eventually drop after a month or so, but this is also related to the number of implants removed.

Dental braces and nickel

According to Thomas Levy, M.D., Orthodontic braces are made of nickel for the most part. 'Nickel is rapidly gaining a reputation for its toxicity, too. Most partial dentures are made of nickel. Approximately 80% of crowns use nickel, even 'porcelain' crowns. Braces usually are nickel. Stainless steel is usually nickel alloy. Nickel compounds have been unequivocally implicated as human respiratory carcinogens in epidemiological studies of nickel refinery workers, and there appears to be a relationship between nickel crowns and breast cancer in women.'[97]

There are a few methods that use gold and plastic, but nickel is still state of the art. Anecdotally, teachers notice a difference with braces. When one of their students has a brace fitted, they anticipate a drop in the student's grade average of about 1 ½ points. That is, from B+ to C minus. This can impact their hopes for college, and may be one of the sources of what is called 'teen age behaviour'. It may, in fact, be just a toxic response to nickel.

According to Dr. David Eggleston, "Nickel is used routinely by national cancer centers to induce cancer in laboratory animals in order to study cancer. The nickel alloys they are using are very similar to those we are using in patients' mouths. Dentists are causing a major health problem."

Eggleston first measured several important immune system components, the T-lymphocytes, in the patients' blood. The normal range for T-lymphocytes is considered to be 70-80% of the lymphocyte population. In one 21-year-old woman with amalgam fillings, the T-lymphocytes comprised 47% of her lymphocyte population. When Eggleston removed her amalgam fillings and replaced them with plastic temporary fillings, the T-lymphocytes rose from 47% to 73% – an increase of 55.3%![98]

Next Eggleston removed the plastic fillings and reinserted amalgam. The T-lymphocytes fell from 73% to 55% (a decrease of 24.7%).

Finally, Eggleston removed the second set of amalgam fillings and inserted gold inlays. After this procedure, the T-lymphocytes bounced back up to 72% (a rise of 30.9%).

Patient No.2 was a healthy 20-year-old white male. When a composite filling was removed and replaced with a nickel-based crown, his T-lympho-cytes dropped from 63% to 56.7%. They rebounded to 73% when the nickel crown was removed and re-placed with gold.

---

97 Thomas Levy, M.D. http://www.best.com/~cnorman/blazing/dental.html
98 Eggleston DW: Effect of dental amalgam and nickel alloys on T-lymphocytes: Preliminary report. *Journal of Prosthetic Dentistry* 51:617-23, May 1984.

Patient No.3 was a 35-year-old white woman, with symptoms of advanced multiple sclerosis. After nine amalgam fillings were removed, her T-lymphocyte level rose from 60% to 71%. It is not known what other long-term results may have occurred, although obviously such information would be interesting.

Although the public is not aware of it, this nickel crown experiment is highly suggestive. Many dental crowns are formed on a nickel base. But nickel is a known carcinogen. Industrial studies of worker exposure to nickel dust and alloys show that such exposure "Will markedly increase the incidence of cancer" (Quicksilver Associates).

"An abnormal T-lymphocyte percentage of lymphocytes or a malfunction of T-lymphocytes can increase the risk of cancer, infectious diseases and autoimmune disease" (Dr. Eggleston).[99]

Nickel is not nearly as active as mercury, however, it corrodes and is far more carcinogenic. One of the most severe known reactions to nickel toxicity is described by Dr. Eggleston. A patient presented herself to the Long Beach Memorial Hospital with kidney disease. She was diagnosed as having idiopathic glomerulo-nephritis. They called it 'idiopathic' because they did not know what was really the cause of the kidney ailment. After examining the patient, her family physician suggested that she be checked with electro-diagnosis. When this was done it was found that she was highly reactive to nickel.

John Lucecki, D.C. reported the following case: "he doctor asked her if she had any dental work done within the past seven years. She said that she had three porcelain crowns put in by her dentist. The doctor explained that porcelain crowns have metal jackets (made of a nickel alloy) underneath the porcelain and suggested that she have these crowns removed immediately. After the removal of the three crowns the patient lost all symptoms of kidney failure. This was one case in a million which was diagnosed properly. Her kidney problem was primarily due to the nickel toxicity. This was poisoning her system."

---

99 Strauss FG, Eggleston DW: IgA nephropathy associated with dental nickel alloy sensitization. *American Journal of Nephrology*, 5:395-7, 1985

Children at risk

There is an even larger problem. The combination of amalgam (mercury) and braces. Mercury alone has been found to create what is called floating suicidal thoughts in adults. It has been observed by the media that suicide is the number one cause of death in teenagers. Is it reasonable to assume that teens are somehow immune to this attack, especially when compounded with the challenge offered by nickel?

Immature minds may not be able to resist these thoughts of unknown origin, and teens are not willing to discuss this abnormal thought behaviour with their parents, teachers, religious leaders, or even their friends. Adults for the most part will not discuss suicidal thoughts until asked, 'Can you identify with floating suicidal thoughts?' Well over 80% of the adult patients with amalgams can and do identify with this immediately, often with a sigh of relief. There is a toxic reason for the thoughts. These unwelcome thoughts generally disappear within 2 to 3 days of the application of the total protocol treatment.

Dr. Mike Godfrey (a medical doctor in New Zealand) and Hal A Huggins, DDS and spokesperson for TERF, examined a 23 year old girl in New Zealand for a 60 Minute television program. She was very weak, could not attend school, work, or adequately take care of herself. She had a nickel retainer cemented behind the 6 lower front teeth that had been there for years. (Many people have retainers cemented, and, years later think nothing of it. There is no orthodontic recall to remove them). They had to canvass four dentists before one was found willing to remove the nickel retainer. Within a few days, it was evident that she was recovering. Within a month she was a normal young adult full of energy.

This shows that although nickel may be cheap in the beginning, the subsequent problems created by nickel in the mouth far outweigh the few dollars saved. Millions of these are placed every year. TERF believes that dentistry should begin to show some respect for the developing, trusting minds of children, and their parents as well. The profession needs to find something non-carcinogenic and non-toxic to replace nickel.

It is in the best interests of society as a whole to leave the children alone to develop into happy, healthy young adults.

At the DaVinci Natural Therapy Centre all people undergoing a full diagnostic "IDEL Diagnostic Programme" will be asked to bring in a panoramic X-ray or Panorex. As you can see from the image below, the Panorex is a large, single x-ray film that shows the entire bony structure of the teeth and face. It takes a much wider area than any intra oral film showing structures outside of their range including the sinuses, and the Temperomandibular Joints. It shows many pathological structures such as bony tumors, cysts, abscesses as well as the position of the wisdom teeth.

The teeth are then checked using Autonomic Response Testing (ART) to identify any tooth foci that will not be visible on the Panorex – these could be related to bacteria producing lethal toxins that block the acupuncture meridians. These foci can then be treated with low intensity lazer therapy (LILT).

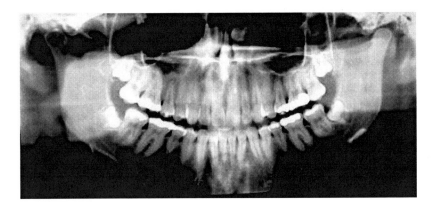

Panorex X-ray

We also get our patients to use the Soladey titanium oxide ionic toothbrush as it is extremely effective at killing bacteria and removing plaque that harbour them, all without toothpaste.

Soladey Toothbrush – No Toothpaste!

Dental plaque is biofilm (usually colourless) that builds up on the teeth. If not removed regularly, it can lead to caries or periodontal problems such as gingivitis.

The microorganisms that form the biofilm are almost entirely bacteria, mainly Streptococcus mutans and anaerobes, including fusobacterium and Actinobacteria. Plaque can also make our teeth less attractive as they turn a brown colour and can cause bad breath.

Why do ordinary hand and electric toothbrushes often leave plaque on tooth surfaces no matter how carefully you brush or floss? Why do you have plaque/tartar when you visit the dentist for a check-up, even though you brush carefully? Because plaque attaches to teeth by an electrostatic bond, friction by itself is not enough to break this bond. This bond is due to plaque having a positive polarity and teeth having a negative polarity.

Instead of using friction or sound (sonic) waves to try to "blast apart" this bond, there is now a patented IONIC technology that changes the polarity of the tooth surfaces from positive to negative.

This is the Soladey titanium oxide ionic brush - as you brush, plaque material is actively repelled by your teeth and drawn to the negatively charged bristles, even in hard-to-reach areas of your mouth. Unlike regular toothbrushes which require toothpaste - an abrasive compound - to help to remove plaque - the IONIC action works with or without toothpaste, making it gentler on the gums. It is probably the simplest but most advanced toothbrush in the world.

How does it work? There is a light-activated titanium rod (semiconductor) inside the handle. When exposed to any light source (a fluorescent bathroom light, a plain light bulb, or sunlight), the photo-sensitive titanium rod inside Soladey converts light into negatively-charged ions (electrons). The rod releases these ions, which blend with saliva to attract positive (hydrogen) ions from the acid in the dental plaque on your teeth.

In the presence of light, saturated low energy electrons in the wet semiconductor are transformed into high energy electrons resulting in a reduction reaction as shown below:

$$H+ + O_2 + e - = HO_2 \qquad 2H+ = + 2\,e - = H_2$$

$$2HO_2 = H_2O_2 \qquad H_2O_2 = 2HO$$

This reaction results in the reduction of H+ ions from the organic acid in the plaque causing its decomposition. The reaction has an effect on plaque formation.[100,101] There is also evidence that the toothbrush has a bactericidal effect against Escherichia coli and Streptococcus mutans.[102]

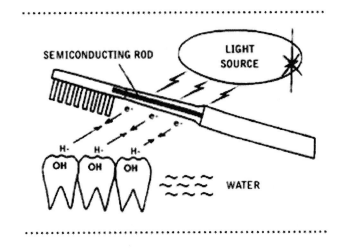

Soladey toothbrush with titanium semiconducting rod

A blind, two-way crossover clinical trial has shown that when the Soladey ionic brush was compared with an ordinary toothbrush with toothpaste as well as a placebo group it was far superior at removing plaque in a shorter time period.[103]

100 Kusunoki, K., Oku, T., Koni, H., Nakaya, K, Mori, T, Hiratuka, V, Taguchi, M, Watanabe, Y and Miyake, T. A study on the effect of the solar energy conversion toothbrush on the control of dental plaque. *Journal of the Osaka Odontological Society* 49, 550-559, 1986.
101 Niwa, M and Fukuda, M. Clinical study on the control of dental plaque using solar energy conversion toothbrush equipped with a TiO2 semiconductor. *Odontology* 77, 598-606, 1989.
102 Moriaoka, T., Saito, T., Nara, K and Onoda, K. Antibacterial action of powdered semiconductor on a serotype g Streptococcus mutans. *Caries research* 22, 230-231, 1988.
103 Hoover, JN, Singer DL, Pahwa, P and Komiyama, K. Clinical evaluation of a light energy conversion toothbrush. *J Clin Periodontol* 19:434-436, 1992.

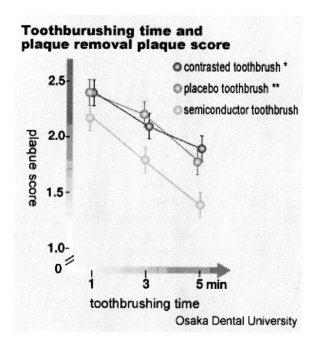

Plaque removal using Soladey brush

This brings us to the end of this chapter on the dangers of modern dentistry. The next chapter will take a deeper look at bioenergetic and informational medicine, another important aspect of holistic health.

Chapter 9

Bioenergetic and Informational Medicine

Scientists, particularly medical doctors, have always found the concept of Energy Medicine extremely controversial and confusing. The belief is that serious scientists do not concern themselves with concepts of 'life force' and 'healing energy' as this is not "evidence-based medicine." I will not go into the arguments of what is or is not evidence-based medicine, as most of what is presently practiced by modern medicine is far from evidence-based; e.g. interactions of a cocktail of drugs given to the same patient, many surgical procedures are experimental, treating chronic disease using drugs, chemotherapy and radiation and much more – none of these are based on the 'Gold Standard' double-blind, placebo controlled trials that pure scientists often wrongly worship.

If you are such a scientist, thinking only in terms of evidence-based medicine, then please do not skip over this chapter – I challenge you to open your mind and heart and read with interest – there is a lot of evidence-based research that has made Bioenergetic and Informational Medicine a true science, even though there is much more that we have to learn. I promise you that by implementing a miniscule amount of what follows in your clinical practice, it is going to make you into a better practitioner, with ever grateful patients.

Bioenergetic and Informational Medicine covers a wide array of multiple disciplines ranging from the biological sciences, ecology, physiology, psychology, anatomy of organs, tissues and cells, as well as the physics of molecules, atoms and subatomic particles. In the human body all these sciences come together to teach us the properties of 'wholeness' which is the integration of the parts working together as a successful unit – this is the premise of this book on 'Holistic Medicine.'

I strongly believe that bioenergetic and informational medicine is going to be the medicine of the future – these discoveries on energetics are now gradually percolating into the consciousness of medical practitioners - researchers and healthcare professionals and the general public are realizing that these energetic healing modalities are here to stay. Many times in clinical practice I have used various energetic diagnostic and healing modalities that have completely cured difficult chronic diseases, where more orthodox approaches could not help.

A little history

From as early as 2750 BC, people were exposed to shocks produced by electric eels – this was one of the earliest examples of using electricity to heal.[1] During the 1700's and 1900's various electric healing devices were developed and used by physicians for treating a range of ailments.[2] By 1884 it was estimated that 10,000 physicians in the USA were using electricity every day for therapeutic purposes without the science to back it. Figure 1 shows an electromagnetic healing device described by the Frenchman d'Arsonval in 1894.

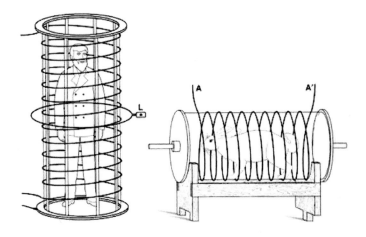

Fig 1 Electromagnetic Healing Device described by d'Arsonval in 1894

Duchenne in 1867 (Figure 2) published his famous studies of the 'muscle points,' otherwise known as motor points – these are points on the body that when stimulated by electrodes can determine the proper workings of the muscles – this is now the modern study of electromyography.

---

[1] Kellaway, P. The part played by electric fish in the early history of bioelectricity and electrotherapy. *Bulletein of the History of Medicine*. 20:112-132, 1946.
[2] Geddes, LA. A short history of the electrical stimulation of excitable tissue including electrotherapeutic applications. *Physiologist* 27 (1):S1-S47, 1984.

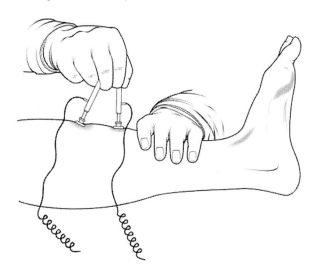

Fig 2 Duchenne in 1867 began the science of electromyography

In 1923, George's Lakhovsky[3], a Russian engineer working in France, built a simple apparatus capable of registering microvoltage measurements from human cells, plants and microbes. In his studies of normal and diseased cells, Lakhosvky found that there were marked differences in their oscillation patterns. Each group of cells emitted frequencies specific to its organ or tissue of origin. Cancerous cells emitted a different, abnormal pattern. Lakhovsky also discovered that harmful factors such as faulty nutrition, environmental pollutants such as toxic chemicals or heavy metals, bacteria or viruses weaken and distort cellular electro-magnetic fields prior to the onset of illness and death.

A little later, Professor Harold Saxton Burr[4] of Yale Medical School carried out his own investigation of human-energy related phenomenon. His systematic measurements of the electromagnetic fields emitted by different body tissues and organs confirmed Lakhovsky's findings concerning the difference in the electrical emissions of healthy and diseased organs and tissues. He called these the 'L-fields' with 'L' representing "Life." Thanks to the controlling L-fields, new molecules and cells in the body are constantly being rebuilt, arranging themselves in the same pattern as the old ones.

---

[3] Lakhovsky, G. The Waves Which Cure (Gauthier-Villars and Co), 1929.
[4] Burr, H.S. Bluprint for Immortality, Neville Spearman Publishers, 1972.

With the advancement of scientific research technology, the number of discoveries regarding the human energy field grew. In 1967, the magnetic field around the human heart was observed and recorded using a sophisticated Superconducting Quantum Interference Device (SQUID) at the Massachusetts Institute of Technology in Cambridge, Masachusetts by Zimmermann and his colleagues.[5,6]

Professor Tiller[7] believes that the magnetic elements in living cells are repositories for voluminous amounts of information, the pathological content of which contributes to the development and sustainment of chronic diseases. All of the major assaults that the body is not able to overcome (toxins, infectious agents and physical or emotional traumas) become imprinted onto these cellular recordings in a CD-like fashion and then continuously feed back into the body's chemistry, altering it adversely.

German physicist Professor Herbert Frohlick[8] of the University of Liverpool, a world-renowned authority on human energy research, summarized his fifty years of research in the field by concluding that every structure in the body, including the entire chemistry of the body, down to the chromosomes, is energy-operated and driven by electromagnetic fields that are created by flows of charged ions. He received the Max Planck Medal, the highest award for physics in Germany.

How Does the Body Work Energetically?

When students of medicine and biology study the cell, the diagrams that they study are very simplistic in the sense that they only look at the structural components – the different organelles contained inside the cell and their function. However, in order to be able to understand the energetic systems of the body, we need to understand the basic anatomy of the body's Living Matrix. It is the living matrix or extracellular matrix (ECM) that communicates with each and every cell of the body forming a

---

[5] Zimmermann, J.E. Josephson effect devices and low frequency filed sensing. *Cryogenics* 12:19-31, 1972.

[6] Zimmermann, J.E., Thiene P, Harding J T. Design and operation of stable rf-biased superconducting point-contact quantum devices, and a note on the properties of perfectly clean metal contacts. *Journal of Applied Physics.* 41:1572-1580, 1970.

[7] Tiller, W. Energy Fields and the Human Body. Frontiers of Consciousness, edited by J. White. New York, Avon Books, 1974.

[8] Hyland, GJ and Rowlands, P (ed). *Herbert Frohlich FRS: A Physicist Ahead of his Time.* (2nd edition), UK: University of Liverpool, 2008.

complex web of interconnectedness. Figure 3 is a summary of these interconnections – notice how the tissues surrounding the digestive tract, nerves, bones, blood vessels, muscles and underlying the skin contain a sparse but active number of generative cells the form and continuously modify the extracellular matrix and play an important role in injury repair and defence against disease.

All of these cells are part of a structural, energetic and informational continuum. This fibre system is now recognized by many scientists as an important communication system that affects all metabolic systems as well. It is part of a semiconducting, oscillatory continuum that allows all parts of the biological organism to communicate with each other. One research scientist, Adey in 1993 refers to this as "whispering between cells."[9]

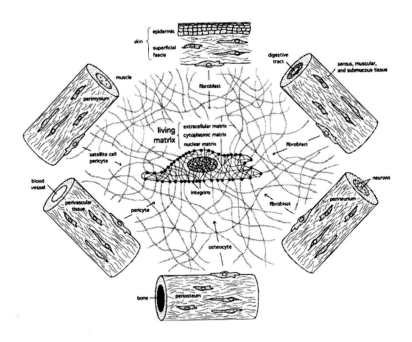

Fig. 3 The Living Matrix

In trying to understand the energy dynamics of the living matrix, the field of physics plays an important role. In the structure of the living matrix

---

[9] Adey, WR. Whispering between cells: electromagnetic fields and regulatory mechanisms in tissue. *Frontier Perspectives.* 3:21-25, 1993.

there is a degree of coherent crystallinity – this is like an ordered crystal matrix that is very important to the structure-energy-communication model of living tissue. Interestingly, many of the key molecules that make up the living matrix such as collagen, elastin, keratin, DNA, actin and myosin are all helical, much like a helical spring. If we can understand how the helical spring can convert energy from one form to another, then we will better understand how the living matrix is able to respond to different energies.

This system is comprised of two main structures: the visible and invisible connective tissue that extends from the molecular level of our body throughout our energy field and the element of water. In "The Hidden Messages in Water", author Masuru Emoto[10] talks about water's crystalline nature. He has observed through his unique process of freezing water, then photographing the crystals, that water not only responds to the vibration of words and pictures but also remembers these vibrations. Words that are hurtful or derogatory, such as "You fool," create a condition where the water can't form crystals. Words such as "love and gratitude" created extraordinarily beautiful crystals.

It was back in 1941 that Albert Szent-Györgyi,[11] who had received the Nobel Prize in 1937 for the synthesis of Vitamin C, gave the Korányi Memorial Lecture in Budapest, Hungary. He said, "if a great number of atoms is arranged with regularity in close proximity, as for instance, in a crystal lattice, the electrons cease to belong to one or two atoms only, and belong to the whole system...A great number of molecules may join to form energy continua, along which energy, viz., excited electrons, may travel a certain distance."

What this means is that free electrons can move around the body quickly and transfer energy and information wherever in the body they wish. This is clarified further by Dr. Donald Coffey and an eminent group at Johns Hopkins School of Medicine.[12] They were studying the nuclear matrix and its interconnections with both the DNA and with molecules that extend

---

10 Emoto, M. Messages from Water, Vol. 1, Hado Publishing, Japan, 1999.

11 Szent-Györgyi, A. The Study of Energy Levels in Biochemistry) *Nature* 148:157-159, 1941.

12 Presented by James L. Oschman, Ph.D.in a lecture entitled "The development of the living matrix concept and its significance for health and healing in a speech commemorating the London premier of The Living Matrix: a new film on the science of healing and the Science of Healing Conference at Kings College, London on March 13, 2009.

across the nuclear envelope and connect to the cytoskeleton.[13] What this meant was that we could now trace the continuity inward from the extracellular matrix and connective tissues, across the cell surface via the integrins and related molecules first described by Bretscher, throughout the cell cytoplasm via the cytoskeleton, and across the nuclear envelope to the genetic material.

In 1991, the same group produced an inspiring report on the way signals propagate through this matrix, which they termed a tissue tensegrity matrix system.[14] The tensegrity aspect had evolved from the work of Buckminster, Fuller and others.[15] Tensegrity is defined as a continuous tensional network (called tendons) supported by a discontinuous set of compressive elements (called struts).

The 1991 report by Pienta and Coffey gave precise language and experimental validation to the transfer of energy and information through the living matrix: "Cells and intracellular elements are capable of vibrating in a dynamic manner with complex harmonics, the frequency of which can now be measured and analyzed in a quantitative manner...a tissue-tensegrity matrix system...is poised to couple the biological oscillations of the cell from the peripheral membrane to the DNA."

The helical molecules in living systems are piezoelectric semiconductors which have the ability of emitting and absorbing light and converting light energy into vibrations that can travel through the living matrix. Due to the transverse Hall effect, these helical molecules can also respond to magnetic and biomagnetic fields. Whenever a therapist applies any type of stimulus to the living matrix, whether it is by touch on the skin, inserting an acupuncture needle, using a pulsing electromagnetic field such as the PAPIMI that we will discuss below, the vibratory energy from these stimuli will be converted by the helical molecules of the living matrix into signals that will travel throughout the living matrix.

---

13 Berezney, R., Coffey, D.S. Isolation and characterization of a framework structure from rat liver nuclei. *Journal of Cell Biology* 73:616-637, 1977.
14 Pienta K.J., Coffey D.S. Cellular harmonic information transfer through a tissue tensegrity-matrix system. *Medical Hypotheses* 34:88-95, 1991.
15 Tensegrity is a naturally occurring construct first recognized and developed by sculptor Ken Snelson and visionary R. Buckminster Fuller. For a detailed discussion, go to Dr. Stephen M. Levin's web site, http://www.biotensegrity.com

Informational Medicine

There are also many phenomenons in healing that are not governed by quantity, space and time. These phenomenon and related treatment modalities are outside modern-day medicine since they are not covered and explained by modern-day physics. These can be placed into the category of 'Informational Medicine' and would include homeopathy, psychology, emotional freedom technique, distant healing, prayer healing, radionics, Hellinger Family Constellations and more. Of these, homeopathy was the first systemically developed form of informational medicine in recent history.

Informational medicine consists of words, signs, symbols, rituals and pictures – the use of information in all its forms – even though this has not been recognised formally by modern medicine it no doubt exists and is a powerful healing modality that goes beyond the placebo effect. There are many informational modalities that are often misunderstood as being energetic. As these modalities do not use substance or energy to diagnose or heal, there is no way that atomic physicists using quantum mechanics can measure the energy as it does not exist as an energy system but an information system.

Alongside the levels of matter and energy, information forms a third level of existence that is guided by its own laws which differ in many aspects from those of matter and energy. They can, however, co-exist – matter and energy can be transformed into each other and so can information be transformed into energy or vice versa. Information can also be transported via energy, as happens most times.

However, a new aspect that is unknown in modern physics, maybe with the exception of Global Scaling[16], is that information can be transmitted without energy. This is possible because pure information is not ruled by time and space. It may be difficult to conceive, but our world is holographic in its structure, which means that every part contains all other

---

16 The Theory of Global Scaling assumes that matter resonates harmonically at its lowest level of energy. This lowest level global scaling theory is not merely designated the "physical vacuum"; however, the frequency spectrum of the natural oscillations of the vacuum comprises many orders of magnitude and is fractally developed, like a melody. This "melody of creation" is, according to the theory, the cause of the logarithmic-hyperbolic, scale invariant, fractal distribution of frequencies of most varied measure – from the elementary particles to the galaxies.

parts - this implies that any part can affect every other part and can be a measure of every other part.

To illustrate this let's look at an example. It is well known that silver particles in a beaker of water will kill bacteria. What is not so well known is that if the colloidal silver was placed in a nearby gas discharge tube, the electromagnetic emissions from this will also kill the bacteria. If one also closely simulated the silver spectrum using light energy, the electromagnetic radiation from this light source would also kill the bacteria. We can clearly see that it is not the physical contact of the silver ions with the bacteria that are killing them but the **specific information pattern** inherent in the silver atom that is responsible. So manipulating the information aspect of the silver can alter the information aspect of the bacteria in such a way as to 'kill' the bacteria.

Bioenergetic medicine is basically the science of the human energy field. In a few decades scientists have gone from a conviction that there are no such energy fields in and around the human body, to an absolute certainty that they exist. These can take different forms such as magnetic, electricity, light, heat, gravity, kinetic energy and sound.

The diagnostic methods described in this book use the human energy field to derive health-related information. For instance, thermography records the thermal properties of the human energy field. The VEGA EXPERT measures electrical energy flow in specific energy channels of the body, known as meridians which are all connected to the Living Matrix. This will be registered after stimulation with a different energy field (a food item, a medical drug, a toxin, a mineral or a vitamin supplement).

Autonomic Response Testing (ART) is a way of measuring energy changes in the autonomic nervous system, which is connected to the Living Matrix - using this method it is possible to understand what stresses the body on an energetic level.

The treatment modalities mentioned are all energetic. For instance, Homotoxicology works with weak-potency homoeopathic formulae. The ionic footbath removes toxins from the feet by stimulating the energetic properties of the cell walls and provokes them to eliminate their toxins. Infrared sauna therapy applies a specific electromagnetic frequency directly on the body which again helps the body to eliminate harmful toxic metals and other xenobiotics. All the diagnostics and all the treatments described can be viewed as energetic and an exchange of vibratory information, again, through the Living Matrix. Every cell is connected to the Living Matrix – anything that can energetically balance the cells will have a direct balancing effect on the Living Matrix – this is why in some cases the healing effects of energy medicine are so dramatic and lightning fast.

Some people gifted by birth, such as mystics and healers have been speaking and writing about the energetic nature of the human being and the interconnections with the sea of energy around us for thousands of years. Barbara Ann Brennan, one such gifted person, a healer as well as a physicist, bridged her natural gift with the science of physics in her book entitled, *Hands of Light: A guide to Healing through the Human Energy Field*.[17] Many writers have contributed to this body of knowledge as well, some naturally gifted, others less so. Many were ordinary scientists, relying on indirect observation using special instruments or biochemical tests to infer on the impact of energetic treatments.

Vibrational Medicine by Richard Gerber, MD[18], and *Energy Medicine: The Scientific Basis*[19] by James Oschman provide excellent overviews of the scientific basis of energy medicine. The fact remains that many energetic therapeutic interventions work, some of them with exceptional results. The practitioners who employ them do not wait for the blessing of conventional medicine, with all its vices, to be ready to explain the why and the how.

Visual Medicine – seeing the effects of energy on water

Masaru Emoto[20] is a Japanese author known for his controversial claim that if human speech or thoughts are directed at water droplets before they are frozen, images of the resulting water crystals either take on a beautiful geometric pattern or a disorganized, ugly one, depending upon whether the words or thoughts were positive or negative. Emoto claims this can be achieved through prayer, music or by attaching written words to a container of water.

---

17 Brennan, BA. Hands of Light: A guide to Healing through the Human Energy Field. USA: Bantam Books, 1987.
18 Gerber, R. Vibrational Medicine (3rd edition). USA: Bear and Company, 2001.
19 Oschman, J.L. Energy Medicine: The Scientific Basis. UK: Harcourt Publishers, 2000.
20 Emoto, M. *The Journal of Alternative and Complementary Medicine*. February 2004, 10(1): 19-21.

Dr. Emoto is at the forefront of the study of water as he has shown visually by using high-speed photography under high-power microscopy to photography water freezing quickly. He has shown using this "visual medicine" that thoughts and feelings affect physical reality. By producing different focused intentions through written and spoken words and music and literally presenting it to the same water samples, the water appears to "change its expression".

He found that water from clear springs and water that has been exposed to loving words shows brilliant, complex, and colorful snowflake patterns (Fig . In contrast, polluted water, or water exposed to negative thoughts, forms incomplete, asymmetrical patterns with dull colors.

The implications of this research create a new awareness of how we can positively impact the earth and our personal health. The success of his books[21] outside Japan has been remarkable. Dr. Emoto has been called to lecture around the world as a result and has conducted live experiments both in Japan and Europe as well as in the US to show how indeed our thoughts, attitudes, and emotions as humans deeply impact the environment.

A bottle of frozen water crystals is labeled with the words "love and thanks" for 24 hours before being photographed, and in another bottle the same water is labeled with the word "devil" before being photographed. The difference in the crystal lattice of the geometric structure as seen under a microscope is astounding. The frozen water with the word "love" wrapped around it shows a beautiful geometric crystal lattice that is pleasing to the eye. The one with the word "devil" wrapped around it has an ugly shape with no geometry of crystal formation.[22]

The Human Bioenergetic System

Humans consist of more than physical nerves, muscles and bones. We are part of a larger dynamic, multidimensional system of energy and light – we are simply much more than the physical body. Our physiological systems comprising of organs and tissues are not only supported by oxygen,

---

[21] Emoto, M. *Messages from Water, Vol. 1,* Hado Publishing, 1991; Emoto, M. *Messages from Water, Vol. 2,* Sunmark Pub, 2001; Emoto, M. *The Hidden Messages in Water,* Beyond Words Publishing, 2004.
[22] See more of these images on Emoto's official website at http://www.masaru-emoto.net/english/ephoto.html

glucose and other nutrients, but also by higher vibrational energies which provide life to the physical body.

These higher energies are regulated by the chakra-nadi sytem and the physical-etheric interface, which include the acupuncture meridian system – it connects the organic and molecular forms with the organizational energies of the etheric body. The etheric energies provide ways of organizing cellular structure and function.

The fine network of nadis distributes high-frequency energies coming in through the chakras to all the body organs and tissues. This high-frequency energy helps to provide balance and order at the molecular level of expression – it is like higher dimensional homeostatic system. When energetic disturbances occur at these higher frequency levels these will manifest in the physical body as symptoms and disease.

If we could widen our perspective and see humans in their multidimensional anatomy, consisting of higher vibrational bodies, chakras, nadis, and meridians (Fig 5), then it would be possible to explain much of what allopathic medicine cannot explain about disease processes. Humans are not closed physiological boxes but open energy systems in a dynamic equilibrium with a multidimensional electromagnetic environment.

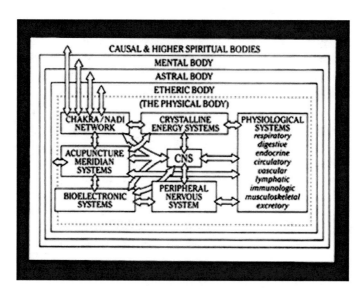

Fig 5 Human Multidimentional Bioenergetic System

The real future of Holistic Medicine will depend on the integration of vibrational medical therapies into clinical practice alongside all the other healing modalities. The holistic physician will need to integrate the physical, emotional, mental and spiritual elements of life in order to truly cure the patient on all these levels. The ultimate approach to healing will be to remove the subtle-energy imbalances that led to the manifestation of illness in the first place.

Even though allopathic physicians have acknowledged for some time that stress contributes to diseases such as stomach ulcers, ulcerative colitis, psoriasis, asthma and more, there have been very few attempts to address the underlying pathogenesis of these diseases – other than using anxiolytic drugs such as valium and the like. These drugs may help in the short-term with acutely stressful situations, but only tend to suppress the symptoms and overlook the primary, underlying causes. It is much more constructive for the holistic physician to integrate and rebalance the elements of the mind and body with the element of spirit.

For many years physicians have looked and treated the physical body as a separate entity to the mind and the spirit. There has begun a paradigm shift away from this dualistic thinking of old into a new model that accepts the health effects of the mind on the physical body. Still, it is early days as the majority of medical doctors are still only trying to direct therapeutic strategies toward particular organ systems instead of treating the whole person. In reality, humans are greater than the sum of their physical organs and physiological systems as the physical body is not a closed system. The physical body interfaces with complex subtle structures and networks that help the life-force and energies of consciousness to maintain a homeostasis required for the health of the physical body.

Many practitioners will ask, well that's all well and good, but how can we measure these 'subtle energies' and help get a better understanding of how they adversely affect our patients? This is an excellent question that can be answered as there are many different technologies and techniques that have been developed over the years for doing just this. However, it must be said that all these technologies are still in the process of development and there is not one system that can purport to measure the subtle energies of the body on all their levels and correlate them with the physical body.

Personally, as a practicing holistic medicine clinician I have had the opportunity of using many of these 'subtle energy measuring devices' –

even though these are not yet fully developed, it is better to get a broader understanding of at least some of the subtle energies that have been responsible for their health problems, as opposed to ignoring these completely. Let us look at some of these modalities that I mainly use in the DaVinci Natural Health Centre and am very familiar with – this is by no means a comprehensive list of all these measuring devices – it would take another book much thicker than this one to list them all. We will examine the Vegetative Reflex Test (VRT) using the VEGA machine, Bioresonance therapy using the BICOM and Rife frequency generators, Infrared Electric Light Sauna Therapy, healing with Low Intensity Lazer Therapy, using Orgone Energy in the Orgone Accumulator, identifying functional problems using Thermography as well as using the energy pathways of the hands and feet in Su Jok Therapies.

The Vegetative Reflex Test using VEGA

One system, which is beginning to grow in popularity among doctors and dentists, is a device known as the VEGA EXPERT VRT device (Fig 6), which was briefly mentioned in chapter 2.

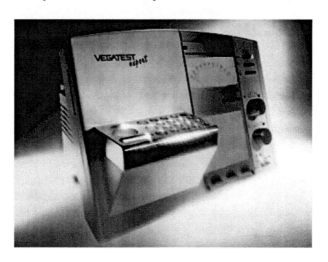

Fig 6 The VEGA VRT device

The VEGA Vegetative Reflex Test (VRT) represents an advanced development of the "Electroacupuncture according to Voll" (EAV)[23]

---

[23] Voll, R. The phenomenon of medicine testing in electro-acupuncture according to Voll. *American Journal of Acupuncture* 8:97-104, 1980.

concept. It features a combination of electronic measurements of skin resistance on specific energy meridian points (acupoints) that disclose vital health information through vegetative (autonomic) reflexes and resonances.

The VEGA device is capable of highlighting the causes of illnesses by using homeopathic bionosodes – this is usually a small portion of diseased tissue from a diseased organ that is ground up and made into a homeopathic remedy. When a particular bionosode that is placed on the honeycomb of the VEGA device induces a resonance reaction in the acupoint, then this infers a relationship between the diseased organ being tested and the related organ of the patient. If the patient does not have a diseased liver, for example, then they will not resonate with a bionosode of a diseased liver placed on the honeycomb of the VEGA device. Even bacteria, viruses, fungi, stealth organisms and more can be tested for resonance with the patient and identified much quicker than any other type of biological testing.

The Vegetative Reflex Test (VRT), or the VEGA bio-dermal testing can help the clinician in the following ways:

- ❖ Discovery of pathophysiologic processes that escape the standard clinical examination.
- ❖ Determination of the existence of focal infections.
- ❖ Determination of sub-clinical infections and energetic functional conditions in different quadrants of the body, as well as different organs.
- ❖ Condition of the immune system and of the immune- related tissues (spleen, thymus and lymph nodes).
- ❖ Determination of emotional stress and disturbances.
- ❖ Identification of the pathogenesis of disease (the root causes and where they began from with their interrelationships.
- ❖ Testing for allergies from environmental factors as well as food intolerances.

Personally, as a clinician, I have found the VEGA equipment very useful in the following cases and circumstances:

When all conventional diagnostic tests (physical and biochemical) reveal no clues to the cause of a patient's complaints, the disorders are most likely functional in nature rather than morphological. The VEGA reveals about 80% of the otherwise undiagnosable cases of migraines, backaches, chronic fatigue syndrome, systemic Candidiasis, bowel distention, IBS, Crohn's disease, sleep disturbance and more.

When conventional examination cannot fully or correctly explain the patient's complaints, the VEGA is highly indicative. It is superbly suited for the diagnosis of functional ailments (about 70% of all patients) and of clinically obscure, sub-clinical disorders. These make up about 20% of all indications.

Up-to-date experience shows that the VRT achieves the greatest rate of diagnostic success in cases of functional disturbances. This is presumably due to the physical basis of the VRT, a diagnostic system that utilizes the phenomenon of biological resonance.

There are about 40% of patients who have many symptoms but conventional laboratory tests yield negative results – these patients are often referred to psychologists or psychiatrists resulting in needless suffering and are a waste of time and money.

The VEGA VRT is capable of going beyond the diagnosis of energetic imbalance levels in particular systems. It is frequently capable of finding the actual causes of the energetic dysfunction, as well as potential cures for the disorders. The manner in which the VEGA Machine is able to carry out this type of analysis is a function of biological resonance.

Bioresonance Therapy

New methods are evolving all the time, which move us closer to the goal of individualized treatment. One such method, BIORESONANCE, also known as BRT (bioresonance therapy), practiced mostly in Germany for over a couple of decades now, can be used to treat a wide range of disorders. BRT has been tested and approved throughout Europe and Canada, and it is in use in 85 countries worldwide. In Germany, where it was developed by Regumed,[24] BRT has been in use for over 25 years.

Bio-resonance promises not only to address the unique needs of each patient, but also, as it becomes more widespread, to provide an answer to

---

[24] http://www.regumed.de

the nagging question: "Why do some individuals do well with one type of medication, while others improve only slightly or not at all?"

At the DaVinci Natural Health Centre we use the BICOM Bioresonance device (Fig 8). The patient's body signals are conducted from the right hand into the input of the device using a BICOM electrode. In the BICOM device the disharmonious frequencies are filtered out and inverted. These inverted therapeutic oscillations are now given back to the patient via the left hand using another electrode.

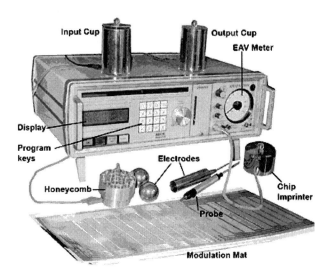

Fig 8 – BICOM Bioresonance Device

Central to its application is the idea that all life is made of energy. Although humans tend to think of themselves as relatively solid creatures, we are actually just a mass of compressed energy. We emit our own electromagnetic fields and, as with all things, we each have our own unique "vibration," or oscillation. This oscillation can easily be measured with electronic equipment. When we are healthy, our bodies produce a smooth, regular oscillation. When the body is under stress, the pattern becomes jagged and irregular.

The treatment of pathological oscillations is to return them back to the body in a modified form- in this case, as a mirror image. This action is based on the principle, as well-known in physics, that oscillations are influenced by their exact mirror image. Returning the oscillation to the patient in this modified form can diminish, or even eliminate, the pathological oscillations of the allergen or toxin, allowing the body's own healthy oscillations to become dominant. If the practitioner decides that medicine would also be useful in treatment, the oscillation of that specific medicine could also be returned to the patient.

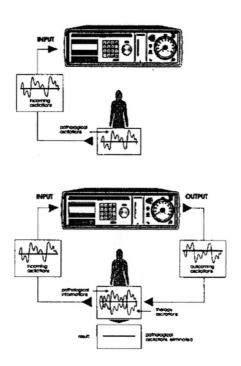

Fig 9 Returning Oscillations of the BICOM

These returning oscillations (Fig 9) help to balance the patient electromagnetically, and are again fed into the BICOM device for further analysis. The process is repeated constantly in fractions of a second. The pathological signals in the body are consequently reduced and finally extinguished, and the physiological endogenous regulatory forces can regulate the biological process unhindered.

There has been a lot of recent media coverage on exposure to electromagnetic fields causing illness by altering the bodies own electric "chemistry". However, practitioners of bio-resonance believe that the reverse is also true; healthy electrical signals transmitted into the body, in this case via hand-held electrodes, can re-harmonize it. In common with homoeopathy and acupuncture, bio-resonance aims to relieve the body of stress factors and improve its regulatory systems.

There is considerable ongoing research in the field of bioresonance and specifically using the BICOM device. One such study was conducted by Machowinski at the Naturopathy Outpatients Clinic of the Carsten's Foundation of the University of Heidelberg under the direction of Prof. Dr. med. I. Gerhard. It was a prospective, randomized controlled study with 28 patients suffering with chronic hepatocellular damage, as reflected by elevated laboratory values of hepatic enzymes such as GOT, GPT and gamma-GT. There were 14 patients in the treatment group using the BICOM and 14 in the control group not receiving any treatment.

On completion of the study the hepatic values of the BICOM-treated group were within normal limits, while the values of the control group were still within the pathological range with no change. The following table shows the percentage decrease in the values:

Hepatic values	Decrease towards normal of excess values (BICOM treatment)	Decrease towards normal of excess values (Control group)
GOT	42 %	4 %
GPT	50 %	5 %
Gamma-GT	38 %	7 %

In the treatment group, the geometric mean values for the degree of improvement were 45% for GOT values (5% for control group), 55% for GPT activity (control group displayed a slight deterioration) and the degree of improvement was 45% for gamma-GT activity (slight deterioration in the control group).

It is clear from the experimental evidence presented that treating minor hepatocellular damage with BICOM therapy in the frequency range between 10 Hz and 150 kHz can bring about reconstitution of damaged hepatic cells.

Infrared Electric Light Sauna Therapy

At the DaVinci Natural Health Centre many patients who are looking at facilitating their detoxification pathways will use the Infrared Sauna[25] (Fig 10) which is based on the energy of infrared light. Infrared electric light sauna therapy is one of the least costly, safest and most powerful ways to eliminate toxic metals, toxic chemicals and chronic infections. The benefits include:[26]

Skin rejuvenation – the skin is one of the largest detoxification organs of the body stretching over two square metres in total area – in most people it is congested, sluggish and toxic due to the use of synthetic clothing, bathing in chlorinated water and exposure to hundreds of chemicals.

Modulating the immune system[27]

Enhanced sweating – many of my patients when they first enter the infrared sauna simply do not sweat. This is an indication of a blocked autonomic nervous system (ANS) and is not a healthy sign. After a few treatments they begin sweating profusely as the ANS becomes activated and the skin begins to clear of heavy metals and toxic chemicals. It is the parasympathetic part of the ANS that is stimulated when using infrared sauna and it is this that facilitates the removal of toxins[28] – when sweating during exercise the sympathetic nervous system is activated which actually inhibits toxin elimination.

Exercise benefits - saunas provide many of the benefits of exercise with much less expenditure of energy. These include enhanced circulation and oxidation of the tissues. Repeated sauna use can lower elevated blood pressure and improve the elasticity of the arteries. Saunas are most helpful for cardiovascular rehabilitation, arthritis, allergies, skin conditions and chemical sensitivity.[29]

---

25 Kauppinen, K., et al. Man in the sauna, *Ann Clin Res.*, 18(4):173-185, 1986.
26 Molchanov, I.S. The effects of low intensity infrared radiation on the organism, *Gig Tr Prof Zabol.*, 12(11)(Nov):46-48, 1968.
27 Kukkonen-Jarjula, K., and K. Jkauppinen. How the sauna affects the endocrine system, *Ann Clin Res.*, 20(4):262-6, 1998.
28 Krop, J. Chemical sensitivity after intoxication at work with solvents: response to sauna therapy, *J Altern Complementary Med.*, 4(1)(Spring):77-86, 1998.
29 Flickstein, A., Infrared Thermal System for Whole-body Regenerative Radiant Therapy, Dascom Graphics, Santa Fe Springs, 1997.

Decongesting the internal organs - heating the body powerfully shunts blood toward the skin to dissipate heat. This decongests the internal organs and greatly stimulates circulation. Sinuses, joints and many other tissues benefit greatly.[30]

The infrared sauna that we use is an infrared electric light saunas which uses incandescent infrared heat lamps for heating. The infrared electric light sauna penetrates deepest, so the air temperature can stay coolest with the same effectiveness. Sweating begins faster and detoxification is increased. Preheating is less necessary, saving time and electricity. While some people like the intense heat of the traditional sauna, many find it difficult to tolerate, especially those who are ill.

The electric light sauna[31] as opposed to the ceramic type also provides the benefits of warming and stimulating colour therapy - red, orange and yellow assist the eliminative organs. Red helps clear the astral or emotional body. Everyone carries around emotional toxins that are every bit as harmful as physical toxins.

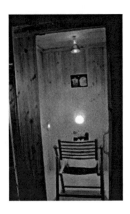

Fig 10 Infrared Sauna

Homeopathy

Homeopathy also works on the human energy system and is a very powerful healing modality when it is used correctly. The energy essence of

---

30 Inoue, S. and M. Kabaya. Biological activities caused by far infrared radiation, *Int J Biometeorol*, 33(3):145-50, Oct 1989.
31 Flickstein, A. Healthmate infrared saunas, *Townsend Letter for Doctors*, 202(May):66-70, 2000.

the homeopathic medicine carries a type of subtle-energy signature of a particular frequency. The homeopathic practitioner will skilfully match the frequency of the homeopathic medicine with the energetic needs of the patient in order to balance the energetic imbalances of the whole body. The physical body tends to resonate at a particular frequency, with minor diurnal and nocturnal variations.

Living tissues contain thousands of different kinds of molecules, each of which is surrounded by water.[32] Until recently, the medical use of direct body spectroscopy has been hampered by the fact that cell and tissue water absorbs the radiations one would like to study. The scientific question is what does the water molecules 'do' with the absorbed information. Do they convert it to random processes (heat)? Or do the water molecules do something more sophisticated? Can water molecules store molecular signatures? Can such information be conducted through the water system? Perhaps the troubling 'artifact' of water absorption actually explains how homeopathic dilutions and the body's water system absorb information from a substance.

In homeopathy, molecular signatures are transferred from a biologically active molecule to the water in which it is dissolved. This happens when the homeopathic physician 'succusses' the sample. Succussion is a method of vibrating or sending a shock wave through a solution. Dissolved molecules are made to vibrate intensely and coherently, and they therefore emit their electromagnetic signatures (emission spectrum).[33]

As Albert Szent-Gyorgyi pointed out, 'Water is the matter and the matrix, the mother and the medium of life.'[34] Without water, life as we know it would be impossible. Yet, water is more complex than the simple chemical formula H_2O suggests.

---

32 The plausibility of homeopathy: The systemic memory mechanism, *Integrative Medicine*. 1: pp. 53-59, 1998.
33 Nuclear magnetic resonance studies of succussed solutions, *Journal of the American Institute of Homeopathy*. 68: pp.8-16, 1975; Anomalous effects in alcohol-water solutions, *Review of Mathematical Physics*. 13: pp.10-12, 1975.
34 Gascoyne, PR, Pethig, R, Szent-Gyorgi, A. Water structure-dependent charge transport in proteins, *Proc NatL Acad. Sd.* USA, Vol. 78, No. 1, pp. 261-265, January 1981, Biophysics.

One plausible mechanism for water memory storage, published by Smith[35], is that hydrogen bonds hold water molecules together in a helical structure that acts like a coil. The magnetic components of fields emitted by the vibrating molecules induce current flows through the water helix. These currents reverberate within the water structure, much like the ringing of a tuning fork.

Even when the sample has been diluted to the point that the original molecule is gone, the signals stored in the water continue to vibrate for a long time.[36] Upon further dilution and succussion, the reverberating signals transfer to other water molecules used to dilute the sample.

At the DaVinci Natural Health Centre we use homeopathic remedies in different ways – from single remedies to strengthen the constitution of the person (whole body), to complex homeopathy where there are different homeopathics mixed together at different potencies (homaccords) – such as is given in homotoxicology. In addition, 'digital homeopathy' is also practiced, as postulated by Dr. Yurkovsky in his Field Control Therapy (FCT).[37]

This entails making homeopathic sarcodes (from healthy organs) or nosodes (from diseased tissue or fluids) or autoisodes (homeopathic remedies prepared from the person's own blood or other body fluid)   at the specific potency that the patient tests for, either through the VEGA diagnostics as mentioned above, or a form of kinesiology testing devised by Dr. Yurkovky that uses muscles in the ankles. Autonomic Response Testing (ART) can also be used to elicit the information. This novel approach to homeopathy really takes the guesswork out of prescribing the correct remedy at the right potency – the body will give this information willingly if you ask it!

There are a number of reasons for why homeopathy can be used to obtain excellent results with a number of "difficult" health issues:

---

35 Smith, CW. Quanta and coherence effects in water and living systems, *J Alt Complement Med* 10 pp. 69–7, 2004.

36 Smith, C. Electrical impedance and HV plasma images of high dilutions of sodium chloride, *Homeopathy*, volume 97, Issue 3, Pages 129-133, July 2008.

37 Yurkovsky, S. Biological, Chemical, and Nuclear Warfare: Protecting Yourself and Your Loved Ones: The Power of Digital Medicine. New York: Science of Medicine Publishing, 2003.

1. When used in low potencies or strengths, there are only extremely small amounts of the original toxins present that will do no harm but will antidote the original toxin in the body by cancelling out its resonant frequency.

2. In higher potencies above 26 C, the homeopathic remedy will contain only the energetic oscillations of the actual toxin that it was initially made from. It is this energetic aspect of the homeopathic remedy that will do the healing work in the body.

3. Homeopathic remedies can easily be prepared by anyone, even laypeople. This enables people to take charge of themselves, their children or other family members, without being dependent on outside help or wasting valuable time that can be crucial for their survival.

The homeopathic remedies offer unparalleled versatility as they can be prepared from contaminated air, water, food, clothing, or even body fluids when the disease process has already begun taking place within the body. This means that even in genetically engineered agents such as bacteria and viruses, it is possible to make a specific "energetic vaccine" against these agents, long before a drug vaccine can be discovered – this could be a life-saver.

In homeopathy, molecular signatures are transferred from a biologically active molecule to the water in which it is dissolved when the remedy is "succussed" or shaken rapidly. This facilitates the vibration of the molecules dissolved in the water so that they can emit their electromagnetic signatures onto the water molecules themselves. This is what is now known as "water memory storage" and does not contradict the laws of biology, physics and quantum mechanics in any way.

One plausible mechanism was postulated by Dr. Cyril Smith in 1985[38] is that hydrogen bonds act like a coil and hold water molecules together in a helical structure. These vibrating molecules emit electromagnetic fields through the water helix and place an "energetic stamp" of the same resonant frequency on them. This is why homeopathic remedies can be made into dilutions where there are no physical molecules left in the solution – beyond Avogadro's number of 10^{26} – and the signal stored in the water helix continues to vibrate for a long time after.

---

38 Smith, CW. Superconducting areas in living systems. In: Mishra, RK (ed), The Living State II. World Scientific, Singapore, pp. 404-420, 1985.

The basic principles of homeopathy can be summarized as follows:

1. The homeopathic approach utilizes minute quantities of medicinal substances to create therapeutic physiological changes through subtle-energy fields.
2. In homeopathic remedies, the energetic signature of the medicinal substance is first transferred to a solvent, such as water. It is the vibrational signature of the substance and not its molecular properties which are utilized for healing benefits.
3. In homeopathy, the more dilute a remedy's molecular concentration, the greater its potency. This is in direct contrast to the pharmacokinetic/drug model, in which there is a greater potency with higher molecular concentrations.
4. Homeopathy is based upon the Law of Similars, whereby a remedy is chosen for its ability to reproduce the symptoms of the sick person in a normal healthy individual. By matching the symptom complex of the patient with the known "drug picture" of the remedy, a correct "vibrational" match between patient and remedy is achieved in order to help the body balance energetically.
5. In homeopathy, a remedy is chosen for its ability to stimulate and rebalance the physical body through supplying a needed frequency of subtle energy. If the remedy's frequency matches the patient's illness state, a resonant transfer of energy will allow the patient's bioenergetic system to effectively assimilate the needed energy, throw off the toxicity, and move to a new equilibrium point of health.

This is a powerful healing modality that can be used successfully in the holistic model.

Low Intensity Lazer Therapy (LILT)

Light is another form of energy that can be very healing and can treat a myriad of conditions. One such technology that uses coherent light is the Low Intensity Laser Therapy (LILT)[39,40,] (Fig 11) which is very often used

---

39 Baxter G D, Diamantopoulos C, O'Kane S, Shields. Therapeutic Lasers Theory and Practice, Churchill Livingstone, New York, NY, 1997.
40 Pöntinen, PJ. Low level laser therapy as a medical treatment modality: A manual for physicians, dentists, physiotherapists and veterinary surgeons. Tampere: Art Urpo Ltd, 1992.

at the DaVinci Natural Health Centre. The device is a small rechargeable 300mW GaA1As laser, 830nm.

The way in which these devices work is really quite fascinating and the effects are both powerful and subtle. Visible light enhances cell proliferation through photochemical changes in the mitochondria, which then set in motion a chain of biological events that ultimately, affect cellular membranes. This, in turn, has an effect on messenger RNA synthesis, which ultimately leads to the observed enhancement of cell proliferation.

Tuner and Hode in their excellent and comprehensive book "Laser Therapy" [41] outline the various mechanisms that laser therapy uses in the body for wound healing and pain relief.

Specifically for wound healing this is the summary of events: the absorption of polarized light in cytochrome molecules such as porphyrins stimulates the creation of singlet oxygen. This increases the increase of ATP-ase and activation of cAMP and enzymes. This will trigger a further series of events such as the activation of macrophages, an increase of procollagen synthesis in fibroblasts, an increase of endothelial cells and keratinocytes, an increase in mast cells – all leading to wound healing.

The mechanisms for alleviating inflammatory processes are a little different: the electrical field across the cell membrane creates a dipole moment on the barshaped lipids, this influences the permeability of cell membranes, which effects Ca^{2+}, Na^+ and K^+ as well as the proton gradient over the mitochondria membranes. This increases serotonin levels in the blood and enhances S.O.D. levels which accelerates in healing of inflammatory processes.

As a consequence of physical changes in the membrane-pore, membranes open and close to let ions, such as calcium, in and out of the cell. Calcium ions act as intracellular messengers in many signal-transducing pathways. The cellular calcium ion concentration can be abruptly raised for signalling purposes by transiently opening calcium channels in the plasma or intracellular membranes.

---

[41] Tunér, J and Hode, L. Laser Therapy: Clinical practice and scientific background. Sweden: Prima Books, 2002.

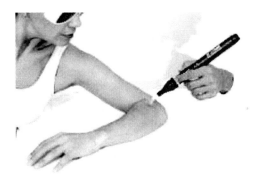

Fig 11 Treating a Patient with LILT

In LILT, Red (633nm) and infrared (830nm) have different effects on molecules. Red (visible) light can produce chemical changes while infrared radiation can only produce physical changes in molecules. In spite of this, both result in clinical improvement.

Specific types of molecules absorb specific wavelengths of light, both visible and infrared. Absorbed radiation produces specific biological effects in tissue, depending upon which types of molecules absorb the light.

Trelles et al[42] reviewed the use of local irradiation with LILT. They found this approach elicited the following types of effects: biostimulatory, analgesic, anti-exudative, anti-haemorrhagic, anti-inflamatory, anti-neuralgic, anti-oedematous, anti-spasmotic and vasodilatory (among others).

Trelles, et al, (1989) and Muxeneder, (1988) also reviewed the effects of LILT in vertebral pain, headaches and local immune responses. They found the main clinical uses included wound healing, pain control, soft tissue injury, arthropathy and osteopathy and treatment of existing scars. They observed local irradiation stimulated extremely rapid healing, even of extensive indolent superficial wounds. It was considered effective and safe. Scarring was minimal.

---

42 Trelles M A, Mayayo E, Miro L et al. The action of Low reactive Level Laser Therapy (LLLT) on mast cells: a possible relief mechanism examined. *Laser Therapy* 1: 27-30, 1989.

According to Mester, et al, (1985)[43] and Muxeneder, (1988),[44] the effects of LILT on wound healing are dramatic. They stated, "many irradiated septic wounds heal as if by first intention."

Having used LILT now for a number of years, I can honestly say that there is probably nothing to match the healing qualities that one sees in cases of swelling and inflammation in superficial muscles, tendons, ligaments, bursae and sheaths as well as skin healing properties[45] - these can all be alleviated by irradiation of the affected areas.

Old scars (surgical or traumatic) can act as trigger points if there are tender areas, keloid formation and adhesions along the scar. Such scars can be associated with chronic, reflex pain, lameness and autonomic effects. LILT of such tissue can produce dramatic clinical improvement in most cases. I also use it for tooth foci with no visible cause on Panoramic X-ray, after testing the teeth using ART – usually three treatments of the LILT is all that is required to alleviate these teeth foci.

Another powerful healing aspect of LILT is in pain relief, often a difficult problem for most practitioners to address. I have seen chronic pain of years duration literally melt away after only one or two LILT treatments – this is really astounding for these types of conditions.[46]

Orgone Accumulator

Some time ago I was reading about a famous revolutionary scientist who had been working with the human energy system back in the 1930's. He had discovered a natural form of energy present in the atmosphere that was

43 Mester E, Mester AF, Mester A. The biomedical effects of laser application. Lasers in Surgery and Medicine 5: 31-39, 1985.
44 Muxeneder R. The conservative treatment of chronic skin alterations of the horse via laser acupunture. *Praktische Tierarzt* Vol 69, Iss 1, 1988.
45 Baibekov, I.M., et al. The effects of low intensity infrared laser radiation on healing of dermatological wounds, *Bull Eksp Biol Med.*, 119(2)(Feb):218-24, 1994.
46 Wolley-Hart A. A handbook for low-power lasers and their medical application. East Asia, London, 1988.

later called Orgone Energy.[47] Wilhelm Reich was born March 24, 1897 in Dobryzcynica, Austria and died in 1957.[48]

In 1940, Wilhelm Reich[49] constructed the first device to accumulate Orgone energy: a six-sided box called an Orgone Accumulator,[50] (Fig 12) constructed of alternating layers of organic materials (to attract the energy) and metallic materials (to radiate the energy toward the centre of the box). Patients would sit inside the accumulator and absorb Orgone energy through their skin and lungs. The accumulator had a healthy effect on blood and body tissue by improving the flow of life-energy and by releasing energy-blocks.

Reich found that organic materials attracted and held orgone energy; and metal attracted and then rapidly repelled it.[51] By designing an enclosure, similar to the Faraday cage, lined on the inside with metal and made with alternating layers of organic and inorganic materials, he discovered that atmospheric orgone energy was accumulated and concentrated inside. He called this device an 'Orgone Energy Accumulator.'[52]

Within the box-like enclosure, the orgone energy given off by an inside metal wall is attracted to the opposite metal wall which again repels it. This creates an oscillation of the orgone energy particles inside. The layering of organic material with metal creates a higher concentration. He experimentally objectified this discovery by observing that the temperature inside an orgone accumulator was higher than inside a control device or outside air temperature.

Also, an electroscope which is a device that can be charged with "static" electricity, discharged more slowly inside of an orgone accumulator than outside. These two experiments confirmed that there was "something

---

47 Reich, W. The Discovery of the Orgone. IJSO, I, (article), (DO II), 1942.

48 Mann, EM. Orgone, Reich, & Eros. Simon and Schuster, 1973; Reich, W. Selected Writings. Farrar, Straus, and Giroux, 1973; Raknes, O. Wilhelm Reich and Orgonomy. Pengiun Books, 1970.

49 Reich, W. Experimental Demonstration of the Physical Orgone Energy. IJSO, IV, (article), (DO II), 1945.

50 The Orgone Energy Accumulator: It's Scientific and Medical Use. Orgone Institute Press, 1951.

51 Reich, W. Orgone Biophysics, Mechanistic Science, and 'Atomic Energy. IJSO, IV, 1945.

52 http://www.orgone.org/articles/ax2001-grnfld-aa.htm

different" about the atmosphere inside of an orgone accumulator that didn't conform to standard physics.

When a person uses an orgone accumulating device, the energy field of the user and the energy field of the device make contact, excite each other, and the two fields luminate, creating an even stronger charge. Since a human being has the higher energy charge, the user attracts and absorbs the energy from the accumulator into every part of their body. The increased absorption of the same bio-energy that is in the body helps the body to expand, thereby reducing the contractive state and promoting natural pulsation.

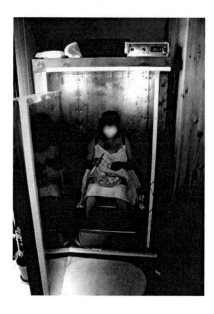

Fig 12 Orgone Accumulator with footbath

The restoration of the parasympathetic response improves the flow of blood to tissues and organs which allow them to function better, resist damage and recover easier from injury; it promotes cellular growth, eases tension and pain, assists digestion and peristalsis, improves appetite when this is impaired, increases core body temperature and can impart an emotional sense of well-being. The orgone accumulator helps the body to help itself by supplying concentrated orgone energy.

In studies using laboratory mice, Reich (and other researchers since) found that the orgone accumulator had a remarkable affect on wounds and burns.

In addition, because of the stimulation of the expansive parasympathetic response, the symptoms of "shock" could be affected.

Orgone energy accumulators can be used by almost everyone. However, Reich noted that people with certain blocked, high energy conditions should either be very cautious or not use an orgone accumulator. The contraindications include decompensated heart disease, high blood pressure, arteriosclerosis or heavy obesity, brain tumours, glaucoma, epilepsy or people who suffer from apoplectic attacks, ALS and MS.

Conditions that can worsen with orgone accumulator use are skin inflammations, rashes, and conjunctivitis.

Within the last twenty years, two double-blind experiments using orgone accumulators were performed at medical universities in Germany and Austria. The results confirmed some of Reich's findings: the subjects using the orgone accumulator recorded both higher core body temperatures and also, initially, a faster heart beat rate. In addition, most reported feeling a sense of well-being and various effects associated with a stimulation of the parasympathetic system.

After using an orgone accumulator for some minutes, warmth, relaxation and sometimes prickliness may be felt. The skin may flush and sweat develops. There is a feeling of a "soft glow", and of well-being. When these sensations are no longer felt, or there is a sudden urge to do other things, the session should end. Some people who have very low energy fields may take a month or more of use before they are recharged enough to feel these effects.

When using an orgone accumulator, a person wears as little clothing as is comfortable so that the energy can more easily penetrate the skin. However, being fully clothed is also just fine as the energy will penetrate the clothing, too; it will just take a little longer for the charge to build.

Ionizing Footbath

Another powerful detoxification tool that uses the human energy system is an ionizing footbath made by a company called Focus (Fig 13). Initially, before looking at this machine I was very sceptical but the DaVinci LifeSciences Research Centre was commissioned to examine how effective the Focus footbath was in removing mercury specifically. After testing a number of patients it was found that indeed the Focus ionizing footbath was capable of removing mercury from the soles of the feet. This captured my attention!

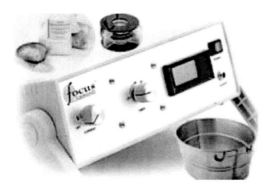

Fig 13 Focus Ionizing Footbath

The 'energetic footbath' is a process application of another medically approved process, Peritoneal Dialysis. This process uses osmosis to remove impurities from the body.

Osmosis is when molecules pass through a semi-permeable membrane like the skin on the soles of the feet – these molecules must be small enough to pass through the semi-permeable membrane, from a low osmotic potential to a higher osmotic potential.

The body's energetic field is stimulated, this tells the cells to release their toxins into the lymphatic system. The waste that is not drawn out, during the 35 minute process, will continue to be dumped into the lymphatic system and will be released during the body's natural elimination process. One can expect stronger urine and more stool from 3 to 5 days after having one 'energetic footbath'.

The addition of a small amount of Himalayan Salt into the footbath provides the electrolyte for the Exciter, as well as the immediate generation of ions. The Himalayan Crystal Salt was chosen because of its balanced crystalline structure, which can be easily metabolized by the body.

Once the Himalayan Salts are introduced into the bath water, the Na+ (sodium) and Cl- (chloride) separate to form negative and positive ions.

The Exciter is configured to maximize the negative ions in the solution. Negative ions will bind with some of the molecules it encounters, effectively giving them a negative charge. The negatively charged material will be attracted to and bound by a positive (or less negatively charged) element. The Exciter also creates two streams of bubbles (hydrogen and oxygen) while actively working within the water. This makes the water heavier, or dense, and accelerates the osmotic effects of the process.

Random samples of 18 clinical patients were used from the Davinci Natural Health Center in Larnaca, Cyprus.[53] These patients had all undergone pre-post provocation testing to determine whether there was mercury stored in their body – this was the case with all these patients. The mercury levels were measured on a PSA Atomic Fluorescence spectrometer, with detection levels of parts per billion.

Pre and post samples of water were taken from the footbath and analysed on the same AF spectrometer. The FOCUS footbath clearly showed that it can eliminate mercury from the body as in nearly all cases there was a mean percentage increase in the post-sample compared to baseline of 54.51% (range of 3.25 to 157.11 percent).

Regular use of the FOCUS bath can achieve:

- ❖ Cellular Cleansing
- ❖ Joint/ Pain Relief
- ❖ Clearer Skin Complexion
- ❖ Increased Circulation
- ❖ Reduced Swelling/Inflammation
- ❖ Activates body's natural elimination system, including lymph node

In 2005, Dr. Chaudhuri[54] conducted a pilot study using another ionizing footbath called the AquaDetox – he took 6 experimental subjects and 3 controls and used Heart Rate Variability (HRV) testing, Arterial Stiffness Indicator, blood pressure and pulse using an electronic meter which averaged 3 readings, meridian stress testing using the Avatar electro-dermal screening device employing the Energetix CMP 48 Point Probe Protocol, Live Blood Microscopy phase contrast and a pH and redox meter

---

53 www.docgeorge.com
54 Chaudhuri, S. *CAM*, Sept 2005, Vol. 5, Issue 2.

to ascertain changes in the treatment water and asked the test subjects to describe how they felt during and after the treatment.

Live Blood Microscopy demonstrated better flowing blood cells due to an improved charge distribution, while blood pressures fell, suggesting a reduction of peripheral resistance. The reduction in pulse, diastolic BP as well as improvement in arterial stiffness and HRV suggested a reduction in sympathetic nervous system activity.

Digital Infrared Thermal Imaging (DITI) or Thermography

The skin is a dynamic organ which under the control of the sympathetics is constantly adjusting to balance internal and external temperature conditions. Thermal imaging is the most efficient technique for the study of skin temperature distribution. By measuring bi-lateral anatomical sites and identifying significant changes thermal imaging is an objective non-invasive diagnostic modality.

The following has been taken from one of the leading manufacturers of thermal imaging – Meditherm:[55]

"Medical DITI (Fig 14) is a noninvasive diagnostic technique that allows the examiner to visualise and quantify changes in skin surface temperature. An infrared scanning device is used to convert infrared radiation emitted from the skin surface into electrical impulses that are visualised in colour on a monitor. This visual image graphically maps the body temperature and is referred to as a thermogram. The spectrum of colours indicates an increase or decrease in the amount of infrared radiation being emitted from the body surface. Since there is a high degree of thermal symmetry in the normal body, subtle abnormal temperature asymmetry's can be easily identified.

Medical DITI's major clinical value is in its high sensitivity to pathology in the vascular, muscular, neural and skeletal systems and as such can contribute to the pathogenesis and diagnosis made by the clinician.

Medical DITI has been used extensively in human medicine in the U.S.A., Europe and Asia for the past 20 years. Until now, cumbersome equipment has hampered its diagnostic and economic viability. Current state of the art

---

55 www.meditherm.com

PC based IR technology designed specifically for clinical application has changed all this.

Clinical uses for DITI include:

- ❖ To define the extent of a lesion of which a diagnosis has previously been made.
- ❖ To localise an abnormal area not previously identified, so further diagnostic tests can be performed.
- ❖ To detect early lesions before they are clinically evident.
- ❖ To monitor the healing process before the patient is returned to work or training.

Skin blood flow is under the control of the sympathetic nervous system. In normal people there is a symmetrical dermal pattern which is consistent and reproducible for any individual. This is recorded in precise detail with a temperature sensitivity of 0.01°C by DITI.

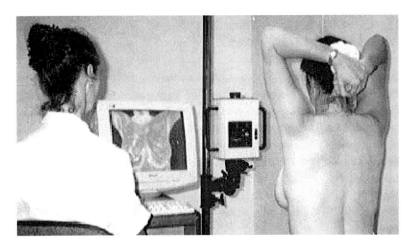

Fig 14 Medical Digital Infrared Thermal Imaging

The neuro-thermography application of DITI measures the somatic component of the sympathetic nervous system by assessing dermal blood flow. The sympathetic nervous system is stimulated at the same anatomical location as its sensory counterpart and produces a 'somato sympathetic response'. The somato sympathetic response appears on DITI as a localised area of altered temperature with specific features for each anatomical lesion."

The mean temperature differential in peripheral nerve injury is 1.5°C. In sympathetic dysfunction's (RSD/SMP/CRPS) temperature differentials ranging from 1° C to 10° C depending on severity are not uncommon. Rheumatological processes generally appear as 'hot areas' with increased temperature patterns. The pathology is generally an inflammatory process, i.e. synovitis of joints and tendon sheaths, epicondylitis, capsular and muscle injuries, etc.

Both hot and cold responses may co exist if the pain associated with an inflammatory focus excites an increase in sympathetic activity. Also, vascular conditions are readily demonstrated by DITI including Raynauds, Vasculitis, Limb Ischemia, DVT, etc.

Unlike most diagnostic modalities DITI is non invasive. It is a very sensitive and reliable means of graphically mapping and displaying skin surface temperature. With DITI you can diagnosis, evaluate, monitor and document a large number of injuries and conditions, including soft tissue injuries and sensory/autonomic nerve fibre dysfunction.

Medical DITI can graphically display the very subjective feeling of pain by objectively displaying the changes in skin surface temperature that accompany pain states.

Medical DITI can show a combined effect of the autonomic nervous system and the vascular system, down to capillary dysfunctions. The effects of these changes show as asymmetries in temperature distribution on the surface of the body – the grey and darker areas on the black and white image (Fig 15) would normally show as red on a colour thermogram.

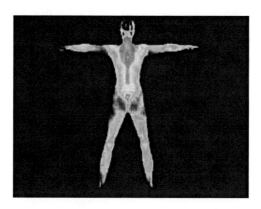

Fig 15 Temperature Distribution on Body with DITI

Thermal Imaging is particularly useful for the monitoring of treatment, whether surgical, physical or pharmacologic.

Inflammation is the precursor to many cancers and other degenerative diseases such as arthritis, heart disease, stroke, diabetes and high blood pressure. Early detection of inflammation using Thermography may help prevent many negative health conditions from developing.

Thermography specializes in: breast imaging,[56] pain diagnostics, early-stage disease detection – it can also visualize pain and pathology, and can assess pain and pathology anywhere in the body. It is very cost-effective, risk free and provides you with instant images.

X-rays, CT-scans, Ultrasound and MRI scans are all tests of 'anatomy' that are assessing the structure of the body - thermography on the other hand is unique in that it measures physiological changes and functioning of the body, not only structural issues.[57]

Thermography also plays an important role in heart disease prevention as it can assess heart functioning and detect inflammation in the carotid arteries which may be a precursor to stroke and blood clots. Early detection of heart problems can save your life!

Thermography can also be used in many other areas of health:[58]

1. Arthritis - can help in its early detection and can differentiate between osteoarthritis and rheumatoid arthritis.[59]

2. Neck and Back Problems[60] - pain and joint degeneration[61] appear very clearly on thermography scans and help to identify the source of the pain in the body.[62]

---

56 McKinna JA; The early diagnosis of breast cancer--a twenty-year experience at the Royal Marsden Hospital. *Eur J Cancer*, 1992.
57 Thomas D. Infrared thermographic imaging, magnetic resonance imaging, CT scan and myelography in low back pain. *Br J Rheumatol*, Aug 1990.
58 Yang WJ. Literature survey on biomedical applications of thermography. *Biomed Mater Eng*, Spring 1992.
59 Darton K. The use of infra-red thermography in a rheumatology unit. *Br J Rheumatol*, Aug 1990.
60 Devulder J. Infra-red thermographic evaluation of spinal cord electrostimulation in patients with chronic pain after failed back surgery. *Br J Neurosurg*, Aug 1996.

3. Dental Issues[63] - thermography can also detect TMJ, gum disease, infected teeth, NICOs and other dental issues that are precursors to many other serious diseases.

4. Sinusitis and Headaches - there is often a relationship between headaches and sinusitis - the thermography scan will show this very clearly.

5. Immune Dysfunction, Chronic Fatigue and Fibromyalgia - when there is inflammation detected by thermography in the Thoracic spine areas of T1 and T2 this correlates well with immune system dysfunction.

6. Carpal Tunnel Syndrome[64] - this is an often misdiagnosed condition - the thermography can help to identify the source of the pain which may be from the cervical spine.

7. Digestive Disorders - thermography can often see IBS, diverticulitis and Crohn's Disease and correlate these with other inflammatory issues in the body.

8. Other Health Issues - these would include bursitis, herniated discs, ligament and muscle tear, TMJ,[65] lupus, nerve problems,[66] whiplash, coronary artery disease,[67] cancer[68] and many others.

Breast thermography[69] (Fig 16) has an average sensitivity and specificity of 90%. An abnormal thermogram is 10 times more significant as a future

61 Greenstein D. Assessment of chemical lumbar sympathectomy in critical limb ischaemia using thermal imaging. *Int J Clin Monit Comput*, Feb 1994.
62 Pawl RP; Thermography in the diagnosis of low back pain. *Neurosurg Clin N Am*, Oct 1991.
63 Gratt BM. Future applications of electronic thermography. *J Am Dent Assoc*, May 1991.
64 Tchou S. Thermographic observations in unilateral carpal tunnel syndrome: report of 61 cases. J Hand Surg [Am], Jul 1992.
65 Gratt BM. Electronic thermography in the assessment of internal derangement of the temporomandibular joint. A pilot study. *Oral Surg Oral Med Oral Pathol*, Mar 1991.
66 Graff-Radford SB. Thermographic assessment of neuropathic facial pain. *J Orofac Pain*, Spring 1995.
67 Lawson W. Infrared thermography in the detection and management of coronary artery disease. *Am J Cardiol*, Oct 1993.
68 Sterns EE. Thermography as a predictor of prognosis in cancer of the breast. *Cancer*, Mar 1991.
69 Head JF. Breast thermography is a noninvasive prognostic procedure that predicts tumor growth rate in breast cancer patients. *Ann N Y Acad Sci*, Nov 1993.

risk indicator for breast cancer than a first order family history of the disease. A persistent abnormal thermogram carries with it a 22x higher risk of future breast cancer. An abnormal infrared image is the single most important marker of high risk for developing breast cancer.

Breast thermography[70] has the ability to detect the first signs that a cancer may be forming up to 2 years before any other procedure can detect it, mainly because it picks up the thermal patterns of the neovascularity (new blood vessels) that are commonly formed by most tumours in order to feed them.

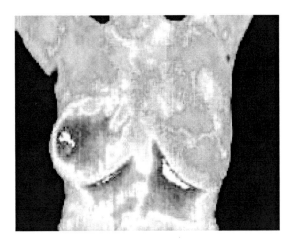

Fig 16 Breast Thermography

Research has shown that breast thermography significantly augments the long-term survival rates of its recipients by as much as 61%.[71] When used as part of a multimodal approach (clinical examination + mammography + thermography) 95% of early stage cancers will be detected.

Dr. Rife Technology

Another famous technology that uses the principle of energy medicine is the frequency generator invented by one of the most incredible geniuses of our time Dr. Royal Raymond Rife, who back in the 1930's had cured 16

70 Williams KL. Thermography in screening for breast cancer. *J Epidemiol Community Health*, Jun 1990.
71 Sterns EE. Thermography as a predictor of prognosis in cancer of the breast. *Cancer*, Mar 1991.

terminally-ill cancer patients with this electronic resonance device. This was an incredible feat, not only then, but also by today's standards. He had invented a Universal microscope[72] (Fig 17) with nearly 6,000 parts that could magnify up to 17,000x without killing the specimen - this is how he identified the cancer virus.[73]

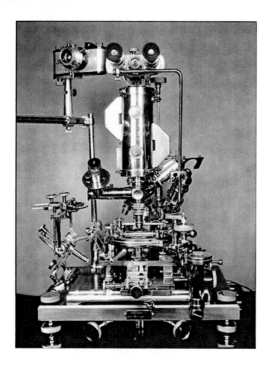

Fig 17 Universal Microscope

Royal R. Rife, born in 1888 (Fig 18), discovered that when a cell was exposed to some form of energy to which it is resonant, this energy would be absorbed by the resonant structure. Should the resonant energy be greater than the cell can effectively dissipate, Dr. Rife found that this cell would fail structurally, often resulting in cell death. A simple way to understand resonance is to think of an opera singer who can break a wine glass with her voice - the wine glass resonates at a certain frequency. If the opera singer can match that natural frequency with her voice, then the glass will absorb this resonant energy and smash.

---

72 Siedel, RE., Winter, EM. The New Microscopes, Annual Report, Smithsonian Institute, USA, pp. 193-220, 1944.
73 Annual Report of the Board of Regents of The Smithsonian Institution, 1944, The Rife's Microscope, The Smithsonian Report, 1944.

This simple principle can be applied to living organisms too, such as bacteria and viruses. This is what Dr. Rife managed to do - he discovered a resonant frequency that he called the mortal oscillatory rate (MOR) for over 55 major bacterial diseases. He also found the MOR for cancer after arduous years of experimentation using the sophisticated Universal microscope that enabled him to see micro-organisms live, without killing them by staining. Using this equipment he isolated the cancer virus that he called the "BX" virus.

In time, Rife was able to prove that the cancer micro-organism has 4 forms:[74]

1. BX (carcinoma)

2. BY (sarcoma - larger than the BX virus)

3. Monococcoid form in the monocytes of the blood of over 90% of cancer patients.

4. Crytomyces pleomorpha fungi

Rife wrote in his 1953 book: "Any of these forms can be changed back to the 'BX' within a period of 36 hours and will produce in the experimental animal a typical tumour with all the pathology of true neoplastic tissue, from which we can again recover the 'BX' micro-organism. This complete procedure has been duplicated over 300 times with identical and positive results'. There is no doubt that Rife was a perfectionist to the greatest degree.

---

74 Rife, RR. History of the development of a successful treatment for cancer and other virus, bacteria and fungi. Rife Virus Microscope Institute, San Diego, USA, 1953.

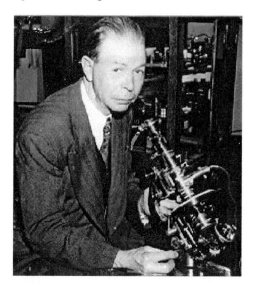

Fig 18 Dr. Rife with his Universal Microscope

What did Rife mean when he said that the other forms could be changed back to the 'BX' form? If we take what Pasteur has taught the world as the absolute truth, then no micro-organisms can change back to other types. Pasteur taught bacteriology based on Monomorphism - there is basically one micro-organism that causes each of the different diseases.

So, for every disease, there is a different bug. However, this is not what Dr. Rife and other researchers such as Beauchamp, Gaessens and Prof. Enderlein saw in their microscopes.[75] Using a darkfield condenser with an iris objective, they could see different forms changing in front of their own eyes. This went directly against Pasteur's theory of Monomorphism, to one of Pleomorphism.

It seems rather remote that all these researchers had reported seeing the same phenomenon of pleomorphism using their microscopes. It is also interesting that monomorphism - one bug for each disease - is still the paradigm that is taught in all medical schools around the world.

By using Live Blood Analysis, it is possible to show that the more toxic the internal mileau of the body, the more these micro-organisms change

---

75 Poehlman, Karl H. Synthesis of the Work of Enderlein, Bechamps and other Pleomorphic Researchers. Explore Vol. 8, No. 2, 1997.

forms to more and more virulent and pathological types which causes degenerative diseases. The ultimate stage would be the 'BX' virus that Rife has not only isolated, or some of the fungal micro-organisms that Prof. Enderlein and others have isolated and are found in over 90% of cancer patients.

As Rife declared in 1953: "These successful tests were conducted over 400 times with experimental animals before any attempt was made to use this frequency on human cases suffering from carcinoma and sarcoma."

In 1934, Dr. Rife opened a clinic, which successfully cured 16 of 16 cases within 120 days. Working with some of the most respected researchers in America along with leading doctors from Southern California, he electronically destroyed the cancer virus in patients, allowing their own immune systems to restore health. A Special Research Committee of the University of Southern California oversaw the laboratory research and the experimental treatments until the end of the 1930s. Follow-up clinics conducted in 1935, 1936 and 1937 by the head of the U.S.C. Medical Committee verified the results of the 1934 clinic. In his 1953 book, Dr. Rife wrote about the cancer clinics on December 3rd 1953:

"The first clinical work on cancer was completed under the supervision of Milbank Johnson, M.D. which was set up under a Special Medical Research Committee of the University of Southern California. 16 cases were treated at the clinic for many types of malignancy. After 3 months, 14 of these so-called hopeless cases were signed off as clinically cured by the staff of five medical doctors and Dr. Alvin G. Ford, M.D. Pathologist for the group.

The treatments consisted of 3 minutes duration using the frequency instrument, which was set on the mortal oscillatory rate for 'BX' or cancer (at 3 day intervals). It was found that the elapsed time between treatments attains better results than the cases treated daily. This gives the lymphatic system an opportunity to absorb and cast off the toxic condition that is produced by the devitalized dead particles of the 'BX' virus. No rise of body temperature was perceptible in any of these cases above normal during or after the frequency instrument treatment. No special diets were used in any of this clinical work, but we sincerely believe that a proper diet compiled for the individual would be of benefit."

Other members of the clinic were Whalen Morrison, Chief Surgeon of the Santa Fe Railway, George C. Dock, M.D., internationally famous, George

C. Fischer, M.D., Children's Hospital in New York, Arthur I. Kendall, Dr. Zite, M.D., professor of pathology at Chicago University, Rufus B. Von Klein Schmidt, President of the University of Southern California.

Dr. Couche and Dr. Carl Meyer, Ph.D., head of the Department of Bacteriological Research at the Hooper Foundation in San Francisco were also present. Dr. Kopps of the Metabolic Clinic in La Jolla signed all 14 reports and knew of all the tests from his personal observation.

Independent physicians utilizing the equipment successfully treated as many as 40 people per day during these years. In addition to curing cancer and other deadly diseases, degenerative conditions such as cataracts were reversed. Rife had been able to determine the precise electrical frequency that destroyed individual micro-organisms responsible for cancer, herpes, tuberculosis, and other illnesses. His work was described in Science magazine, medical journals, and later the Smithsonian Institution's annual report.[76]

Unfortunately, Rife's scientific theories and method of treatment conflicted with orthodox views. His work was stopped and both the research and the treatments were forced underground. The AMA took him and his associates to court - this trial would start Rife on a long road of deterioration, alcoholism and depression .... as the deaths from cancer mounted year after year. While the court case was taking place (and afterwards), the AMA visited all the doctors involved. Those who didn't stop using the Frequency Instrument would lose their medical license.

One of his main co-supporters Milbank Johnson died under mysterious circumstances (possibly poisoned), and records of Rife's work were destroyed. No medical journal was ever permitted to print Rife's work, except one by the Franklin Institute that slipped by the censors. In 1946, Rife's problems forced him to sell off his laboratory piece by piece.

Doctors secretly continued curing cancer patients for 22 years after the original success of the 1934 clinic, but always with opposition from medical and governmental authorities. However, from 1950 to the mid-1980s, a number of research scientists, working independently, have slowly been verifying the scientific principles upon which Rife's clinical cures of the 1930s were based. A body of recognized scientific evidence now overwhelmingly supports the original cancer theories articulated and

---

76 Lynes, B. 1992. The Cancer Cure that Worked. Marcus Books, Ontario, Canada.

demonstrated by Rife 50 years ago. This includes modern AIDS researchers.[77]

Autonomic Response Testing (ART)

The autonomic nervous system (ANS) is the part of the nervous system that we cannot control with our mind. The ANS regulates breathing, heart rate, digestion, immune function, sleep patterns, hormone regulation, blood pressure, blood sugar levels, tissue regeneration, and liver and kidney detoxification. Even though the autonomic nervous system is the chief regulator of most functions of the body, the electrocardiogram is a common test to measure how the ANS is working. The electrocardiogram measures the rate and rhythm of the heart.

Autonomic Response Testing (ART) grew out of the importance of detecting and correcting problems of the autonomic nervous system. ART allows the doctor to correct the problems of the ANS and to help restore the self regulating mechanism of the body allowing the patient to return to a state of health. Autonomic Response Testing (ART) is a system of evaluation and treatment developed by Dietrich Klinghardt, MD, Ph.D[78] and Louisa Williams, DC, ND. Dr. Klinghardt is a German trained physician who also has a Ph.D in neurology. ART uses Applied Kinesiology, Electroacupuncture (EAV), O-Ring testing, Nogier pulse, Chinese pulse, heart rate variability and other techniques to assess the health or dysfunction of the autonomic nervous system.

Dr. Klinghardt believes that many practitioners using kinesiology or muscle testing in their practice are often getting inaccurate information because the autonomic nervous system is not functioning properly. In ART, this condition is called 'blocked regulation' and refers to the inability of the ANS to self-regulate and is caused by 7 common factors. These include: undiagnosed food allergies, heavy metal toxicity, petroleum chemical toxicity, chronic unresolved infections and scars, temporomandibular joint dysfunction (TMJ), unresolved psychological

---

77 Watts, D. Resonant Frequencies – Anti-Viral, Anti-bacterial, Use in Healing. Proc. World Congress on Cancer Aust, April 1994.
78 http://www.klinghardtneurobiology.com

stress, and electromagnetic stress. Dr. Klinghardt has developed specific tests for these factors and treatments to correct them. [79]

There are many issues that can block the ANS such as jewellery, spectacles, quartz watches, beepers, food allergies, psychological issues, spiritual issues, dehydration, nutritional deficiencies, heavy metals, infections, geopathic fields, electromagnetic, synthetic clothing, underwire bras, cell phones, pagers, malocclusion, structural problems, visible scars, tattoos, reverse organ spin, solvents, pesticides, herbicides, toxic nerve ganglia, man-made prosthesis and visual issues.

The basic premise behind ART is to identify accurately that which is causing a stress on a persons system. This is its first mode of application. Thereafter it is also possible to use ART to monitor the effects and changes to the ANS from any prescribed treatment to the findings of the ART diagnosis. This provides and accurate and reliable double edge sword of both diagnostic and treatment therapy.

During the first visit, a doctor using ART will evaluate the patient with special attention on identifying any of the factors that are blocking a patient's ANS regulation. This is accomplished through a review of the patient's medical and dental history and a physical exam that includes kinesiology and nervous system evaluation. Once the blockages have been identified, the doctor will choose a treatment plan that will correct these problems. The "direct resonance phenomenon" also allows the practitioner to scan the body for specific infections, toxins and other "invisible" problems.

A typical visit may reveal that a patient has severe wheat allergies, heavy metal toxicity from the mercury in their teeth, and a scar from a past appendix surgery that are all causing stress on the ANS. The primary treatment for this patient would include scar therapy (using neural therapy, wheat germ oil, or cold laser), dietary advice to avoid wheat and gluten grains, and a referral to a biological dentist to replace the mercury fillings with a bio-compatible material. In addition, the doctor may prescribe natural remedies including homeopathic drainage, vitamins, minerals, herbs, essential fatty acids, amino acids, exercise, meditation etc.

---

79 Klinghard, D, William, L: Autonomic Response Testing, manual, American Academy of Neural Therapy, Seattle, WA, 1996.

A great degree of accuracy is possible with ART. It will even uncover sub-clinical health issues that are not detectable by standard blood tests but may be causing symptoms in the patient. Now with ART, the educated guess is no longer necessary. ART is the finest natural method of guiding the health practitioner to the root of the problem.

ART is different from other forms of muscle testing in that it uses the latest findings of quantum and biophotonic physics to aid in the assessment of the body. This allows for a much deeper level of testing not available before to traditional kinesiologists. Tools such as a polarization filter and signal enhancers are used to get stronger, clearer feedback from the body. ART often finds things that are missed with traditional kinesiology. ART practitioners in general also have the ability to test for a wider variety of root causes of illness, including specific infections, toxins, and emotional disturbances.

ART is used along with traditional tests to determine the root causes of illness. It is not used to diagnose diseases.

ART has been shown to be the most accurate of all kinesiology techniques, with the best reproducibility and inter-examiner reliability.

Su Jok Therapy

Many people are familiar with energy healing modalities such as acupuncture, electroacupuncture or acupressure (shiatsu, reflexology), but not with Su Jok therapy[80]. In an ingenious way, Professor Park Jae Woo[81], a Korean philosopher and scientist, discovered a unique healing method to heal with hands and feet that is easy to apply – we were fortunate to have him as our professor and mentor here on the island of Cyprus that he so much took to.

He demonstrated zones or points on the feet and the hands which are connected to, and have correspondence with, all organs and tissues of the body[82] (Fig 19). There are also other micro systems such as each finger or toe corresponding to all parts of the body[83] (Fig 20). Pathological changes in the organism manifest as abnormalities of these zones or points.

---

[80] Park, JW. A Guide to Su Jok Therapy. Su Jok Academy Publishers, Moscow, 2001.
[81] http://www.smilesujok.com/63083/Prof Park--Jae-Woo
[82] Park, JW. Su Jok for Everybody. Moscow Su Jok Academy, 2000.
[83] Park, JW. Fingertoe Therapy. Su Jok Academy, Moscow, 2002.

Manipulating these areas in various ways, can bring on significant healing effect. In this, Su Jok's underlying philosophy is similar to acupuncture and reflexology.

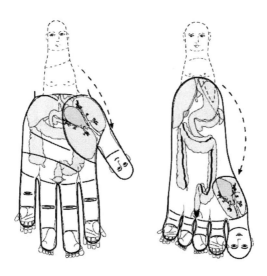

Fig 19 Su Jok – Hand and Foot Basic Correspondence Systems

By finding the "pressure-pain" points on the hand and foot that correspond to the pain in the body, it is possible to stimulate these points of correspondence using a variety of techniques to cure the pain or health problem in question. Since the hand is Yang and the foot is Yin, using hand and foot makes it possible to treat in harmony with Yin and Yang.

We have four clinics on our bodies - 2 hands and 2 feet that can help to cure over 90% of our health problems, if we understand their topography and use it accordingly. This correspondence system opens new understandings and methods to care for human health in general as well as to prevent and cure specific diseases. Knowledge of the principles of this "remote control system" and their health implementation through hand and foot therapy provides an impressive vehicle for health care.

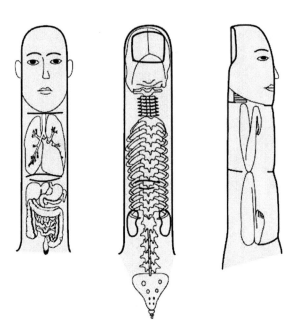

Fig 20 Fingertoe Correspondence Systems

This system of medicine created by Prof. Park is called "Onnuri medicine[84]" – Onnuri stands for the "whole world" as this method covers a number of therapies that are truly holistic. This system of medicine is based on a number of premises such as the Homo-Hetero theory, Triunit theory (Neutro, Hetero and Homo), Six-Origin theory (Six-Ki theory, emotion and reason theories), Eight-Origins theory, and H-particle theory. All these theories come together in the ultimate Diamond energy system that embraces the fundamental laws governing all creation. The Diamond energy system has the capacity to link all the dimensions of all the energy systems together to form a single, unified framework incorporating the core meridians, chakras, border meridians, energy gateways (external chakras) and the 12 meridians of the body and their energy gateways (points). On the strength of this integrated energy system it has become possible to deal with a diverse range of health issues.

There are many correspondence systems to be found in the Homo-system of the human body such as the fingertoe correspondence systems and their therapy (acupuncture); hand and foot correspondence systems and their

---

84 Park, JW. Onnuri Su Jok Therapy. Su Jok Academy Publishers, Moscow, 1999.

reflexotherapy and acupuncture (Su Jok Acupuncture). There are also a myriad of other correspondence systems such as the auricular (ear), limbs, trunk and many more.

When the precise correspondence points are found and stimulated, there is almost always an immediate response of the patient within seconds to a few minutes. The relief of pain is incredibly fast, no matter what the aetiology may be. There is no other natural method of treatment known today that has such a dramatic and efficient effect on pain conditions.

The identified correspondence points can be stimulated in various ways: small micro-needles, natural seeds[85] (good for children and infants), grains, natural stones, artificial stimulators such as metal and magnet stars of various shapes that have been specially designed for Su Jok treatments, rubber bands for haemorrhaging and ball bearings or Tsu balls.

Moxa (heat treatment) can also be used for weakened patients, as well as light impulse devices, solar therapy using the sun's rays or simple plant twigs or other parts of a plant. The therapist can also use metal rollers for more general stimulation of many points and Cayenne plasters to deal with coldness conditions. There are numerous combinations, which can be given to the patient to do as part of the home treatment programme.[86]

There is also a whole system of Su Jok Therapy that has been formulated, and can be used in emergency cases such as heart attacks, external and internal bleeding, and others.[87] The hand is literally a complete hospital with many departments that are on standby to deal with any situation as it arises.

Knowing the exact correspondence points on the hands will enable any practitioner to quickly and effectively stimulate these points using a simple probe, which can be carried easily in your pocket. The beauty of Su Jok Therapy is that it can be practiced without any equipment or remedies anywhere, anytime with anyone. Indeed, in India where there are many Su Jok Therapists, each doctor can see and treat up to 300 patients per day with minimal cost! There are no limitations to the combinations of techniques that can be used effectively - the only restriction will be the creativity of the practitioner.

---

85 Park, JW. Su Jok Seed Therapy. Su Jok Academy, Moscow, 2000.
86 Park, JW. Being Your Own Su Jok Doctor. Su Jok Academy, Moscow, 2002.
87 Park, JW. Su Jok in Emergency. Su Jok Academy, Moscow, 2002.

In emergencies Su Jok Therapy is very fast and effective, and where the therapist does not have a probe they can use keys, branches of trees, nails, stones - I have even used chop sticks and a pencil effectively, even in an airplane! For example, with cardiac cases, a simple massage of the correspondence area of the heart will alleviate pain in minutes. After the initial massage, if there are blood vessel contractions, moxa can be used to effectively relax the blood vessels.

With internal haemorrhage, the therapist can use a rubber band around the correspondence area, as well as stimulating this area using a probe. When there are skin burns it is possible to find and stimulate the correspondent points until the pain decreases, as well as use black seeds to reduce heat, followed by green seeds to help repair the skin. In acute appendicitis, simply find the correspondence points and stimulate them. With kidney stones and colic the therapist can use moxa on the kidney correspondence area, as well as using red kidney beans (the more similar, the more powerful the therapy). Acute coughing can be stopped in minutes by stimulating the "coughing area" of the fingers.

PAPIMI

The PAP Ion Magnetic Inductor or PAPIMI[88] was developed by and named after Greek professor Dr. Panos Pappas now at the Piraeus Technical University in Greece. In 1984 he began working with a colleague on a high-current research project in the laboratories of the Massachusetts Institute of Technology. The device uses a powerful magnetic field to penetrate all over the body, passing right through the skin into the deepest tissues. The pulsing magnetic field is present there only briefly, but with great intensity.

His colleague and close friend was diagnosed with an inoperable cancer with less than three month survival prognosis, but continued to work on the plasma physics project which involved repeated daily, electrical arcing that occurred with the sudden opening of massively high-current circuits in the catastrophic heat failure of various conductors. After finishing the project and returning to Greece, Professor Pappas was astonished to learn that at last examination his friend's cancer had entirely disappeared without a trace. In discussing this phenomenon, they considered that exposure to repeat arcing may have caused this remission.

---

88 www.papimi.com

Prof. Papas decided to return to the drawing board and continuing with animal studies - he found that tumours implanted in laboratory animals consistently shrank and disappeared when exposed to the electromagnetic field pulses of the device he had built for that purpose. In view of a long series of successful animal trials, and as no adverse effects were noted in either the experimental animals or controls, Pappas offered his PAPIMI device for the experimental treatment of human cancer patients at the Papanikolaou Oncology Research Center of the Hellenic Anticancer Institute.

The first of these was perhaps the most dramatic example of what was to follow. In 1990 the patient presented in extremis with stage IVa uterine cancer, vaginal fistula, lymph nodes and severe abdominal haemorrhage, and was not expected to survive. With no other therapy than six months of treatments with the prototype PAPIMI (which has since been greatly improved), she became the only patient in her hospital's records with similar complaints that was discharged in a cured and healthy state.

In continuing to treat more patients, many of whom had other medical problems, some surprising new discoveries began to emerge. In one such patient, the ugly, painful, swollen knuckles of rheumatoid arthritis were visibly reduced in size during a single treatment and the pain disappeared. In another patient with a detached retina in one eye the retina re-attached spontaneously without any other treatment.

An open wound healed with unprecedented speed, and new scar tissue was replaced with normal, healthy cells. An AIDS patient treated for Kaposi's sarcoma suddenly acquired new energy, appetite and an increasing T-cell count. Bacterial infections and even such parasites as tape worms and hook worms were found to disappear with PAPIMI treatments, and new anecdotal reports of such coincidental cures and pain relief continue to come in from wherever the non-invasive PAPIMI devices are used.

Such dramatic evidence of the safety and efficacy of the PAPIMI quickly won official approval of its use in Greece, the European community and Canada. But puzzling questions remained as to how the PAPIMI's short, powerful bursts of magnetic energy could effect such rapid healing and pain relief. In particular, there was the apparent paradox of how they could cause cancer cells and infectious organisms to die on the one hand, and renew vital energy to normal cells on the other. These mechanisms had to be reasonably explained before Professor Pappas' novel therapeutic device would be accepted by the medical and scientific community.

For this reason, he spent three years of sabbatical leave in the U.S. for the vast medical literature and research resources now available to us. His constant and diligent efforts succeeded in developing the evidence to support the explanations and theories, which were used in applying for international patents on the PAPIMI (Fig 21) that have since been granted by many countries, including the U.S.A.

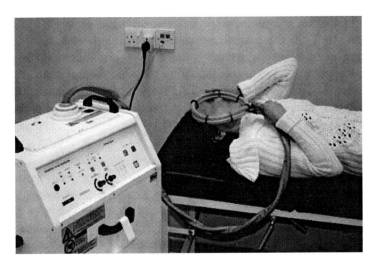

Fig 21 Patient being treated with the PAPIMI for sinusitis

So how does the PAPIMI work? When the probe of the device exposes a tissue, its magnetic field spreads and penetrates into this tissue, like it does not receive any resistance. The penetrating magnetic field changes rapidly. It develops and disappears in a short period of time leaving a cyclic electric field that can penetrate deeply into tissues.

The PAPIMI pulses activate the molecules, and can cause a Nuclear Resonance and Excitation effect. As the pulses are of very short duration they do not contribute to a heating effect of the cells which could cause some type of damage.

The Biological Nuclear Reaction of the French Researcher Louis C. Kervran:[89]

$$11Na\ 23 + 8O16 + energy = 19K39$$

This implies that Sodium plus Oxygen plus (Magnetic) Energy nuclearly transmutes into Potassium.

However, this process is known in biology as the Sodium and Potassium Pump, which is wrongly assumed to be an exchange and not a nuclear transmutation. It is wrongly assumed that Potassium continuously enters in to the cells and Sodium continuously comes out of the cells, which are obviously two impossible processes!

This nuclear process is accomplished with a low heat, in a low rate of thermal decomposition, which is the most important, and the same time, the most commonly found phenomenon of Nuclear Fusion in Biology.[90]

All of the many types of living cells that make up the tissues and organs of the body are tiny electrochemical units. They are powered by a "battery" that is continually recharged by the cells' metabolic chemistry in a closed loop of biological energy.

We are concerned here with that battery, which consists of the membrane that surrounds the cell. The electrical charge, or voltage across the membrane of a normal, healthy cell varies from about 70 to 100 millivolts; this is called the Trans Membrane Potential, or TMP.

When a cell is poisoned, damaged, deprived of nutrients or infected, energy is lost in fighting the problem and the TMP falls to a level where the cell loses its vitality and either struggles to heal itself or dies. The PAPIMI is capable of raising the TMP of sick or damaged cells into a normal range, thus restoring their bio-energy, facilitating the exchange of potassium and sodium ions (the Na/K pump) and restoring their normal rate of production of ATP which fuels the entire process. Normal healthy cells are not adversely affected by PAPIMI because, as in recharging any

---

89 Kervran, CL. Biological Transmutations. Happiness Press, 1980 (Reprinted 1998).
90 Vysotskii, V.I., Kornilova, A.A., and Samyolenko, I.I. Experimental Discovery and Investigation of the Phenomenon of Nuclear Transmutation of Isotopes in Growing Biological Cultures," Infinite Energy, 2, 10, 63-66, 1996.

battery, the membrane-batteries of living cells in particularly will not accept an overcharge.

Put in terms of physical chemistry, rather than biological terms, another parallel phenomenon appears to occur: the acceleration of adenosine triphosphate (ATP) synthesis and other aspects of the cell's biochemical anabolism. The electrons drawn to the inner membrane by elevating the TMP increase the ionic charge in the interior. This raises the internal degrees of freedom at a molecular level, catalyzing dormant biochemical reactions that would not otherwise proceed as quickly due to lack of available energy. Entropy is reduced and the cell's metabolic rate increased, enabling the cell to heal itself and attain an optimum functional level.

Medical literature over the past few decades offers ample proof that the induction of tiny currents of electricity is remarkably effective in healing, regenerating and revitalizing cells damaged by trauma.[91] Many of the earlier techniques developed from this research involved implanting fine electrodes at the boundaries of the injured tissue, and causing a tiny current to flow through the affected area from low-voltage batteries. Subsequently, it was found that these healing currents could also be induced by relatively weak magnetic devices placed close to the trauma and kept there for days or weeks.[92]

Thus the healing effects of micro-currents generated or induced in the conductive pathways of the body have been well established and this application is an accepted clinical procedure.

There remained for Professor Pappas to discover that a weak pulsed magnetic field, hundreds of times faster than had ever been used, applied for a millionth of a second at a time within a frequency spectrum never before used in medical devices, could accomplish much more within a few minutes what other stronger magnetic induction devices required days or weeks to affect - and to do so with much more efficient and far-reaching therapeutic results.

---

91 Adey, WR. 1990. Electromagnetic fields and the essence of living systems: modern radio science. Oxford University Press, Oxford.
92 Becker, RO. 1990. Cross currents: the perils of electopollution, the promise of electromedicine. Jeremy P. Tarcher, Los Angeles, CA.

Using this electromagnetic process for healing is simple. You place the treatment probe (the loop) on whichever part of the body that has a problem and keep it there for about eight minutes. Standard protocols recommend the usage of the machine for three such sessions per day.

What are some of its technical specifications? The device produces a train of extremely short bursts of very high frequency oscillations by periodically exciting a gaseous plasma chamber at its natural resonant frequency.

Special precision circuitry in the PAPIMI makes each burst or pulse of oscillations last 0.1 microseconds in duration by a thyratron-type of control. The nanosecond rise and decay time of each pulse of oscillations is so steep that a wealth of third order harmonics are generated in each pulse, which makes it difficult to characterize the resulting pulse frequency as other than an effectively narrow but complex frequency spectrum.

The remarkable aspect of this novel plasma-resonance method of generating such pulses of radio frequency energy is the extremely high amplitude (on the order of many kilovolts) they attain, resulting in massive current flow through the low-impedance load circuit. In this respect, and also by virtue of its complex frequency spectrum, the PAPIMI is unique among the large family of Pulsed Electromagnetic Field (PEMF) devices of which it is a member.

Also, unlike other PEMF devices that produce continuous trains of much wider and more closely-spaced, heat-generating pulses at MHz rates in a "woodpecker" effect, the pulse repetition frequency of the PAPIMI is extremely low with relatively very long intervals between pulses. Variable control circuits output pulses of the PAPIMI to between two and five pulses per second at most therapeutic settings.

For this, and another reason connected with the manner in which the energy is delivered, the PAPIMI has little or no heating effect on living tissue; it is considered to be an athermal PEMF device capable of delivering an effective and beneficial form of bio-energy to living cells.

It is noted that in over 100,000 PAPIMI treatments for a variety of medical problems, no adverse effects or incidents have been reported in patients or in technicians exposed to PAPIMI pulses for many hundreds of hours a year.

This device can aid any disease process. It has been proven valuable in chronic diseases where micro blood circulation is significantly impaired. Based on my experience, few, if any, medical devices have the penetration power of this machine and can access deep and chronic problems with tissues and bones. It is phenomenally beneficial for stimulating and regenerating any part of the skeleton. It has also been found miraculous in the healing of bone fractures.

Hermann Maier, the world champion Austrian alpine skier, nicknamed the "Herminator" for his strong, fearless skiing, had a terrible motorcycle accident in 2001 that almost severed his leg. Doctors and laypersons alike feared he would never walk again. He started PAPIMI treatments early January 2003, after recommendations from his doctors.

Two weeks later, he started ski racing again for the first time. His comeback became the sensational news in Europe. To the disbelief of both the medical profession and the enthusiasts of the winter sport, Maier returned to professional skiing in 2003, and a year later he was crowned world champion again.[93] This was one of the biggest sensations in Austria and Western Europe.

Prof. Pappas is certain the PAPIMI was the only reason for Maier's recovery. To this day, the medical community remains bewildered by the event. Few bothered to investigate in depth this extraordinary demonstration of healing.

Here are a few case examples of patients that were treated only by the PAPIMI at the DaVinci Natural Health Centre in Cyprus:

Case 1 (26-year old female) – Pain of 6-month duration in the external part of the ear which disappeared after only 3 PAPIMI treatments (100% cure).

Case 2 (51-year old male) – Presbyopia for 3 years wearing +1.75 glasses completely cured (100% cure) after only one treatment of the PAPIMI – has been without glasses now for 2 months and can read font style 8 clearly close-up. Also treated chronic haemorrhoids requiring surgery in only one treatment.

---

93 http://www.papimi.gr/herman_maier.htm

Case 3 (44-year old male) – this man was diagnosed with Multiple Sclerosis (MS) in 1991 and had many symptoms when recently seen such as loss of sensation on both hands (40%), pain in the back of the head (85%), sinusitis (40%), short-term memory loss (37%), loss of balance (100%) and his clarity of thinking was diffuse (50%). He also walked very slowly, could not carry any shopping baskets and had a general depression and apathy. The percentages above indicate the percentage improvement in these symptoms after 12 treatments on the PAPIMI within 15 days. His wife also reported that he walked much quicker – he was now 50 metres ahead of her, instead of being 200 m behind, and his apathy and depression had converted to enthusiasm and excitement for life. His energy levels were much improved.

Case 4 (45-year old female) – this lady presented with pain in the gums and mouth after major dental surgery for periodontal disease, as well as a painful cyst on the sclera of the eye. In only 3 PAPIMI treatments the acute dental pain had completely subsided (100% improvement) and the pain in the eye cyst had disappeared completely with a shrinking of the cyst. Her dental surgeon commented on the rapid healing of the mouth after surgery and said that he had not seen such rapid healing in his entire career.

Case 5 (56-year old female) – this lady presented with a number of symptoms related to connective tissue and cartilage degeneration, as well as dizziness (100%), burning sensation of stomach (66%), thoracic back pain (57%), numbness in the right foot (70%), Sjogren's syndrome (a chronic, inflammatory, autoimmune disorder characterized by dry mouth (xerostomia) and dry eye (keratoconjuctivitis sicca) – there is no known allopathic cure for this disorder), (70%), difficult and painful movement in the right arm (80%), pain in knee related to related to severe degeneration of the lateral meniscus with displacement of the fragments (40%). These percentage improvements were achieved with only 10 PAPIMI treatments, but the most striking improvement was for the incurable Sjorgen's Syndrome which was considered incurable by top ophthalmic surgeons in Israel and Cyprus. A recent assessment by an ophthalmic surgeon showed a dramatic improvement – this attracted the attention of the surgeon who has booked an appointment at the Centre to investigate this phenomenon.

Case 6 (34-year old) – diagnosed with Multiple Sclerosis in 1998. Had a total of 6 PAPIMI treatments, with the following percentage improvements in neck pain (100%), pain in left shoulder (28%), pain in shoulder blade (57%), pain in maxillairy sinuses (66%), pain above eyes (100%), burning and itching in the left hand (60%), weakness in the left arm (62%) and general energy levels increased by 60%. He continues to have maintenance sessions of about one weekly and has not seen an MS relapse in over a year.

Perhaps one remarkable case that has been documented by Dr, López Peral and reported by Laurent Schidler on 23/01/2007 was of a woman with breast cancer who began PAPIMI treatments – average of 20 monthly sessions, 18 minutes duration each session. An X-ray also showed bone necrosis in the upper jaw (see Fig 22 – the red rings mark these areas). The only solution was bone grafting as modern medicine has not other solution for bone necrosis. She began a series of PAPIMI treatments for the upper jaw and 2 months later another X-ray was taken (Fig 23) showing the regression of the bone necrosis in the upper jaw. Figure 24 shows an enlargement of one of the upper incisors before and after PAPIMI treatment. Moreover, all her blood values were in the normal range and her cancer was in complete regression, without using any allopathic treatments.

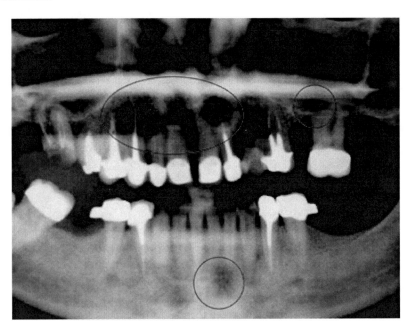

Fig 22 showing bone necrosis in upper jaw

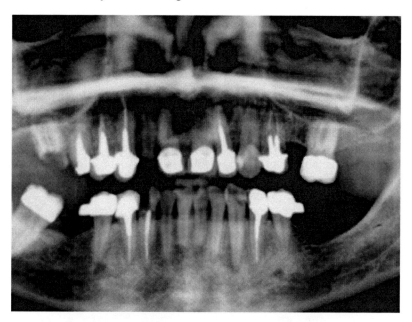

Fig 23 Bone necrosis of upper jaw regressing after PAPIMI treatments

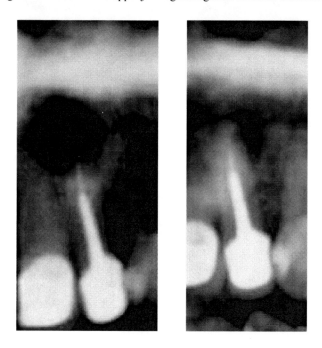

Fig 24 Bone necrosis (left) and after PAPIMI treatment (right)

There are many other remarkable cases that have been helped by this powerful, but gentle healing device – most of these can be reviewed on the official websites of PAPIMI.

Matrix Regeneration Therapy (MRT)

We are constantly being bombarded with various environmental toxins which adversely affect our health. Initially, the body can detoxifying these toxins, but as they increase and build up in the tissues, they begin causing disease or pathology.

It is crucially important that these toxins that accumulate in the connective tissues and mesenchyme be removed. One of the ways to remove these deeply-buried toxins is by using the MATRIX REGENERATION THERAPY. This device consists of three synergistic components (Fig 25):

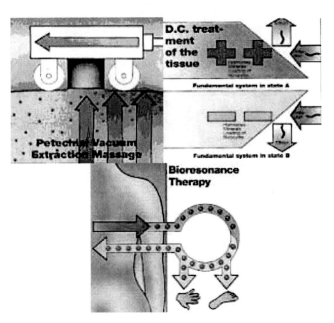

Fig 25 Three synergistic components of MRT

1. Petechial Suction Massage - this uses a suction electrode to generate a partial vacuum in the tissues mechanically loosening clogged deposits and toxins in the tissues and diverting them via the lymph capillaries. As in cupping, worn-out and toxin-laden blood is drawn to the surface, therefore helping to purify the tissues and eliminate toxins.

2. A Direct Current – a weak direct current is introduced into the tissues using the roller electrode on the device that shunts off excess charge from the diseased tissue. This helps the repolarized tissue to become alkaline again which is a precondition for normal metabolic functioning.

3. Bioresonance Therapy - the neutralization of pathological energy fields is the domain of Systems Information Therapy, a further development of bioresonance therapy. Via the suction electrode, liberated toxin information is detected and transmitted to the control unit for processing, where these pathological frequency patterns are transformed into therapeutic signals and routed back to the patient Subtraction Loesch Therapy (SLT). Self-healing powers can thus be activated by means of resonance effects, and the healing process initiated.

How is treatment conducted? The patient lies on their stomach (Fig 26) in a relaxed state. There are four clip-on electrodes that are attached to the hands and feet and the DC counter-electrode is placed under the stomach. The suction probe with the two rollers will be rolled over the left and right side of the body for about 20 minutes. The spinal column is also rolled with the electrodes from cervical to sacral ends. There are also cases where the thighs are also covered to help remove cellulite – this is about one of the most efficient and successful ways of dealing with cellulite and varicose veins, as attested by hundreds of successful cases at the DaVinci Natural Health Centre.

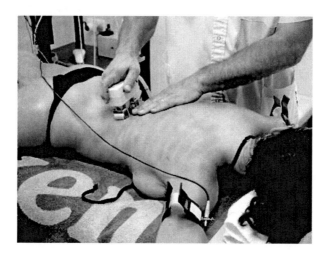

Fig 23 Patient receiving MRT treatment

As treatment progresses, the tissues in the treatment region become stronger and firmer and pain sensitivity diminishes markedly. It is amazing how a stressed patient with tension headache can walk out after half an hour free of pain and no need to take medication.

Personally, the enormous healing effects of MRT can really be a life-saver for many chronically ill patients, including metastatic cancer which requires blockades to be removed quickly in order to achieve regulation, as well as activating and stimulating the immune and lymphatic systems and haematopoiesis, through cytolysis. All of these positive effects will happen simultaneously during each treatment – there is no other form of therapy that I am aware of that can achieve all this so simply with very little effort.

Let's move into another realm of healing that is at the apex of the pyramid, healing the soul.

Chapter 10

Healing the soul

'Beyond living and dreaming there is something more important...waking up.'
Antonio Machado

Introduction

Just before starting to write this chapter I thought of its structure – my initial intention was to write about how the mind can influence the emotions and consequently influence our physical body – there is a lot of scientific research that has proven these connections. When I sat down to write I had 'writer's block' – the words would not flow easily and after a few clumsy paragraphs I thought again.

There was a deeper gut feeling that was telling me not to reiterate all the science behind psychoneuroimmunology, which is the study of how the nervous and immune systems connect with our psychoemotional states, but to look at a deeper level – the level of the soul. After all, it is the soul or spirit or Higher Consciousness that is at the top of the pyramid, as discussed in Chapter 1. If you can heal the soul, you will pretty much heal the rest of the body on all its levels. Conversely, if you try healing the other levels of the body when there are spiritual issues outstanding, then you will achieve little overall healing. I have seen this occur in a number of patients over time and I will share such examples in the text below.

In many religions, spiritual traditions and philosophies, the soul is the spiritual or immaterial part of a living being, often regarded as eternal. It is usually thought to consist of one's consciousness and personality, and can be synonymous with the spirit, mind or self.

The more I work in the field of holistic health, the more I realize just how important is the healing of the soul. Often, using energy testing, I see patients who are completely blocked on the heart chakra because of past events and experiences and have perpetual relationship problems. I have also witnessed a number of patients who had a subconscious wish to die – this was made very clear with words and actions, but defied logic. It was exactly because of these subconscious forces related to systemic entanglements[1] with other family members, that the person had no control over the consequences. We will discuss more about systemic entanglements below.

One of the most powerful therapies that I have encountered in all my training, that can help to heal on this very important and deep level, is 'Hellinger's Family Constellations' or as I have called it on my website: 'Hellinger's Soul Healing.' We were fortunate here in Cyprus, to have had a gifted facilitator and trainer, Stephen Victor,[2] who spent about 18 months with a group of us – training us, but more importantly healing us; helping us to release constraints and open doorways to elegantly grow, change, expand; awaken and open our hearts to love – which is important in enabling one to become a facilitator to these family constellations[3].

It is crucially important that a facilitator of either gender can set aside their intellectual understandings and what they believe, and instead submit themselves to the 'Knowing Field'[4] as it is from this field that he or she is informed, guided and directed as how to proceed in the identification and resolution of an issue.

Hellinger's soul healing constellations work

It is often difficult to describe in words the work of Bert Hellinger[5] and his Family Constellations, which we have called 'Soul Healing' as ultimately this is what this work boils down to. It is a powerful tool that bypasses the mind and goes right into the deeper soul. Family Constellations is the brainchild of German psychologist Bert Hellinger, and the outgrowth of

---

1 Systemic entanglements are traumatic or unresolved issues that had been hidden by the family system such as a murder, an abortion or miscarriage, an infidelity, the premature death of a parent or child, incest, a secret related to inheritance issues or some other injustice. Hellinger says these entanglements disturb our lives and manifest in the form of sudden illness or accidents, depression or feelings of isolation, physical and mental illness, and persistent relationship conflicts and dysfunction.

2 http://www.stephenvictor.com

3 A constellation is the placement of family members in a field of energy so that family patterns and entanglements can be played out and reviewed.

4 The term, knowing field, was initially coined by Dr. Albrecht Mahr in 1997 at the first international conference on Family Constellations in Wiesloch, near Heidelberg, Germany.

5 Hellinger, B. Acknowledging What Is: Conversations with Bert Hellinger. Zeig, Tucker & Co., Inc., Phoenix, Arizona, 1999.

years of pioneering work integrating systems theory (see below), psychotherapy, family and group therapy and phenomenology.[6]

The family system or soul

At a deep level we are connected with everything, especially our family legacy – including our ancestors, whether we recognize it or not. Constellation work is based on a simple but profound idea: our well-being is tied to the well-being of our Family System, or 'Family Soul,' which includes the living, the dead and the generations that preceded us. It invokes an ancient practice (honouring the ancestors) with a post-modern spin (temporarily re-creating our 'tribe'). Constellation work approaches individual pain or wounding in the larger context of the Family Soul, to which we are entangled, without even being aware of it. Moreover, we are often loyal to these family members, whether they are alive or dead, regardless of the consequences on our own lives.

This soul healing work goes way beyond, and differs from, psychotherapy as it is not the individual therapist's skills that are imperative, to work with the individual person. Unlike psychotherapy, where the success of the outcome is very much correlated with the degree of training of the psychotherapist and whether these techniques which have been learned, are applied correctly in the appropriate case.

Psychotherapy addresses the psychological and emotional makeup of the person, but rarely touches the level of the soul – it is possible for people to spend months and years talking to a psychotherapist and still not address the level of the soul. Family constellation work utilizes the language of the soul – there is no real interest in the person's story on the level of the personality, but it focuses on the heart of the matter with pin-point accuracy. I have seen more achieved in one family constellation than I could have achieved as a psychotherapist in 6 months.

---

6 In phenomenological inquiry one has to be non-judgemental of any particular person - this requires an inner state devoid of pre-conceptions, intentions and judgements, particularly as they relate to feelings, ideas, beliefs and behaviours. One has to be open to the dynamics of the situation without focusing on the individuals, with a readiness to act, but paradoxically refraining from action. In the dynamics of these paradoxes there is an intensity of perception where central themes emerge with a deeper truth and the next step emerges. This can only happen when we open our hearts and transcend all the morality that has been inculcated by family, church and society in general.

In the soul healing constellation, the outcome is not determined by my own skills or relationship with the client, but more on tapping into the extended Soul of the family unit that is interconnected with the individual soul who is partaking in the constellation. It is the trust in this Greater Soul that will gradually find a resolution – so in that respect the person in the constellation can do without the individual therapist. The only role of the therapist is to tap into the Field nurturing this Greater Soul and facilitate the process in order to achieve the forgiveness, love and reconnections of the various souls who were alienated over time. This ability to bow to the Greater Soul does not require academic, university education or individual psychotherapeutic skills but humility of spirit to completely trust the guiding forces of this Greater Soul with whom one lives so intensely in the constellation.

How can we explain this Greater or Family Soul? One way to think about it is as a field of energy that we are all enveloped in, and are interconnected with, encompassing both the living and dead. The biologist Rupert Sheldrake,[7] found in his research that related people, places, and animals exist in a 'morphic field[8]' of energy which has both influence and memory. This invisible morphic field of energy links all family members much like it does a flock of birds, and any painful event within this family system will ultimately affect every single family member and will stretch across generations, including all the deceased family members who may have died many years ago.[9]

As a result, people often carry these painful events of their ancestors through the generations, which often affect their beliefs, attitudes and behaviours. It is not that there is an external force that is determined to 'punish' us for the deeds of our ancestors, but more that energy cannot be created nor destroyed – however much we want to exclude something – it will be included, to bring things back into some type of balance. All soul systems work hard to maintain this balance, often to the detriment of the personalities involved.

---

7 www.sheldrake.org
8 The morphogenetic field would provide a force that guided the development of an organism as it grew, making it take on a form similar to that of others in its species.
9 There is a Biblical quote from Exodus, Chapter 34, Hebrew Scriptures: "The sins of the father will be visited on the children and on the grandchildren to the third and fourth generations."

Systemic entanglements

Hellinger called these emotional wounds I mentioned, 'systemic entanglements' – these are traumatic or unresolved issues that have been hidden by the family such as a murder, an abortion or miscarriage, an infidelity, the premature death of a parent or child, incest, a secret related to inheritance issues, some other injustice or a painful event. Specifically, circumstances that can cause a systemic entanglement are those whereby a family member:

- ❖ Died at a young age, at childbirth or maybe lost a parent or sibling. Suffered illness, disability or had their life at risk due to childbirth. Committed or attempted suicide.
- ❖ Died in action as a soldier or killed others in wartime.
- ❖ Committed a serious crime or was a victim of a crime, and went to prison.
- ❖ Had a stillborn child, abortion or miscarriage.
- ❖ Had an 'illegitimate' child or a child that was abandoned or given up for adoption.
- ❖ Had a former spouse, fiancé, partner or lover of the opposite gender.
- ❖ Had a serious or long-lasting illness.
- ❖ Had a physical or mental disability.
- ❖ Died in the Holocaust or was interned in a prisoner-of-war camp.
- ❖ Went missing or disappeared for long periods.
- ❖ Joined the clergy or entered a monastery; or lived an unusual life. Lost a fortune, become disinherited or disowned.
- ❖ Became a serious scapegoat; was ignored, rejected, slandered or cast out.
- ❖ Suffered severe trauma, mental illness, sexual abuse or life-threatening events.
- ❖ Had serious symptoms or difficulties repeated across generations.
- ❖ Had a child with serious problems.
- ❖ Immigrated to another country.
- ❖ Had a shameful family secret.
- ❖ Experienced anything that might be considered tragic or highly unusual.

If any of your family members, whether dead or alive, went through any of the abovementioned circumstances, then it is very possible that they are systemically entangled.

Hellinger says these entanglements disturb our lives and manifest in the form of sudden illness or accidents, depression or feelings of isolation, physical and mental illness, as well as persistent relationship conflicts and dysfunction.[10]

As all systems seek wholeness and balance then often we unwittingly identify with an ancestor's pain or issue and take it on as our own, or we may recreate this ancestor's trauma in our own lives in order to try and heal it. However, the family system can only reach a balance if every person, dead or alive, has a respected place within it.

This is what underlines the premise of systemic entanglements where our fate or destiny can become entangled with the fate or destiny of an ancestor, simply because they are part of our family system on a soul level. Anything that blocks the flow of love through the generations such as someone in the family system being ignored, rejected, exiled, forgotten; or if the order of the family is disturbed and the child does not take their place in this hierarchy and becomes the parent, or the eldest child becomes the youngest, then again this will block the flow of love through the generations.

In Hellinger's Soul Healing the family system is comprised of a number of people such as: all the children, including the deceased and the still born; the parents and their siblings; the grandparents; the great grandparents, including even more distant relatives who suffered a particularly difficult or unjust fate; non-relatives who through their death or misfortune, someone else in the family benefited; previous partners of the parents and grandparents.

There is a fundamental principle that applies to all family systems – it simply says that all members have an equal right to belong. Whenever a member of the family system is alienated, this is the condition which causes another member of the family to develop a systemic entanglement that is beyond their logical, conscious understanding. It could be an uncle who committed suicide and this act stigmatized the family and so he was

---

10 Hellinger, B. Love's Own Truths: Bonding and Balancing in Close Relationships. Zeig, Tucker & Thiesen, Inc., Phoenix, Arizona, 2007.

never talked about; an illegitimate child that no-one mentions or the traumatic death of a biological child that was too painful to remember; an abortion that was covered-up and never talked about due to the shame and guilt involved. These are a few examples but there are many more that may involve one's profession, nationality, skin colour or gender.

Or, sometimes when a child dies young, the parents give the next child the same name. They effectively tell the deceased child, 'you don't belong any more. We have a substitute for you.' The deceased child can't even keep his or her own name. In many families such children are neither counted among the children, nor are they mentioned. Their fundamental right to belong is injured and denied to them and usually another member of the family becomes systemically entangled with them to make amends and reconnect on a soul level – this may mean that another child becomes anorectic and finally dies, to honour and acknowledge the deceased sibling.

This may sound bizarre if it occurred on a conscious level, but this is not the case – it is clearly on a subconscious, systemic level and a way that the system balances itself. As the fundamental family dynamic is that all family members have an equal right to belong, this cannot tolerate injury or injustice. The way that the family system balances when someone is excluded, is another family member will become subconsciously loyal to the excluded member.

Let's take an example of a systemic entanglement – an uncle dies suddenly of cancer without warning and silence descends over the family due to the shock. The niece develops cancer and even though her chances of survival are good she does everything in her power to avoid all sorts of treatment – there is a deeper wish to die. She really wants to reconnect with the uncle who has been disconnected on a soul level from the family system – she wants to go into the grave and honour him and be loyal to him – it is an act of deep, deep love for the uncle, even though it involves her own sacrifice. These dynamics are often seen by therapists working with chronically ill patients, particularly cancer, and are part of the systemic entanglements that need to be resolved for there to be deeper healing on all levels.

Another example may be a married man who fell in love with another woman and told his wife that he did not want her and rejected her based on capricious reasoning. There followed children with his new partner but there were many problems with his daughter who demonstrated a hatred towards him that was difficult to understand, as he truly loved and cared for her. In the family system, the daughter had become systemically entangled with the previous wife and felt the same hate that the wife had felt towards her ex-husband. This may even occur without ever meeting the previous partner as it is a hidden systemic compensatory force that is avenging the injustice done by other family members, securing justice for the earlier members and causing injustice for the younger.

Resolution of systemic entanglements

In the family constellation there are many healing statements made with the guidance of the facilitator. These statements are the 'Language of the Soul' and are important for helping people overcome systemic entanglements. Words can be very hurtful, but they can also be very healing. They can create a perceptible shift in the energy of the constellation – I have often witnessed a whole group of people sigh together when healing statements have caused an energy shift in the room. These healing statements need to emanate from the level of the soul in order for them to be effective, it cannot be just any words. When the words come from the soul there is often a feeling of 'there is no more to say.' Words from the level of the personality are often superfluous and lack the deeper truth that detracts from the goal of resolution. These words will then allow the soul to acknowledge what is, and deal with the simple truths.

This is an important point as it often has implications when we are trying to apologise to those that we have hurt in real life. Let's take a couple of examples of statements – one is the language of the soul and the other is from the personality – see which is which. The case is of a girl who has deeply hurt her sister by sleeping with her boyfriend. 'I'm really sorry, I apologise for this as I did not mean it to happen. He was flirting with me a lot and I had just been hurt by my boyfriend, who left me – I was vulnerable and I let it happen. I'm really sorry and I ask for your forgiveness.' Or, 'I am deeply sorry, I've wronged you. I no longer have the right to call myself your sister.' Which of these two statements do you think is the language of the soul?

When the language of the soul is heard by the ears of the soul, it penetrates the heart, and the need for punishment, revenge or recompense most often dissolves. We cannot challenge the power of words: they can both heal and hurt, as well as creating freedom of expression. The language of the soul does not look at what is right or wrong, what is just or blameworthy – it looks at facts in the presence of truth – when we touch the presence of truth, we touch grace in the presence of the Divine. When we experience the language of the soul, it becomes a deeply spiritual experience.

The fundamental order of the family will be reconstituted when the excluded members are taken back into the family system on a soul level and given the respect that is due to them. In the example of the ex-wife and daughter given above, it may be that in the constellation the second wife honours the first wife by bowing to her and saying: 'I honour you as you came first, and I second. You made room for me to be here now.' As we submit to the truth of what is, our place and position within the new family system is automatically elevated.

The ex-husband could also bow to his previous wife and say: 'I honour you as the mother of our children and I give our children permission to take after you as you are an honourable woman. I release you and I let you go with love.' I have often seen in constellations how the ex-wife's face mellows and changes as she has now been respected and has been accepted back into the family system where she rightly belongs.

What could then follow in a typical constellation is where the children from both sides stand in front of the parents in order of birth and prostrate themselves in front of them, honouring them as their parents. The troublesome daughter could also stand in front of her father and say to him: 'You are my father and I am your daughter. Take me as your daughter. Can I have your blessing?' He could then say to her: 'Daughter, take only my love and leave the rest. You have my blessing.' These sentences when authentically spoken can restore the fundamental order of a family. She could then prostrate herself in front of the father, honouring him as her father.

In the first case of the niece who is systemically entangled with the dead uncle, it would be appropriate in the constellation to have a representative of the uncle lying on the floor dead. The young niece would then kneel and hold the uncle's hand and say: 'I didn't want you to go, I miss you. But it was your time to go, but mine to stay – I will be with you later, but not for a while yet. You are in my heart always.' She then gets up after reconnecting with the uncle who on a soul level now comes back into the family system – this is enough to break the systemic entanglement and remove the negative thoughts that she has about his dying.

More serious entanglements can be caused by not feeling that you belong in a family system, a fundamental right. For example, when a child dies in a family at a young age, the other children tend to feel guilty that they are still alive while their sibling is dead. They feel that that they are advantaged and their deceased sibling is disadvantaged, edging them to feel that they should not belong to the family system. They are then tempted to compensate by subconsciously arranging to fail at everything, or to become ill, or in extreme cases wanting themselves to die, without knowing the reason – this could be via anorexia, drugs, addictions and the like, as mentioned above.

This systemic entanglement can be resolved in a typical constellation where the deceased brother's representative lies on the ground 'dead,' and the sibling crouches down by him and says: 'You are my brother, I see you, I see you. It was your time to go and mine to stay – I will join you later but not for a while yet. You have a very special place in my heart. I ask for your blessing.' These words pay respect to the deceased brother who gives their sibling the blessing required to continue living without feeling guilty.

I will give another example of a patient who I saw about 6 months ago – a 62-year old lady who was severely depressed and was taking a cocktail of medications comprising 13 different drugs, amounting to 30 pills per day! She was totally dependent on the husband and her 4 daughters for every type of support including cooking, cleaning, shopping, washing and the like. She also had a multitude of other health issues that had over the years been suppressed by the myriad of drugs she was taking.

During the initial assessment, apart from having difficulties staying awake and concentrating on my questions, she had difficulty sitting in the chair without falling over. When I asked her when her problems began, she immediately responded: 'When I was 29 years old.' I asked her why 29 and she went on to explain that at that age, when her young boy was 4 years old, he was taking a ride on her husband's tractor and fell over, and was crushed by the heavy tire. Since this time she has been 'locked-in' with her young boy in a delayed grieving reaction, literally lying next to the child in the grave where she felt she belonged. She saw no one, as one of her daughters bitterly complained: 'we never had a mother, ever.' This mother felt so guilty about her child's death that she stopped living herself and became loyal to her child's grave, not seeing or hearing anyone else.

One of her 4 daughters came to a Hellinger Family Constellation workshop and set up a constellation about her mother not seeing her and never paying much attention to her. The representative for the dead young child was placed on the ground and as soon as the mother's representative saw the child in the grave she immediately went down and embraced the child very tightly, crying and wailing at the top of her voice – even though she was not the actual mother. This continued for over 20 minutes and no attempts to separate them was possible.

The lack of freedom and strength to get on with her life due to her failure to 'consent to what is' became very apparent, and literally when asked whether she could see her 4 daughters who were standing right in front of her around the grave, she said that she could not. Eventually she calmed down and managed to say to her deceased child: 'I see you, I see you, I see you. It was your time to die, this was your fate which I now bow to and accept. My time will come too, but not for a while yet. I hold you in my heart and love you dearly. I shall live my life fully in honour of you.'

Six months have now gone by and this lady has reduced her medication from 13 different kinds to only 3. She is doing all her household chores, walking to her daughter's houses, which is over an hour's walk, as well as swimming every morning in the sea. She has overcome her depression and her husband is delighted with his new-found wife, the one he so much remembered all those years ago when they married. It would have been difficult to achieve so much in so little time if she had not dealt with the guilt of her deceased child – the retrieval and healing of the soul from the grave in this case was probably the key factor that led to her amazing recovery, and this was all done in her absence by her daughter, who set up the constellation.

This is also one of the mysteries of the Field, that the healing effects when family members are reconstituted back into the family system, can affect people who were not even present in the same room and that the representative somehow took onboard the emotions and mental state of the mother and became the catharsis for healing in absentia. I explain this phenomenon in the section 'The constellation process.'

Opening up to love

By honouring the role and the fate of every family member we can reconnect with our own path and reclaim our own destiny. This soul healing work enables us to clear these blockages and systemic entanglements so that love flows freely again. There is nothing that is more powerful as a healer of wounds than free love. Many indigenous cultures understand on a deep level that in healing the ancestral family soul we ultimately heal ourselves. The Bible talks about the sins of the fathers are visited upon the sons. Many earth-people cultures have a ritual of 'feeding' the dead ancestors and honouring them so that they do not feed on us. These systemic entanglements from our ancestors can cause serious problems and behaviours in us that inevitably we feel are our own, even though they do not originate within us.

This makes it very difficult to heal these problems when they transcend us and go beyond our conscious awareness. In the many soul healing workshops that I have attended in my own training as a facilitator, it never ceases to amaze me the relief in people when they realize that often their individual traumas are not of their own doing. After a personal constellation we tend to perceive family members differently and accept them with compassion knowing full well that their wrongdoings are also entanglements of their previous ancestry. Understanding better the roots of their pain and struggle it is much easier to lovingly connect with them.

Family constellations are about simple truths – we are really looking at small particles of matter amongst the many that make up the whole. The simplest truth for all human beings is the truth of love – unconditional love. John Payne in his book 'The Language of the Soul: Healing with Words of Truth' says the following: 'One example of this was a client making an inner movement towards accepting her alcoholic father. There were a number of simple truths. First, 'My father is an alcoholic and there is nothing I can do to change it,' second, 'Much of my life has been spent resisting this truth, wanting to change fate.' The third truth is: 'This is my father, the one and only, I have no other.' The fourth truth, the one that we can access when we can overcome our arrogance and resistance is: 'I love my father deeply.'[11]

It is often amazing in a constellation session how simply submitting to unconditional love can free us and liberate us beyond all that we have known. Simple truths belong to the realm of the soul and the rewards can be huge.

---

11 Payne, JL. The Language of the Soul: Healing with words and truth. Findhorn Press, UK, 2006.

The constellation process

The constellation process takes place in the 'Field' or the 'Knowing Field' which is a safe and confidential circle where the people present have invited their personal divine beings whether they be saints, the Virgin Mary, Mary Magdalene, a holy mountain or sacred place, a power animal or any other divine spirit they elicit a deeper meaning from. People usually sit in a circle with the women on one side and the men on the other side in the chronological order of their birth – this 'taking one's place' in the hierarchy of life creates a gentle flow of energy that is soothing and powerful.

When someone is ready to set their constellation (see below) they sit next to the facilitator and express what is on their heart. There is no need to take a detailed account of personality descriptions or to say much about the story of one's life; the most important elements are:

❖ *Who* is a member of the family system? and
❖ *What* specifically happened?

Then the person chooses people from around the group to represent their family members, including themselves, or other entities that may be an important part of their constellation. The client then places these representatives in the Field in a standing pattern that has meaning to them, allowing their heart to guide them, not their intellect. These people are placed in the constellation floor space in a way that represents a picture of how the family feels for them – they then return and sit next to the facilitator.

There are often times that the therapist will also choose representatives at random, adding further to the constellation – often these additional representatives can be 'entities' representing a goddess, a saint, the moon, the sun, fear, low self-esteem, money or whatever else the' 'Field' is asking for.

What is truly amazing is that each representative takes on the role of those that they represent – information begins to come through the Knowing Field to the representatives in a way that affects their feelings, thoughts and actions, often to the surprise of the representatives themselves. If we switch off our brains and our intellect and allow our bodies to tap into this Field with its spiritual and emotional intelligence; breathing through our hearts and not our lungs, then it is truly amazing how the representative takes on the qualities of the person they have been chosen to represent. An angry 'grandfather' may come on to the floor swearing in anger, just like the real person they are representing. Sometimes they may have pain in a limb, just like the real person had pain in the same limb, due to an accident. There is definitely a mystery in the way that this happens.

Personally, I have been chosen to represent many different family members and have played many different roles. Often, the feelings that you have are so strong that you truly cannot understand where they are coming from. I have often felt strong feelings of love and compassion for people in the Field that I knew nothing about, only to find out when the constellation was over that the person I was representing really did have a deep affection and loving relationship with this person, even though they may have been married to someone else.

There have been a number of occasions when I have had a deep feeling of wanting to preserve the secret that the family was carrying which eventually comes to light in the constellation. I have learnt to trust these feelings and let them guide me in the Field, even though sometimes my intellect tells me that there is no sense in these feelings. I have proven my intellect wrong and my heart and perceptual capacities correct on many occasions. What is important is to stand back and respect that the Knowing Field belongs to something that is far greater than ourselves and that we do not need to understand it intellectually, simply to trust in it.

Repeatedly, what begins with a simple constellation involving two or three people evolves into a complex labyrinth that may include representatives of the soil of our birth (the country we were physically born in) fate, disease, death or war. As these 'Knowing Fields' inform the 'Knowing representatives,' surprising new perspectives on ourselves and our family history begin to emerge. The facilitator merely guides by asking the representatives how they feel and interpreting the developments, to help understand the underlying family dynamics. The facilitator must also be guided by the Fields and not by their own intellect.

In constellations there is no time and space and often logic is not the logic of the person that is being represented in the Field. It is highly recommended that these constellations not be analyzed, as when you begin defining something as meaningful as this you often confine it too. There is a time when we must completely trust in this timeless dimension called the 'mystery' and let the soul heal on the deepest level.

Constellation work addresses a variety of issues including:

Unexplained sadness, grief, anger and shame; addictions and other destructive behaviours, relationship failures and confusion (with parents, siblings, partners, or children); depression and unhappiness; business failures and money problems; illnesses and chronic health problems; organizational confusion; adoption issues; loss of direction and purpose and repeating 'accidents.'

The goal of the constellation is to show the client a resolution picture of the family system, a new way to envisage one's self and the family dynamics. Often at the end of the constellation, the client is allowed to stand in his or her own place, to experience the balanced family system. The client may experience immediate change as a result of the constellation or it may take some time for these very deeply ingrained patterns to work themselves out. In either case, it is left to the client to take the patterns revealed in the constellation and let them unfold naturally within the soul.

This way of working is phenomenological in nature. Hellinger works with what he observes in the constellation. While there are certain patterns that are often observed, each situation is different and the dynamics of each constellation must be uncovered anew. Clients are often surprised to see the dynamic that is operating within their family system and the resolution is often a 'surprise' as well. Sometimes even years of psychotherapy won't totally reveal the true origins of a person's issues, much less the resolution. In fact, the focus on pathology may very well keep clients bonded to their problems, rather than moved toward a solution.

I can only say that I have also found deep healing through the family constellation work that I have participated in. It's surprising to see that our stories do not really differ that much – we all suffer loss and experience love. We all lose our way from time to time. In family constellations we have a unique opportunity to stand in each other's shoes and to see a reflection of ourselves in the eye of others. We then begin to realize that we are all interconnected, a part of the Greater Soul and the greater extended family where we all belong to each other.

The important thing is that the constellation reveals the dynamics operating within the client's family system and presents us with ways of resolving those dynamics. This revelation of the pathological and disturbed dynamics that have caused an imbalance in the family system is often enough to initiate a resolution of the problem.

In the constellation, the client is not told what to do to resolve the problem. The picture presented needs to be processed by the client's soul in order to determine the next steps – this is why it is often advised not to discuss with details after each constellation as it can block this important 'soul processing' and make it into a more conscious, psychodynamic process. This is one of the most challenging and most profound tasks for the client – to trust in the constellation process and stay with these images while a natural unfolding takes place.

Acknowledging and accepting what is!

Hellinger in his books and lectures has talked about 'acknowledging what is' or 'accepting what is' as being an important component of resolving family dynamics and systemic entanglements.[12] This is a very profound and deep notion that should not be underestimated as I have seen it work miracles in constellation work. Hellinger also uses the German word *Gelassenheit* which literally means 'letting-be-ness.' This is akin to the feeling of 'serenity,' even though there is no exact English equivalent. 'Letting' means moving on, transformed, and the experience only becomes meaningful when one leaves it behind.

When we let something be, we stop rationalising, explaining, moralising, imposing our own interpretations, and instead perceive and acknowledge what really is, without necessarily consenting to it. This really opens up the possibilities of transformation.

Most of our problems come from being involved either in the business or fate of another. In the family system this can happen when one member carries the burden and feelings of another member as their own. This unconscious entanglement can be out of loyalty, a sense of superiority or the feeling that 'I am more capable than the other of carrying the burden.'

---

12 Hellinger, B. On Life and Other Paradoxes. Zeig, Tucker and Theisen, Inc., Phoenix, Arizona, 2002.

One of the most powerful healing forces that I have witnessed in a family constellation is when a victim of a tragedy such as a rape or incest; or a war crime, bows to the person representing 'fate' in the Field. This 'consenting to what is,' without necessarily accepting or sanctioning it, is the force required to move on with our lives.[13] When a person is confronted with a tragedy in life, there is often a tendency to feel anger, rage, depression and other negative emotions.

Indeed, they may spend a lifetime immersed in these emotions which tarnish all aspects of their lives. They may also spend a lifetime 'beating up' fate – saying that it should never have happened to them and mulling on how unfortunate and unlucky they have been. This attitude of 'life sucks' does not help them move forward spiritually one inch – they are usually well-rooted in the mud of life without helping themselves to move forward, grow and mature.

When a person in the Field can stop beating fate up and actually bow to fate, the energy transition in the room at that moment in time is often breathtaking! This acknowledgment of fate, which is their life circumstances up to that point in time, is all that is required to help them move out of the negative patterns of life into a more fulfilling and spiritually rewarding existence. If all of us can 'acknowledge and accept what is' without fighting and arguing with fate, we would all be better people with far fewer problems. It is common, however, for people to resist with much suffering, conditions and business that is not theirs. We can either focus on the things that we can change in our lives, or focus on what cannot be changed, therefore shifting our energies onto that which is not wanted.

It is often a lot easier to harbour negative emotions for our family of origin, rather than 'submit' – this word usually conjures up feelings of weakness, giving one's power away, and resistance becomes inevitable. It is often difficult to understand and accept that the life we have, and therefore our destiny, is unavoidably tied up with, and owing to our family of origin. This is our life, there is no other, our mother is the only one for

---

13 The distinction between "consenting to what is" and "accepting or sanctioning what is" is not simply semantics. The distinctions are the difference that makes the difference energetically. Hellinger did not care whether the client or patient accepted reality (language of the personality) but if reconciliation was to occur, the client or patient had to consent (language of the soul) to reality. This is the punch line, the centre, the crucial aspect of all constellation work - receiving the benefits of reality changing, resulting from the acknowledgement that can only occur through consent.

us, and our father is the only one for us – this cannot be changed, however much we resist. But how can an abusive parent, or a missing parent, an alcoholic parent, or one that deserted the family for another partner, the parent that died when the child was young – how can all these parents be the perfect ones, the one and only? The simple answer lies in the simple truth that we ARE our parents – we inherit their gifts and talents, we inherit their knowledge and experiences and our life is because of them.

When parents give life, they act in deepest accordance with their humanness, and they give themselves as parents to their children exactly as they are. There is nothing that they can add to, nor can they leave anything out. Father and mother, consummating their love for one another, give to their children the whole of what they are. A child cannot leave anything out from the life he or she was given, or does wishing it were different change anything. Our parents are the only possible ones for us. Imagining anything else to be possible is an illusion.

When we submit to our parents we receive the gift of life fully, as it was passed down to us, in its entirety. We open our hearts to receive the blessings of life, as well as acknowledging and submitting to the mystery of life. When we do not submit, we find that whatever we achieve in life feels empty, nothing in life is complete, all of it carries a sense of something missing – we need to submit to become our parent's child in order to receive the blessing of life. Jesus said 'Honour thy mother and father' – when we reject or feel superior to our parents we say 'no' to life and cut ourselves off from the creative life force of the cosmos.

Imagine yourself bowing deeply before your parents and telling them, 'The life you gave me comes to me at the full price it has cost you, and at the full price it has cost me. I take it at its full value, with all its limitations and opportunities.' At the moment that this language of the soul is authentically spoken, we acknowledge life as it is and our parents as they are. The heart opens – whoever manages this affirmation feels whole and at peace.

Family constellation work can take us to a deeply spiritual experience when we bow in submission to our fate, in totality. This humble gesture and bodily movement has the essence of living the prayer 'Thy will be done.' Whenever I have witnessed this in the many constellations I have attended, with the awesome silence that often prevails; it is truly the presence of Grace.

The intrinsic order - the orders of love in family systems

There are certain natural phenomena that have been observed in family systems through constellation work. There is an intrinsic and distinct order that states who belongs, and who does not belong to the family system, as well as to the larger whole. Individuals seem to have three levels of consciousness: firstly, the consciousness that we have as individuals that incorporates the elements of right and wrong, our responsibilities and how we behave in certain circumstances. In addition, we belong to the collective conscious of our biological family that can span back many generations, and finally we participate in the consciousness of our ethnic and national groups, whether we are white, black, Jewish, Greek Orthodox, Catholic, Muslim, German, Greek, English and so forth.

These Orders of Love are important as when they are disrupted, as is often seen in family constellations, we see an undeniable effect on the family system. The Orders of Love stipulate who comes first and who after that, and describes a natural flow of love from the great-grandparents, to grandparents, to parents to children. It can go back many generations, but generally have the greatest influence in Systems work three to seven generations back.

The Orders of Love can become disrupted when a family member becomes excluded on a soul level, either intentionally or as a result of family members not being able to embrace the difficult fate of any family member, such as an abortion, murder, suicide, a child born out of wedlock and the like. In the Orders of Love, one of the overriding principles is that love is born at conception as parents give life, and their children receive life. When a child, no matter at what age, decides to place themselves equal or higher than a parent, this will lead to disruptive life patterns in the child.

This simple but profound notion is easily embraced by many psychotherapists such as myself and provides a basis to work with 'difficult' clients that traditional psychotherapy has difficulty helping. However, the Orders of Love goes beyond what traditional psychotherapy teaches into the dominion of the soul. At the heart of the soul is the acknowledgment and acceptance of what is, which is the basis and power of love. When resolutions for the disruption of the Orders of Love are amended, all members of the family system, including the nation, belong equally together, regardless of life's circumstances – whether they are suicidal, alcoholics, died at a young age or whatever. We respect each other's fate and bow to it – this is what restores the Orders of Love.

Physical illness and disease

I have seen a number of clients attending family constellations for chronic illnesses such as cancer. These people can be greatly helped in their journey to health by setting family constellations, even though the objective is not to find a cure as such, but to look at the system to which the client belongs.

Usually in such chronic illnesses, there lurks a magical belief system that works its mischief. Namely, that we can release those we love from their suffering and misfortune when we take it upon ourselves. For example, the child's (living) soul often tells her terminally ill mother, 'I'd rather be ill, than have you suffer. I'd rather I die myself than have you die.' Or when a mother is being pulled away from life by systemic forces, it sometimes happens that a child commits suicide in the magical belief that her sacrifice will free her mother to stay. Often when a client is entangled with the fate of a family member who has suffered, it is an energetic drain on their physical organism that leads to the weakening and pathology of the physical   body.

Anorexia often has this dynamic - an anorectic child slowly shrinks away, until they die. It quite often turns out to be the case that in the souls of such anorectic children, they are saying to their father or mother, 'its better if I disappear than if you go.' On the level of the soul, this is a deep, innocent love, but has dire consequences in real life. The reconciliation in the family constellation would involve the child facing the parents and telling them, 'It is better if I disappear than if you go' – the parents must then acknowledge this entanglement by replying, 'Child, I will stay and you have my blessing to lead a rich and full life, away from illness.'

Family constellations provide the platform for clients to come face-to-face with those that have died so that a resolution to their systemic entanglements can be found. If there is resolution, this will have a positive influence on their overall energy field and help them recover from their illness. In the healing process it is imperative that the clients relinquish their unspoken loyalty to the ones that have died, which in turn restores peace and balance to the Greater Soul.

CHAPTER 11

VIEWING CANCER HOLISTICALLY:

THINKING OUTSIDE THE BOX

When a new cancer patient steps into my office, the first question that goes through my mind, no matter what type or stage of cancer they have, is: "What are the causes of this person's cancer?"

Discovering the cause of the cancer is the first and most important step in its cure. It is also important to understand something about the physiology and behaviour of the average cancer cell, as this understanding is going to be very important in facilitating the cancer cure. As we will see before the end of this chapter, cancer is not really a disease but an adaptation by the body to an imbalanced and toxic internal milieu. It is a desperate attempt of the body to try to maintain homeostasis in a hostile environment. It may surprise you to know that cancer cells were once part of the normal cells of your body – they are not the enemy, something else is! It is not the cancer tumour that will kill you, per se, but the causes that initially were responsible for creating the cancer cells. Indeed, cancer is a SURVIVAL MECHANISM.

When I begin testing cancer patients to determine the causative factors, using the IDEL Diagnostic Programme[1] (see Chapter 2), I usually find between 15-20 or more causative factors. The testing is comprehensive and takes about 5 hours of clinical time, but it can be the difference between life and death – any other way is guesswork.

Cancer is multidimensional

Cancer is certainly multi-dimensional with interconnecting causes on different levels. Cancer is related to a change in the biochemistry of the normal cell – factors such as nutrition, pernicious agents (including medicinal drugs) and radiation can all directly affect the cell. On the physical level nutritional deficiencies, chronic inflammation caused by microorganisms such as viruses, bacteria, fungi and parasites, food intolerances as well as congested detoxification pathways, pH, redox and

---

1 See www.docgeorge.com/IDEL-Diagnostic-Programme.html

resistivity changes, toxic metals and organic xenobiotics, geopathic, electromagnetic, mobile phone and ionizing radiation stress can all be involved.

On a psychoemotional and spiritual level suppressed negative emotions, emotional traumas, negative beliefs, systemic entanglements (Hellinger)[2] and blocked or distorted bio-energy flows - as found in the acupuncture meridians (teeth and scar foci) - are also contributing factors – most of these have been discussed in chapter 2 and other chapters of this book.

These are all trigger factors that can make cells divide uncontrollably. It must be stressed that it is never one cause but a myriad of causes all interacting over time to cause the cellular degeneration. Even though oncologists and cancer researchers place emphasis on the genetics of cancer, this is a small component of this cascade that is usually responsible for no more than 7% of pathogenesis.[3]

Besides, a series of papers written by Ilmensee, Mintz and Hoppe in the 1970-1980's showed that replacing the fertilized nucleus of a mouse ovum by the nucleus of a teratocarcinoma did not create a mouse with cancer. Instead, the mice when born were cancer free.[4] These studies support the theory that abnormalities in other cell structures outside of the nucleus, such as the cell membrane and the mitochondria, as well as functional disturbances in cellular energy production and cell membrane potential, are also involved in cancerous transformation.

Moreover, oncogenes can be altered by their environment, the cell's internal terrain and surroundings and generally abnormal cellular oxygen metabolism ("dysoxygenosis").[5] Given that the gene pool has not really changed for thousands of years, why is it that cancer was a rare disease 40-50 years ago. If you were a medical doctor working in a large hospital in the 40's and 50's you would be lucky to see just a few cases of cancer per year. Why have the genes changed so drastically and decided to kill so many people now? Maybe we should be looking at other more significant causes?

2 Hellinger, B. To the Heart of the Matter. Carl-Auer-Systeme Verlag, Germany, 2003.
3 Lichtenstein, P, Holm, N, et al. Environmental and heritable factors in the causation of cancer. *NEJM*. 343: 78-85, 2000.
4 Seeger, PG. and Wolz, S. Successful biological control of cancer by combat against the causes. *Neuwieder Verlagsgesellschaft*, Neuwied, Germany, 1990.
5 Ali, M. Oxidative regression to primordial cellular ecology: Evidence for the hypothesis and its clinical significance. *J Integrative Medicine*. 2:4-49, 1998.

Cancer is not a disease!

Andreas Moritz, a holistic practitioner, researcher and author has made this profound statement in his book, "Cancer is Not a Disease:"[6]

"Cancer does not cause a person to be sick; it is the sickness of the person that causes the cancer."

The crucial goal in cancer cures is to eliminate all the cancer cells in the body, not simply the tumour. In order to achieve this one must work on many levels to bring the body back into balance, eliminating the causative factors and using non-toxic, natural remedies to halt the rapid proliferation of cancer cells, while modulating the immune system. This is the premise of the Holistic Model of Cancer that I am espousing here.

Holistic Medicine sees cancer as a disease of the total organism, not just a localised event. It is a systemic disease that is multifactorial in its causes. It is therefore crucial to understand the workings of cancer cells – how do they respire, what are their by-products, how do they differ from normal cells and why? It is this understanding that I believe will lead to thinking 'outside the box' – something that is imperative if we are going to have half a chance at curing the patient.

Treatments like chemotherapy and radiation can certainly poison and kill cancer cells, but the problem is that these treatments also kill good, healthy cells too, such as in the bone marrow, gastrointestinal tract, liver, kidneys, heart, lungs, immune system and more. Once these organ systems become damaged, it may be impossible to reverse this damage and then the cancer cells will proliferate at a higher rate and further upset the homeostasis of health. These poisonous, toxic treatments also cause much inflammation in many cells of the body to the point that hair follicles cannot hold onto the strands of hair on your head.

How can a real cure for cancer occur at the expense and destruction of other parts of the body? Tumour regression and removal does not cure the underlying causes of the cancer – this is where the main focus of any therapy must be, to address the underlying causes of the cancer which is

---

6 Moritz, A. Cancer Is Not a Disease, It's a Survival Mechanism. (3rd edition). USA: Enerchi Wellness Press, 2005.

the main sickness. And let's not forget the first sentence of the Hippocratic Oath that both medical doctors as well as naturopathic physicians swear to:

Primum, Non Nocere (First, Do No Harm)!

Chemotherapy and radiation – is this the solution?

Cytotoxic chemotherapy agents can cause a host of adverse effects, ranging from short-term, self-limiting adverse reactions to death. Many chemotherapy agents are themselves carcinogenic, or may increase the risk of secondary tumours due to immunosuppression. For example, 2 to 12% incidence of acute leukemia has been observed 2 to 10 years after treatment of Hodgkin's disease with chemotherapy.[7]

Even with the extensive use of chemotherapy, and often its over-prescription, there is very little change in mortality rates over the last 50 years. Modern radiotherapy and chemotherapy were not applied widely until about 1965. In fact, mortality rates in the chemotherapy era have gone up. Between the years 1950 and 1989, the age- and population-adjusted mortality rate for all races, males and females increased 10%. Overall, the advent of chemotherapy has not greatly affected mortality rates.[8]

In 1986, McGill Cancer Center[9] scientists sent a questionnaire to 118 doctors who treated non-small-cell lung cancer. More than three quarters of them recruited patients and carried out trials of toxic drugs for lung cancer. They were asked to imagine that they themselves had cancer, and were asked which of six current trials they themselves would choose. Of the 79 respondents, 64 (81%) said they would not consent to be in a trial containing cisplatin, a common chemotherapy drug. Fifty-eight or 74% of the oncologists found all the trials using any type of chemotherapy unacceptable. What reasons did they give? Basically, they quoted the ineffectiveness of chemotherapy and its unacceptable degree of toxicity.

---

7 Calabresi, P., Schein, P. Medical Oncology Second edition. New York: McGraw-Hill, Inc., 1993.
8 Boik, J. Cancer and Natural Medicine: A textbook of basic science and clinical research. USA: Oregon Medical Press, 1996.
9 Robbins, J. Reclaiming Our Health. USA: HJ Kramer, 1996.

In 1990, the highly respected German epidemiologist, Dr. Ulrich Abel[10] from the Tumor Clinic of the University of Heidelberg, conducted the most comprehensive investigation of every major clinical study on chemotherapy drugs ever done. Abel contacted 350 medical centers and asked them to send him anything they had ever published on chemotherapy. He also reviewed and analyzed thousands of scientific articles published in the most prestigious medical journals.

It took Abel several years to collect and evaluate the data. Abel's epidemiological study, which was published on August 10, 1991 in *The Lancet*, should have alerted every doctor and cancer patient about the risks of one of the most common treatments used for cancer and other diseases. In his paper, Abel came to the conclusion that the overall success rate of chemotherapy was "appalling." According to this report, there was no scientific evidence available in any existing study to show that chemotherapy can "*extend in any appreciable way the lives of patients suffering from the most common organic cancers.*"

Abel points out that chemotherapy rarely improves the quality of life. He describes chemotherapy as "*a scientific wasteland*" and states that even though there is no scientific evidence that chemotherapy works, neither doctor nor patient is willing to give up on it. The mainstream media has never reported on this hugely important study, which is hardly surprising, given the enormous vested interests of the groups that sponsor the media, that is, the pharmaceutical companies. A recent search turned up exactly zero reviews of Abel's work in American journals, even though it was published in 1990. I believe this is not because his work was unimportant - but because it is irrefutable.

Another more recent research study has been published in the journal *Clinical Oncology*. This meta-analysis, entitled "The Contribution of Cytotoxic Chemotherapy to 5-year Survival in Adult Malignancies"[11] set out to accurately quantify and assess the actual benefit conferred by chemotherapy in the treatment of adults with the commonest types of cancer. All three of the paper's authors are oncologists. Lead author Associate Professor Graeme Morgan is a radiation oncologist at Royal North Shore Hospital in Sydney; Professor Robyn Ward is a medical

---

10 Abel, U. Chemotherapy of Advanced Epithelial Cancer: a critical review, *Biomedicine and Pharmacotherapy*, 46: 439-452, 1992.
11 Morgan G, Ward R, Barton M. The contribution of cytotoxic chemotherapy to 5-year survival in adult malignancies. *Clin Oncol* (R Coll Radiol). 16(8):549-60, 2004.

oncologist at University of New South Wales/St. Vincent's Hospital. The third author, Dr. Michael Barton, is a radiation oncologist and a member of the Collaboration for Cancer Outcomes Research and Evaluation, Liverpool Health Service, Sydney. Prof. Ward is also a member of the Therapeutic Goods Authority of the Australian Federal Department of Health and Aging, the official body that advises the Australian government on the suitability and efficacy of drugs to be listed on the national Pharmaceutical Benefits Schedule (PBS) – roughly the equivalent of the US Food and Drug Administration.

Their meticulous study was based on an analysis of the results of all the randomized, controlled clinical trials (RCTs) performed in Australia and the US that reported a statistically significant increase in 5-year survival due to the use of chemotherapy in adult malignancies. Survival data were drawn from the Australian cancer registries and the US National Cancer Institute's Surveillance Epidemiology and End Results (SEER) registry spanning the period January 1990 until January 2004.

Wherever data were uncertain, the authors deliberately erred on the side of overestimating the benefit of chemotherapy. Even so, the study concluded that overall, chemotherapy contributes just over 2 percent to improved survival in cancer patients.

Yet, despite the mounting evidence of chemotherapy's lack of effectiveness in prolonging survival, oncologists continue to present chemotherapy as a rational and promising approach to cancer treatment. Associate Professor Graeme Morgan says: "Some practitioners still remain optimistic that cytotoxic chemotherapy will significantly improve cancer survival. However, despite the use of new and expensive single and combination drugs to improve response rates...there has been little impact from the use of newer regimens."

The Australian authors continued: "...in lung cancer, the median survival has increased by only 2 months [during the past 20 years, ed.] and an overall survival benefit of less than 5 percent has been achieved in the adjuvant treatment of breast, colon and head and neck cancers."

Basically, the authors found that the contribution of chemotherapy to 5-year survival in adults was 2.3 percent in Australia, and 2.1 percent in the USA. They emphasize that, for reasons explained in detail in the study, these figures "should be regarded as the upper limit of effectiveness" (i.e., they are an optimistic rather than a pessimistic estimate).

Often statistics are manipulated based on false statistics, as well as misunderstandings regarding terminology.[12] According to Dr. Ralph Moss,[13] cancer researcher and author of many books such as *The Cancer Industry:*[14]

"If you can shrink the tumour 50% or more for 28 days you have got the FDA's definition of an active drug. This is called a response rate, so you have a response....(but) when you look to see if there is any life prolongation from taking this treatment what you find is all kinds of hocus pocus and song and dance about the disease-free survival, and this and that. In the end there is no proof that chemotherapy in the vast majority of cases actually extends life, and this is the GREAT LIE about chemotherapy, that somehow there is a correlation between shrinking a tumour and extending the life of the patient."

The cancer establishment is really bent on shrinking tumours, even though there is no relationship to survival benefit. **An article in the British Medical Journal concurred - it observed that while tumour shrinkage is the usual way to measure the efficacy of chemotherapy, "radiological shrinkage of solid tumours . . . often has little or no survival benefit . . . . Unfortunately, few studies have compared chemotherapy with supportive care alone."**[15]

A 1984 review of 80 studies of chemotherapy for breast cancer found that 76 of them had looked only at tumour shrinkage, not at effects on survival or quality of life; and three of the remaining four had found no survival advantage for the drugs.[16]

One of the nation's top statisticians in the field of cancer is Hardin B. Jones, Ph.D., former professor of medical physics and physiology at the University of California at Berkeley. After years of analyzing clinical

---

12 Enstrom, J.E. & Austin, D.F. Interpreting Cancer Survival Rates, *Science*, 195: 847-851, 1977.
13 Moss, R.W. Questioning Chemotherapy, New York: Equinox Press, 1995.
14 Moss, RW. The Cancer Industry: The Classic Exposé on the Cancer Establishment. New York: Equinox Press, 1999.
15 Mead, G. Chemotherapy for solid tumours: Routine treatment not yet justified, *British Medical Journal* 310:246, 1995.
16 Oye, R et al. Reporting results from chemotherapy trials: Does response make a difference in patient survival?, *JAMA* 252(19):2722-25, 1984.

records, this is the report he delivered at a convention of the American Cancer Society:[17]

"In regard to surgery, no relationship between intensity of surgical treatment and duration of survival has been found in verified malignancies. On the contrary, simple excision of cancers has produced essentially the same survival as radical excision and dissection of the lymphatic drainage."

What, then, is the statistical chance for long-term survival of five years or more after surgery?[18] That, we are told, depends on the location of the cancer, how fast it is growing, and whether it has spread to a secondary point. For example, two of the most common forms of cancer requiring surgery are of the breast and the lung. With breast cancer, only sixteen percent will respond favourably to surgery or X-ray therapy.

With lung cancer, the percentage of patients who will survive five years after surgery is somewhere between five and ten percent - these are optimistic figures when compared to survival expectations for some other types of cancers such as testicular chorionepitheliomas.[19]

An objective appraisal, therefore, is that the statistical rate of long-term survival after surgery is, on the average at best, only ten or fifteen percent. And once the cancer has metastasized to a second location, surgery has almost no survival value. The reason is that, like the other therapies approved by orthodox medicine, surgery removes only the tumour. It does not remove the cause.

Radiation and/or radiomimetic poisons will reduce palpable, gross or measurable tumefaction. Often this reduction may amount to seventy-five percent or more of the mass of the growth. These agents have a selective effect - radiation and poisons. They selectively kill everything except the definitively neoplastic [cancer] cells. For example, a benign uterine myoma will usually melt away under radiation like snow melting, but the active neoplastic cells in the tumour will remain. The size of the tumour

---

17 Jones, HB. A Report on Cancer, paper delivered to the ACS's 11th Annual Science Writers Conference, New Orleans, March 7, 1969.

18 Benjamin, D.J. The Efficacy of Surgical Treatment of Cancer, *Medical Hypotheses*, 40 (2): 129- 138, 1993.

19 Johnstone, FRC. Results of Treatment of Carcinoma of the Breast Based on Pathological Staging, *Surgery, Gynecology & Obstetrics*, 134:211, 1972.

may thus be decreased by ninety percent (known as the "response rate") while the relative concentration of neoplastic cells is thereby increased by ninety percent.

As all experienced clinicians know - or at least should know - after radiation or poisons have reduced the gross tumefaction of the lesion the patient's general well-being does not substantially improve. To the contrary, there is often an explosive or fulminating increase in the biological malignancy of his lesion. This is marked by the appearance of diffuse metastasis and a rapid deterioration in general vitality followed shortly by death.

From the data available it would seem that the use of post-operative irradiation has provided no discernible advantage to patients in terms of increasing the proportion who were free of disease for as long as five years.[20] This is an embarrassingly difficult fact for a radiologist to face, for it means, quite literally, that there is little justification for his existence in the medical fraternity. Consequently, one does not expect to hear these facts being discussed by radiologists or those whose livelihood depends on the construction, sale, installation, use, or maintenance of the multi-million-dollar linear accelerators.

A 1987 review of eight trials from around the world found that the risk of death after ten years for women who had not been treated with radiation after their breast surgeries was 26 percent lower than for women who had gotten.[21] "The majority of cancers," wrote Dr. John Cairns of Harvard in 1985, "cannot be cured by radiation because the dose of X-rays required to kill all the cancer cells would also kill the patient."[22]

The potential risks involved in handling cytotoxic agents have become a concern for health care workers. The literature reports various symptoms such as eye, membrane, and skin irritation, as well as dizziness, nausea, and headache experienced by health care workers not using safe handling precautions. In addition, increased concerns regarding the mutagenesis and teratogenesis [deformed babies] continue to be investigated. Many

20 Fisher, B., et. al. Postoperative Radiotherapy in the Treatment of Breast Cancer; Results of the NSAPP Clinical Trial, *Annals of Surgery*, 172, No.4, Od. 1970.
21 Cuzick, J et al. Overview of randomized trials of postoperative adjuvant radiotherapy in breast cancer, *Cancer Treatment Reports* 71(1):15-29, 1987.
22 Cairns, J. The treatment of diseases and the war against cancer, *Scientific American* 253(5):51, 1985.

chemotherapy agents, the alkylating agents in particular, are known to be carcinogenic [cancer -causing] in therapeutic doses.[23]

In a courageous letter to Dr. Frank Rauscher, his boss at the National Cancer Institute, Dr. Dean Burk condemned the Institute's policy of continuing to endorse these drugs when everyone knew that they caused cancer. He argued:

"Ironically, virtually all of the chemotherapeutic anti-cancer agents now approved by the Food and Drug Administration for use or testing in human cancer patients are:

- ❖ highly or variously toxic at applied dosages;
- ❖ markedly immunosuppressive, that is, destructive of the patient's native resistance to a variety of diseases, including cancer;
- ❖ usually highly carcinogenic [cancer causing].

These now well established facts have been reported in numerous publications from the National Cancer Institute itself, as well as from throughout the United States and, indeed, the world. Furthermore, what has just been said of the FDA-approved anti-cancer chemotherapeutic drugs is true, though perhaps less conspicuously, of radiological and surgical treatments of human cancer.

If it is true that Orthodox chemotherapy is (1) toxic, (2) immunosuppressant, (3) carcinogenic, and (4) futile, then why would doctors continue to use it?[24] The answer is that they don't know what else to do. Patients usually are not scheduled into chemotherapy unless their condition seems so hopeless that the loss of life appears to be inevitable anyway. Some doctors refer to this stage, not as therapy, but experimentation, which, frankly, is a more honest description.

Another reason for using drugs in the treatment of cancer is that the doctor does not like to tell the patient there is no hope. In his own mind he knows there is none, but he also knows that the patient does not want to hear that and will seek another physician who will continue some kind of treatment,

---

23 Skeel, RT. and Lachant, NA., Handbook of Cancer Chemotherapy, Fourth Edition New York: Little, Brown and Company, p.677, 1995.
24 Peto, J. & Easton, D., Cancer Treatment Trials - past failures, current progress and future prospects, *Cancer Survey*, 8: 513-533, 1989.

no matter how useless. So he solves the problem by continuing the treatment himself.

An interesting study would be to compare the effectiveness of chemotherapy and radiation with no treatment at all. Would the cancer patient live longer if they received no treatment whatsoever?

One of the few studies that had made this comparison was conducted by Dr. Hardin Jones, professor of medical physics and physiology at the University of California, Berkeley.[25] He told an ACS panel:

"My studies have proven conclusively that untreated cancer victims actually live up to four times longer than treated individuals. For a typical type of cancer, people who refused treatment lived for an average of 12 ½ years. Those who accepted surgery and other kinds of treatment lived an average of only three years. . . . I attribute this to the traumatic effect of surgery on the body's natural defense mechanism. The body has a natural defense against every type of cancer."

Dr. Jones was speaking fourty years ago, but more recent data are lacking, because studies comparing treated and untreated patients are no longer being done. To fail to treat potentially curable patients with "proven" methods is now considered unethical. Most drug studies merely compare the effects of two treatment regimens, both more or less equally toxic, on the size of tumour growth.

In a 1991 study in which chemotherapy was compared to no treatment in 250 women with metastatic breast cancer, the drugs not only did not improve survival but significantly decreased the quality of life.[26]

According to Dr. Cairns, chemotherapy prevents death in only 2 to 5 percent of cancer cases. The chance the drugs themselves will kill the patient is about the same: somewhere between 2.5 percent and 5 percent.[27]

With early breast cancer, on the other hand, a modest survival benefit has been found. A 1992 British review of 31 randomized trials involving

25 Jones, HB. *A Report on Cancer*, paper delivered to the ACS's 11th Annual Science Writers Conference, New Orleans, Mar. 7, 1969.
26 H. Muss, et al. Interrupted versus continuous chemotherapy in patients with metastatic breast cancer, *New England Journal of Medicine* 325:1342-48, 1991.
27 Culliton, B. The rocky road to remission, *Science* 244:1432, June 23, 1989.

11,000 women found a slight increase in overall survival after 10 years for patients given "polychemotherapy" (more than one drug for more than one month). The women's chances of being alive 10 years later, however, were still only 51.3 percent with the drugs, versus 45 percent without them a mere 6.3 percent survival benefit. And this grim prognosis was for women with breast cancer in the early, "treatable" stages.[28]

Despite these very modest benefits, the National Cancer Institute has recommended chemotherapy for all breast cancer patients, whether or not they have visible signs of cancer after surgery. The theory is that projected over thousands of women, a significant number of lives will be saved.[29]

The same year, the General Accounting Office issued a report on the effectiveness of chemotherapy in breast cancer. It focused on patients with cancers of the type thought to benefit most from the drugs. The GAO found no detectable increase in the survival of these patients, despite a threefold increase in the use of chemotherapy since 1975.[30]

The problem especially for the 93.7 percent who aren't benefited is the drug's crushing side effects. Virtually all chemotherapeutic drugs are toxic and immunosuppressive. Being unable to distinguish between cancerous and normal cells, they wind up killing both. Most also cause secondary cancers, which can show up many years after "successful" chemotherapy.[31]

---

28 Early Breast Cancer Trialists' Collaborative Group, Systemic treatment of early breast cancer by hormonal, cytotoxic, or immune therapy, *Lancet* 339(8785):71-85, 1992.
29 The recommendation was based on a series of 1989 studies finding a "significant prolongation of disease-free survival" from drug treatment. However, the studies did not find a significant increase in actual survival. "Disease-free survival" was a term of art meaning a period of time without new tumours. See B. Fisher, et al., "A randomized clinical trial evaluating sequential methotrexate and fluorouracil in the treatment of patients with node-negative breast dancer who have estrogen-receptor-negative tumours," *New England Journal of Medicine* 320(8):473-78, 1989; Ludwig Breast Cancer Study Group, Prolonged disease-free survival after one course of perioperative adjuvant chemotherapy for node-negative breast cancer, *New England Journal of Medicine* 320(8):491-96, 1989; E. Mansour, et al., "Efficacy of adjuvant chemotherapy in high- risk node-negative breast cancer," *New England Journal of Medicine* 320(8):485-90, 1989.
30 See "GAO report on breast cancer," *World Research Foundation News* (3rd & 4th quarter 1990), page 7.
31 R. Walters, op. cit. See also H. Vorherr, "Adjuvant chemotherapy of breast cancer: Reality, hope, hazard?", *Lancet* (December 19/26, 1981), pages 1413-14: "Data on five-year survival [show] the benefit from adjuvant [independent] chemotherapy of breast cancer is only 4% . . Mortality due to chemotherapy may be as high as 4.4% . . In view of

If the conclusion from the research that we have examined so far is that surgery, chemotherapy and radiation have little to offer the cancer patient in terms of a cure, then we need to look elsewhere. Again, I would like to bring your attention back to the real causes of cancer, and not the symptoms which is basically the tumour. We need to understand the basic physiology of a cancer cell in order to better comprehend why a normal cell decides to convert into a cancer cell. It is basically a survival mechanism in order to adapt to a polluted environment where oxygen levels have dropped to such a degree that the aerobic cell becomes asphyxiated. Let's look closer at some of the research that has been done to demonstrate this.

Cancer and mitochondrial dysfunction

We have already looked at a multitude of causative factors that can trigger the healthy cell to undergo a biochemical change and become a cancer cell. It was once believed that most of this triggering takes place in the nucleus and the genetic material that it contains, but Dr. Seeger found that these pernicious agents and energies affect mostly the cytoplasm. P.G. Seeger[32] in Germany, published 290 scientific works and was twice nominated for the Nobel Prize (in 1979 and 1980), showed that in cancer cells the respiratory chain was blocked by the destruction of important enzymes, such as cytochrome oxidase.[33]

It was also shown that cancer cells convert glucose into lactic acid[34] to produce energy - Seeger and others found that cancer cells utilise only between 5 to 50% of the oxygen of normal cells and produce up to 40 times as much lactic acid as normal cells. The lower the oxygen levels, the more virulent become the cancer cells. In 1957, Seeger[35] successfully transformed normal cells into cancer cells within a few days by blocking

the many uncertainties and controversies about adjuvant chemotherapy, which itself has serious health hazards, no patient should be routinely subjected to this kind of 'treatment."
32 Seeger, P.G. Fundamental importance of cell respiration for cell metabolism. *Zahnarztl Mitt.* 58 (20):1085-90, Oct 16 1968.
4 Jung, H., Seeger, PG. Metabolism of malignant tumours. Arztl Forsch. 10;10(10):1/489-92, Oct 1956.
34 Seeger, PG. Cell respiration and cancer. *Dtsch Gesundheitsw.* 14;14:893-8, May 1959.
35 Seeger, PG. Experimental results in the biology of cancer: comparative measurement of respiratory intensity of normal & cancer cells & the activation of respiration by means of various substances. *Hippokrates.* 30(11):413-9, Jun 15 1959.

the respiratory chain using chemicals. He also discovered after thousands of experiments that certain nutrients from the vegetable kingdom could restore cellular respiration in cancer cells and transform them back into normal cells.[36]

So what is destroying these very important cytochrome enzymes? There is no question that the heavy metals and xenobiotics in our environment are the prime cause as they target and destroy cardiolipine, a lipid contained in the inner mitochondrial membrane, to which the cytochrome enzymes of the respiratory chain are attached. When the cardiolipine is destroyed by these pernicious agents, the oxidative processes are adversely affected.[37]

The destruction of this enzyme cytochrome oxidase (Cytochrome a/a3) is what triggers the cell to begin dividing as a cancer cell.[38] This is really important to understand in order to be able to reverse these degenerative, cancerous cells by utilizing specialized enzyme-active nutritional substances and select vegetable and fruit hydrogen acceptors. These enzyme-rich nutritional substances include: Saccharomyces cerevisiae (live fluid yeast strain), red beet juice, raw blueberry juice, bromelain (pineapple enzyme), raw pineapple juice, raw red grapes, raw red cherries, carotene (specifically beta carotene from carrot juice). Others would include barley Grass powder, Kamut Grass powder and Chlorella. It is no coincidence that cancer patients attending holistic cancer centres are asked to consume quantities of these natural products.

Cancer and Anaerobic Respiration

Dr. Otto Warburg (1883-1970)[39] was Director of the Max Planck Institute of Cell Physiology in Germany. The holder of many international honours, Dr. Warburg was considered by Dr. Dean Burk, head of the Cytochemistry Department of the US National Cancer Institute at the time, to be the world's greatest biochemist. In 1931 Warburg won the Nobel Prize in Medicine for his discovery of the oxygen transferring enzyme of cell respiration, and was voted a second Nobel Prize in 1944 for his discovery

---

36 Seeger, P.G. and S. Wolz: Successful biological control of cancer by combat against the causes. Neuwieder Verlagsgesellschaft, Neuwied, Germany, 1990 (only book available in the English language).
37 Green, DR., & Kroemer, G. The Pathophysiology of Mitochondrial Cell Death. *Science* Vol. 305. no. 5684, pp. 626 – 629, 30 July 2004.
38 Schlager, SI & Ohanian, SH. Correlation between lipid synthesis in tumour cells and their sensitivity to humoral immune attack. *Science* 197: 773-776, 19 August 1977.
39 Warburg O. On the origin of cancer cells. *Science* 123:309-14, 1956.

of the active groups of the hydrogen transferring enzymes. Conferred honorary degrees by the universities of Harvard, Oxford and Heidelberg, he was a member of the Royal Society of London, a Knight of the Order of Merit founded by Frederick the Great, and was awarded the Great Cross with Star and Shoulder Ribbon of the Bundesrepublik.

Warburg's research spanned more than sixty years, and he was the author of over 500 published research papers and five books. His description of the experiments in which he transformed normal cells into cancer cells was contained in his lecture at the meeting of Nobel-Laureates on 30 June 1966 at Lindau, Germany.[40]

Prof. Otto Warburg summarized his many years of research very succinctly:

"Cancer has only one prime cause. It is the replacement of normal oxygen respiration of the body's cells by an anaerobic [i.e., oxygen-deficient] cell respiration."

Dr. Majid Ali, M.D.,[41] a medical doctor and cancer researcher also aptly states:

"The state of the oxygen in the body, not chemotherapy or radiotherapy, determines the long-term health and quality of life of the patient".

He further purports an Oxygen Model of Cancer that has three basic aspects: Acidosis (too much acidity) leading to Oxidosis (too much oxidation) which further leads to Dysoxygenosis (lack of oxygen) – this sequence of events is what is required to trigger the growth of cancer cells. Dr. Ali continues to say: "Chemotherapy drugs significantly contribute to oxidosis (too much oxidative stress), acidosis (too much acidity), and dysoxygenosis (oxygen dysfunction) in many ways. It is for these reasons that nearly all cancers become much more aggressive and grow rapidly when they return following chemotherapy."[42]

---

40 This lecture, titled "The Prime Cause and Prevention of Cancer", was reproduced in English by Dr Dean Burk and published by Konrad Triltsch, Wurzburg, Germany.
41 Ali, M. The Crab, Oxygen and Cancer: The Dysox Model of Cancer. Canary 21 Press, USA, 2004.
42 www.majidali.com

Apart from living in an oxygen-deficient environment, cancer cells also have a voracious appetite for sugar – they use 18 times more glucose than normal cells and produce only 2 molecules of ATP (energy units) as opposed to the 38 molecules of ATP produced by a healthy, normal cell. Cancer is therefore caused by an oxygen-deficient, glucose-rich (sugar) environment.

These observations provide us with important clues to how we should treat a cancer patient – first, DO NOT feed cancer cells SUGAR, which is their primary food. Second, make certain that the body obtains plenty of OXYGEN to facilitate the respiratory chain and unblock important enzyme systems. We will soon see how another famous scientist; Dr. Johann Budwig managed to do just this.

Reoxygenation of Cancer Cells

Even though Prof. Otto Warburg won two Nobel prizes for his work on oxygen and cancer cells, demonstrating that a reduction of oxygen by 35% was enough to trigger a healthy cell to become a partially anaerobic cancer cell. One thing that he could not seem to solve, however, was how to get the oxygen back into the cancer cell. He knew that fatty acids on the membrane of the cancer cell had something to do with this, but it was Dr. Johanna Budwig,[43] a German biochemist, pharmacologist, physicist and fat researcher (1908 – 2003), whose research found that phosphatides and lipoproteins were highly deficient in cancer patients and were crucial for the oxygenation of the cancer cell. She also showed that commercially processed fats and trans fats can destroy the cell membrane and lead to many chronic diseases.

By using liberal amounts of high-quality flaxseed oil (Linum usitatissimum), mixed with cottage cheese or quark which are rich in the sulphur-amino acids cysteine and methionine, the respiratory chain was reactivated and cancer patients recovered.[44] The chemical reaction makes the oil "water soluble" and is able to absorb through the cell membrane of the cell. This is now known as the *Budwig Diet* and consists of adding Flaxseed oil to Quark or Cottage cheese.

---

43 Budwig, J. Flax Oil As a True Aid Against Arthritis Heart Infarction Cancer and Other Diseases (3rd Edition), 1994.
44 Budwig, J. Cytostatic or cytodynamic control of cancer? *Hippokrates* 27 (19): 605–612, 1956.

Dr. Budwig found that in about three months on her flaxseed oil-quark combination, cancer patients began to improve. Tumours shrunk in size, patients' strength returned, and further blood analysis showed that the greenish-yellow substance in the blood disappeared. Phosphatide and lipoprotein levels returned to normal, and red blood cells and haemoglobin returned to normal levels.

After over 10 years of clinical research, Dr. Budwig's combination of 2 tablespoons of organic flaxseed oil combined with one quarter cup of cottage cheese has been used successfully in Europe to treat a variety of diseases in addition to cancer, including arteriosclerosis, eczema, stomach and intestinal disorders, arthritis, and strokes. It is now an obligatory dietary protocol in most of the cancer patients that are seen at the DaVinci Centre and supervised nutritionally.

All this scientific research and its practical results continue to be ignored by the Cancer establishment and despite the evidence to the contrary, they still maintain that cancer originates in the nucleus; that it cannot be reversed but only treated by killing all cancer cells; that curing cancer with nutrition is impossible, and those who do it anyway are frauds and quacks, and must be prevented from practising. Cured cancer patients have praised the Lord on many occasions for the 'quacks' that have helped them cure their cancer!

To further facilitate our understanding, let's look briefly at the different steps in the development of a cancer cell.

Steps in the Development of a Cancer Cell

Cancer cells do not just grow of their own accord without reason. The first step in the pathogenesis of the cancer cells is the attachment of carcinogenic type molecules to the membrane surface. This involves two factors: (a) the presence of carcinogenic-type molecules primarily of the polycyclic type, and (b) a chronic inflammation from other factors such as disturbed pH that will change the polarization of the cell as well as its Trans Membrane Potential (TMP).

Electrically charged particles such as ions, and proteins, accumulate on both sides of the various membrane interfaces of a cell, and create an electrical potential. Normal cells and cancer cells have many different physiologic qualities, which include those of their TMP and electrochemistry. A normal cell has a TMP of about 70 to 100mv.[45] This is equal to an electrical potential of between 10 and 20 million volts per metre. The mitochondrial membranes of a normal cell maintain an electrical potential of almost 40 million volts per meter.[46]

When a cell becomes cancerous, plasma membranes degenerate and depolarize,[47] and the electrical potential across the membrane drops drastically. Seeger in the 1990's worked for over 50 years on cancer research – in summary, his findings are: that cells become more electronegative in the course of cancerization, that *membrane degeneration* occurs in the initial phase of carcinogenesis first in the external cell membrane and then in the inner mitochondrial membrane, that the degenerative changes in the surface membrane causes these *membranes to become more permeable to water-soluble substances* so that potassium, magnesium, calcium migrate from the cells and sodium and water accumulate in the cell interior, that the degenerative changes in the inner membrane of the mitochondria causes *loss of anchorage of critical mitochondrial enzymes*, and that the mitochondria in cancer cells degenerate and are reduced in number.[48]

As the distribution of ions shift, cancer cells tend to become very electronegative, and the tissue areas surrounding the cancer cells become quite electropositive. This electropositivity has been used for detection of cancer.[49] The combined effects of the low plasma membrane electrical potential, and ionic imbalance, assists in the conversion of a normal cell's aerobic based metabolism to that of a cancer cell with an anaerobic based

---

45 Cone CD. Variation of the transmembrane potential level as a basic mechanism of mitosis control. *Oncology* 24:438-470, 1970; Cone CD. The role of surface electrical transmembrane potential in normal and malignant mitogenesis. *Ann NY Acad Sci* 238:420-35, 1975; Cone CD. Transmembrane Potentials and Characteristics of Immune and Tumour Cells. Boca Raton, Florida: CRC Press, 1985.
46 Brown G. The Energy of Life: The Science of What Makes Our Minds and Bodies Work. New York, NY: The Free Press, 1999.
47 Marino AA, Morris DM, Schwalke MA, Iliev IG, Rogers S Electrical Potential Measurements in Human Breast Cancer and Benign Lesions. *Tumour Biology* 15(3):147-52, 1994.
48 Seeger PG, Wolz S. Successful Biological Control of Cancer: By Combat Against the Causes. Gesamtherstellung: Neuwieder Verlagsgesellschaft mbH,1990
49 Marino AA, Iliev IG, Schwalke MA, Gonzalez E, Marler KC, Flanagan CA, Association Between Cell Membrane Potential and Breast Cancer. *Tumour Biol.* 15(2):82-9, 1994; Marino AA, Morris DM, Schwalke MA, Iliev IG, Rogers S Electrical Potential Measurements in Human Breast Cancer and Benign Lesions . *Tumor Biology* 15(3):147-52, 1994.

metabolism. Conversion to anaerobic glycolysis (fermentation) as a primary mechanism for energy production results in excessive accumulation of organic acids and acidic pH alterations in cancerous tissues.

In addition, pernicious agents attach to cardiolipine and block the Cytochrome oxidase enzymes, therefore competing with oxygen and not allowing it to enter the cell in optimal amounts, even though glucose is still allowed to enter. The cell will then begin to convert from aerobic respiration to anaerobic respiration. The next step in the absence of oxygen is for the glucose to undergo fermentation to lactic acid. The cell's pH will inevitably become acidic, finally dropping to pH 6.5 or lower.

In this acid medium the DNA loses its positive and negative radical sequence which changes the amino acid sequences entering the cell. Ultimately the RNA is changed and the cell becomes apoptotic, completely losing its control mechanism. It is highly likely that chromosomal aberrations will occur at this stage. Making the cell alkaline and oxygenating it will help it to produce enough energy to activate the p53 gene to produce the proteins that can cause apotosis.

Finally, in the acid medium the various cell enzymes are completely changed. Von Ardenne[50] has shown that lysosomal enzymes are changed into very toxic compounds. These toxins kill the cells in the main body of the tumour mass. A tumour therefore consists of a thin layer of rapidly growing cells surrounding the dead mass. The acid toxins leak out from the tumour mass and poison the host. They thus give rise to the pains generally associated with cancer. They can also act as carcinogens. The high acidity and low oxygen environment also triggers vascular endothelial growth factor (VEGF) leading to angiogenesis that feed the growing tumour.

So as you can see, cancer is a destructive behaviour of cells, incited and perpetuated by many factors that cumulatively lead to anomalous oxygen signalling. It has six other principal characteristics:

1. Respiratory-to-fermentative (RTF) shift in ATP production

---

50 Von Ardenne M., P. G. Reitnauer and D. Schmidt. Theoretische Grundlagen und in vivo Messungen zur Optimierung der selekiven übersäurung von Krebsgewebe. *Acta Biol Med Germ* 22: 35-60, 1969.

2. Production of abnormal quantities of organic acids, lactic acid and others.

3. Creation of an insulate of coagulated proteins (sialo-glycoproteins) around malignant cells to repel leukocytes.

4. Uncontrolled cellular replication that disrupts local tissue architecture.

5. Colonization of distant tissues in which the destructive behaviour of neoplastic cells continues.

6. Under certain conditions, a cancer cell can be coaxed to alter its behaviour.

Cancer cells severely punish healthy cells that get in their way. They smear the surfaces of noncancerous cells with their toxic acids, blocking their membrane channels, receptors, and pumps. They clot proteins in the fluids that bathe noncancerous cells, and so rob them of their nourishment.

The process of protein clotting also reduces blood and lymph flow in healthy tissues, so devitalizing them. By those and other nefarious activities, cancer cells also cause mutations in genes of noncancerous cells. The cumulative results of all those phenomena are deoxygenation of normal cells causing cancer-like metabolic changes in noncancerous cells, which literally cannibalizes them.

So how can we reverse this extreme acid environment of a cancer cell, which is one of the key factors in the series of events that make the cancer cells more and more virulent?

Reversing acid pH in cancer cells

There are many natural substances known that can effectively kill cancer cells. One that is well researched by Dr. Keith Brewer[51] and is very useful in metastatic cancers that can swiftly reverse an extremely acidic cancer cell into an alkaline one, is Cesium chloride - a natural mineral found in the earth, that has a pH of 8.0 and can freely enter the cancer cell. Cesium

---

51 Reprinted from Pharmacology Biochemistry & Behavior, v. 21, Suppl., 1, by A. Keith Brewer, Ph.D.," The High pH Therapy for Cancer, Tests on Mice and Humans," pp. 1-5, Copyright 1984.

ions are taken into the cell via the sodium-potassium pump, substituting for potassium, and are trapped there. They also block the exit of the potassium ions by blocking the potassium channel proteins in the cell walls - one reason why it is crucial for patients to also take potassium along with the Cesium.

Cesium raises the cancer cell pH to the range of 8.0, neutralizing the lactic acid produced by the cancer cell and stopping pain within 12 to 24 hours.[52] A pH range of 8.0 is a deadly environment for the cancer cell. The cancer cell dies within a few days and is absorbed and eliminated by the body.

The accumulation of Cesium and potassium ions in the cell negates the voltage potential across the cell membrane. This voltage potential is required to energize the sodium-glucose co-transport system that feeds the cell. The cell thus starves and will eventually lyse. The sodium-potassium pumps of cancer cells operate 20 times faster than normal cells, and will therefore starve much quicker than normal cells due to the fast uptake of Cesium.[53]

There are certain factors which may enhance the Cesium therapy. The Cesium penetration into the cancer cell can be increased by the following two methods:

1. The first approach resides in broadening the electron donor capacity of the cancer cell membrane by the application of cyanide, an electron donor radical as found in nitriles ($C_{20}H_{27}NO_{11}$), a glycoside initially isolated from the seeds of the tree *Prunus dulcis*, also known as bitter almonds.

2. By the use of DMSO. The second approach enhances the potential gradient across the cancer cell membrane by the utilization of weak acids like ascorbic acid (Vitamin C) and retinoic acid (Vitamin A).

Perhaps the most well known physician to use Cesium to treat cancer is Dr. H. E. Sartori.[54] He began his Cesium (Cs) cancer therapy program in April 1981 at Life Sciences Universal Medical Clinics in Rockville,

---

52 Brewer, A. K. Cancer: Comments on the physics involved. *Am Lab* 5: 12-23. 1973.
53 Brewer, A. K. and R. Passwater. Physics of the cell membrane. V. Mechanisms involved in cancer. *Am Lab* 8: 37-45, 1976.
54 Sartori, HE. Cesium therapy in cancer patients, *Pharmacology Biochemistry and Behavior*, Volume 21, Supplement 1, 11-13, 1984.

Maryland, where 50 patients with "terminal" metastatic cancer were treated.

Cesium chloride was given to patients, along with vitamin A, vitamin C, vitamin B17, zinc, and selenium. The diet consisted primarily of whole grains, vegetables, and linolenic acid rich foods such as flaxseed, walnut, and wheat germ. To increase efficiency of the treatment and improve the circulation and oxygenation, the patients received the chelating agent EDTA and DMSO. The study included 10 patients with breast cancer, 9 with colon cancer, 6 with prostate cancer, 4 had pancreatic cancer, 6 had lung cancer, 3 had liver cancer, 3 had lymphoma, 1 had pelvic cancer, and 8 had cancer from an unknown site of origin.

The results demonstrated an impressive 50% full recovery from various metastatic cancers that were given zero percent prognoses. A consistent finding in these patients was the disappearance of pain within the initial 3 days of Cs-treatment, probably due to the rapid neutralization of the lactic acid.

By normal standards, the results were impressive. Approximately 50% of the metastatic patients with breast, colon, prostate, pancreatic, and lung cancer survived for at least 3 years, despite the fact that conventional doctors gave them only a few weeks to live! Thirteen patients died in the first two weeks of therapy. Autopsy results in each of these thirteen disclosed reduced tumour size from the cesium therapy. Pain also disappeared in 100% of the patients within 1 to 3 days after initiation of cesium therapy.

Please bear in mind that these were stage IV metastatic cancers with a zero prognosis by the medical fraternity, so a stage I or II cancer would certainly expect far higher success ratings closer to 80-90%. The cure rate for similar advanced cancer patients by orthodox medicine is close to zero percent.

Cesium is best used transdermally by mixing with DMSO. This method was introduced in the 1960's by a research team headed by Stanley W. Jacob, M.D.,[55] at the University of Oregon Medical School. A study was conducted in which DMSO was mixed with a haematoxylon (a purple dye) and injected into patients with cancer. The purpose of the study was to

---

55 E. J. Tucker, A. Carrizo, Haematoxylon Dissolved in Dimethylsulfoxide [DMSO] Used in Recurrent Neoplasms, June 1968.

determine which cells would "attract" the DMSO. They learned that DMSO has an affinity for cancer cells. As a matter of fact, some of the cancer patients were cured during this study, even though DMSO was only being combined with a dye!

Other minerals are also used along with the Cesium such as Germanium, for stimulating natural killer cells and T-suppressor cells; Indium enhances food and mineral absorption by the body; Manganese makes up part of a molecule known as mucopolysaccharides, used to form collagen that builds tissues throughout the body; Molybdenum is instrumental in regulating pH balance in the body - for each pH point increase (e.g., 6.1 to 6.2), the oxygen level is increased ten times, so this is crucial; Selenium is essential for building glutathione peroxidise enzymes as well as immune modulation.

Mass spectrographic and isotope studies[56] have shown that potassium, rubidium, and especially cesium are most efficiently taken up by cancer cells. This uptake was enhanced by Vitamins A and C as well as salts of zinc and selenium. The quantity of cesium taken up was sufficient to raise the cell to the 8 pH range. Where cell mitosis ceases and the life of the cell is short. Tests on mice fed cesium and rubidium showed marked shrinkage in the tumour masses within 2 weeks. In addition, the mice showed none of the side effects of cancer.

Tests have been carried out on over 30 humans. In each case the tumour masses disappeared. Also all pains and effects associated with cancer disappeared within 12 to 36 hr; the more chemotherapy and morphine the patient had taken, the longer the withdrawal period. Studies of the food intake in areas where the incidences of cancer are very low showed that it met the requirements for the high pH therapy.

There were a number of other studies that were done in the mid-80's using cesium on animal models of cancer that demonstrated impressive results.[57,58,59,60,61,62,63,64]

---

56 Pinsky, C and Bose, R. Pharmacological and toxicological investigations of Cesium, *Pharmacology Biochemistry and Behavior*, Volume 21, Supplement 1, Pages 17-23, 1984.
57 Messihab, FS. Biochemical aspects of cesium administration in tumor-bearing mice, *Pharmacology Biochemistry and Behavior*, Volume 21, Supplement 1, Pages 27-30, 1984.
58 Messiha, FS. Effect of cesium and ethanol on tumor bearing rats, *Pharmacology Biochemistry and Behavior*, Volume 21, Supplement 1, Pages 35-40, 1984.

There was more research that took place at the beginning of the century to try to understand the behaviour of the cancer cell. This research was known as the Trophoblastic Theory of Cancer and is very significant in understanding how the cancer cell protects itself from the immune system and what can be done to overcome this.

Trophoblastic Theory Forgotten

If someone were to tell you that the pancreas is an extremely important organ that helps to prevent the spread of cancer in the body, you would probably ask "why?" This question was answered at the beginning of the century!

John Beard, Ph.D. was a Scottish Embryologist who formulated the Trophoblastic Theory of Cancer in 1902.[65] Beard, who taught at the University of Edinburgh until his death in 1923, was not a physician but a research biologist whose main interest was the placenta. He published his first book "The Enzyme Treatment of Cancer" in 1911.

What he discovered was that cancer cells are virtually indistinguishable from pre-embryonic cells called "trophoblast cells" – these are cells that grow very quickly during the initial stages of pregnancy in order to stimulate the development of the placenta and umbilical chord.

Placental cells not only look like cancer cells under the microscope, Beard realized, but even more significantly, the trophoblastic cells behave like cancer cells. These placental cells are called trophoblasts and are the first

---

59 Messihab, FS and Stocco, DM. Effect of cesium and potassium salts on survival of rats bearing Novikoff hepatoma, *Pharmacology Biochemistry and Behavior*, Volume 21, Supplement 1, Pages 31-34, 1984.

60 Neulieb, R. Effects of oral intake of cesium chloride: A single case report, *Pharmacology Biochemistry and Behavior*, Volume 21, Supplement 1, Pages 15-16, 1984.

61 Sartori, HE. Nutrients and cancer: An introduction to cesium therapy, *Pharmacology Biochemistry and Behavior*, Volume 21, Supplement 1, Pages 7-10, 1984.

62 Brewer, AK. The high pH therapy for cancer tests on mice and humans, *Pharmacology Biochemistry and Behavior*, Volume 21, Supplement 1, Pages 1-5, 1984.

63 Tufte, MJ, Tufte, FW, Brewer, AK. The response of colon carcinoma in mice to cesium, zinc and vitamin A, *Pharmacology Biochemistry and Behavior*, Volume 21, Supplement 1, Pages 25-26, 1984.

64 Messiha, FS. Cesium: A bibliography update, *Pharmacology Biochemistry and Behavior*, Volume 21, Supplement 1, Pages 113-129, 1984.

65 Beard, J: "The Action of Trypsin..." *Br Med J* 4, 140-41, 1906; Beard, J: "The Enzyme Treatment of Cancer" London: Chatto and Windus, 1911.

cells to differentiate from the fertilized egg. The most highly malignant exhibitions of cancer known are the chorionepitheliomas comprised of frank trophoblast cells - cytologically, endocrinologically and otherwise indistinguishable from normal pregnancy trophoblast cells.

Researchers have identified a number of differences between cancer cells and normal cells, such as:

1. Cancer cells are invasive; such cells produce a host of enzymes that enable them to break down tissue barriers and spread through normal tissue with deadly efficacy.
2. Cancer cells and malignant tissues develop their own blood supply - through the process known as angiogenesis - allowing the tumour to grow effectively wherever it chooses to grow.
3. Cancer cells and tumours, unlike normal tissues and organs, grow without restraint or inhibition – their apoptotic mechanism has 'switched off'; normal tissues grow as needed and when needed but only as appropriate.

It is interesting to find that cancer cells, like trophoblast cells, do not induce any immunological reaction. A prime reason for this was discovered in this century by Currie and Bhagshawe[66] who showed that the trophoblast was surrounded by a coating (sialo-glycoprotein) including a molecule that gave it a negative charge. The molecule can be likened to mucilage and has been termed the sialo-mucinous coat.

A negative charge is also found on the white blood cells responsible for immune reactivity. Since two like charges repel, we have delineated the primary reason for lack of rejection based on immune responses. This same type of coating is found on the cancer cell. In fact, it is one of the chief reasons for classifying all cancer cells as "trophoblastic."

Another observation was that the placental trophoblasts seem to take a downturn in activity around the time of the activation of the foetal pancreas, which occurs around the 56th day. This ties in with modern research which has shown that these trophoblast cells secrete a hormone called Human Chorionic Gonadotropin (HCG or CGH), and the quantities of this hormone rise until around the 56th day and then begin to taper off.

---

66 Currie GA, Van Doorninck W, Bagshawe KD. Effect of neuraminidase on the immunogenicity of early mouse trophoblast. *Nature*. 13;219(5150):191–192, Jul 1968.

It is this very hormone that coats the trophoblast and cancer cell to make them both immunologically inert. This pregnancy hormone is expressed in all types of cancers. Dr. Manual Navaro[67] in the 1960's and 70's found that measuring CGH in the urine was 95% accurate in the early detection of cancer, but this was improved by Dr. Emil K. Schandl, a Clinical Biochemist and Oncobiologist with Metabolic Research, and *American Metabolic Laboratories.*[68] Dr. Schandl has developed a battery of blood tests designed to predict the risk of developing cancer long before detectible symptoms may occur. These tests have proven to be excellent for monitoring individuals receiving non-toxic or toxic treatments. In order to be able to realize actual therapeutic progress, it is recommended to perform the Profile before, during, and at the conclusion of a certain therapy. If the markers decrease, that is a very good sign of healing.

The CA Profile[©69] includes intact HCG and HCG-beta, core, and fragments, PHI (phosphohexose isomerase), GGTP (gamma glut amyl transpeptidase) enzymes, CEA (carcinoembryonic antigen), TSH (thyroid stimulating hormone), and DHEA-S (dehydroepiandrosterone). The HCG hormone (human chorianic gonadotropin) and its fragments are generally made by the embryonic origin trophoblast cells. It is present in a high percentage of any type of cancer.

Two different methods are being used to confirm the validity of the often very low amount of the hormone in the blood. One is *immunoradiometric assay,* i.e. IRMA and the other one is *chemiluminescence,* i.e. IMM. Both of these methodologies are extremely sensitive and will detect very minute quantities of the hormone. Dr.Schandl named this tumour marker the *pregnancy and "malignancy hormone."* HCG suppresses the immune system and generally it is produced under anaerobic cellular conditions by the trophoblast.

The CA Profile[©] may yield 85-93 positives out of 100 pathologically established malignancies. Because of its capacity to foretell the development of cancer years before a tumour is apparent, a positive finding may be a serious warning sign of a developing cancer. The CA Profile[©] test also can be used to monitor the response of cancer patients to

---

67 Navarro, M. Elevation of urinary hCG can be detected much earlier than when the tumour becomes apparent, *Jour. Philippine Med. Assoc.* 36, 425-432, 1960.
68 http://www.caprofile.net
69 Schandl, E.K., The Cancer Profile, *American Assoc.Bioanalysts*, Abstract, Las Vegas, NV, May 13-15, 2004.

various therapies: an increasing or decreasing value of a tumour marker may indicate the futility or benefits of a therapy.

After the trophoblast cells have built the placenta and embedded themselves in the endometrium, they have no further function. On the 56th day the embryo's pancreas begins to produce pancreatic enzymes which break down the sialo-glycoprotein coat and allows the phagocytes to engulf the trophoblast cell.

Treating Cancer with Systemic Enzymes

So what is the significance of this regarding the treatment of cancer? Simply that using pancreatic enzymes, which are known as 'systemic enzymes' helps to digest this sialo-glycoprotein coat of the cancer cell, therefore changing the charge from negative to positive. This inevitably facilitates the attraction of leucocytes which have a negative charge.

Professor Beard believed that when the health of the pancreas becomes impaired and the output of pancreatic enzymes declines or stops, any malignant cancer cell that begins dividing, grows out of control.

If indeed this is the case, then an interesting question is raised – why is it possible to get pancreatic cancer when there are so many enzymes to digest the sialo-glycoprotein coat of the cancer cell?

The answer lies in the fact that for the pancreatic enzymes to be activated, they need a highly alkaline environment such as pH 8.0. This is only present in the small intestine in the initial part of the duodenum. Cancer of the initial part of the small intestine or duodenum is rare. It must also be noted that pancreatic enzymes as used for digesting food, are not adequate for treating cancer as they do not contain the activating factors trypsin and chymotrypsin, which are imperative.

Enzyme formulas have now been created containing both trypsin and chymotrypsin – the most popular of these is Wolf/Benitez "WoBenzyme®" systemic enzyme formula, which is reportedly the second-best selling OTC product in parts of Europe – after ordinary aspirin. A typical high-quality formula of systemic enzymes, like Wobenzyme-N® would have the following ingredients: Rutin (Rutoside) (150 mg) Papain (Papaya Enzyme) (180 mg) (492 FIP-unit), Bromelain (135 mg) (675 FIP-Unit),

Iodine (60 mcg) (Potassium Iodide), Pancreatin (300 mg) (56,000 USP), Trypsin (72 mg) (2,160 FIP-unit), Chymotrypsin (3 mg) (900 FIP-Unit).

Indeed, Dr. Gonzalez is presently conducting a phase II clinical trial using systemic enzymes to treat metastatic pancreatic cancer, with a 60% success rate. This began with an initial pilot study in ten patients suffering inoperable adenocarcinoma of the pancreas where the standard survival for the disease is very poor. An expectation of a survival time of one year for three of ten patients would be considered a positive result.

Nestec (the Nestle Corporation) agreed to fund the trial, which began in January 1994.[70] Of 11 patients followed in the trial, 8 of 11 suffered stage IV disease. Nine of 11 (81%) lived one year, 5 of 11 lived two years (45%), 4 of 11 lived three years (36%) and two lived longer than four years. In comparison, in a trial of the drug gemcitabine, of 126 patients with pancreatic cancer not a single patient lived longer than 19 months.

Nutrition and Cancer

The major factor underlying the cancer process is improper diet. The incidence of all kinds of cancer is related more to the high intake of cooked food containing fat, protein, cholesterol, salt and preservatives than to anything else, although anything at all detrimental to the purity of the bloodstream must one way or another contribute to the problem. The deprivation of oxygen to the cells is caused not only by high blood viscosity, poor circulation and low oxygen levels, but also by the absence of the enzymes needed to process the oxygen. The respiratory enzymes may be absent because of nutrients missing from the diet, or the respiratory enzymes may be inhibited by carcinogens in the bloodstream derived from sources such as food, smoking, alcohol, putrefaction in the colon and poisons from infected teeth.

About 40% of cancer patients die of malnutrition, not the cancer.[71] High-dose nutritional supplementation can help prevent this. High-dose supplementation can also bolster immunity.[72] Finnish oncologists used

---

70 Gonzalez NJ, Isaacs LL. Evaluation of pancreatic proteolytic enzyme treatment of adenocarcinoma of the pancreas, with nutrition and detoxification support. *Nutr Cancer* 33(2), 117-124, 1999.
71 Grant, JP. *Nutrition*, 6,4, 6S, July 1990 suppl.
72 Bendich, A. Chandra, RK (eds). Micronutrients and Immune Function, New York Academy of Sciences, p.587, 1990.

high doses of nutrients along with chemo and radiation for lung cancer patients. Normally, lung cancer is a "poor prognostic" malignancy, with a 1% expected survival at 30 months under normal treatment. In this study, however, 8 of the 18 patients (44%) were still alive 6 years after therapy.[73]

Oncologists at West Virginia Medical School randomized 65 patients with transitional cell carcinoma of the bladder into either the "one-per-day" vitamin supplement providing the RDA levels, or into another group which received the RDA vitamin plus higher doses of vitamin A (40,000 IU), vitamin B6 (100mg), Vitamin C (2,000 mg), Vitamin E (400 IU), Zinc (90mg). At 10 months tumour recurrence was 80% in the control group (RDA supplement only) and 40% in the experimental "metavitamin" group. Five year projected tumour recurrence was 91% for controls and 41% for megavitamin patients. Essentially, high-dose nutrients cut tumour recurrence in half.[74]

Researcher at Tulane University compared survival in patients who used the macrobiotic diet versus patients who continued with their standard Western lifestyle. Of 1,467 pancreatic cancer patients who made no changes in diet, 146 (1%) were alive after one year, while 12 of the 23 matched pancreatic cancer patients (52%) consuming macrobiotic diets were still alive after one year.[75]

In examining the diet and lifespan of 675 lung cancer patients over the course of 6 years, researchers found that the more vegetables consumed, the longer the lung cancer patient lived.[76] It appears that research does support the belief that by adding an aggressive nutrition component to a patient's cancer treatment protocol, it is possible to improve the chances of a complete remission or regression, as well as significantly add to the quality and quantity of life.

Personally, I have heard a number of oncologists recommending to their patients that they should not take any antioxidants while on chemotherapy or radiation treatments. Is it true that nutritional therapy reduces the effectiveness of chemotherapy or radiation treatment? Most of the

---

73 Jaakkola, K., et al. Treatment with antioxidant and other nutrients in combination with chemotherapy and radiation in patients with lung cancer, *Anticancer Res*, 12,599-606, 1992.
74 Lamm, DL, et al. Megadose vitamin in bladder cancer, *J Urol*, 151:21-26, 1994.
75 Carter, JP. Macrobiotic diet and cancer survival, *J Amer Coll Nutr*, 12:3:209-215, 1993.
76 Goodman, MT. Vegetable consumption in lung cancer longevity, *Eur J Ca*, 28:2:495-499, 1992.

scientific literature[77,78,79] supports the fact that nutrition and antioxidants can help and not hinder the use of chemotherapy and radiation. The reason for this is that antioxidants are absorbed by aerobic or healthy cells and not anaerobic or cancer cells. Antioxidants will therefore protect healthy cells against damage from the toxic chemotherapy and radiation. Authors that reviewed famous intervention studies (studies taking nutrients over a course of time to determine outcome) stated: "Overall there is evidence for protective effects of nutrients from supplements against several cancers."[80]

We have already mentioned above that sugar and all related products will feed cancer cells[81] and help them become more virulent, by decreasing further their oxygen supply. However, there are other foods such as meat that should also be cut out altogether. Why?

Meat is rich in Glutamine, another essential food for cancer cells which will promote tumour growth. Please also bear in mind that high glutamine levels are also found in wheat. Cooked meat is also likely to contain Heterocyclic Amines (HCA's), known carcinogens that are produced during the cooking process of many animal products including chicken, beef, pork, and fish. Smoked meats and cured meats usually contain nitrosamines, nitrites and nitrates and colour enhancers that can cause liver, stomach, brain, bladder and kidney cancers. Meat is also known to contain hormones such as Diethylstilberterol (Des) which can cause cancer of the uterus, breast and other reproductive organs, and is not good if you already have a hormone-sensitive breast cancer. Consumption of high saturated fat found in most meats, can increase certain hormone levels as well as inflammation in the body.

Eating plenty of fresh vegetables and their juices is always a good idea in cancer, along with some fresh fruit, but not a lot, and certainly not fresh fruit juices that are heavily laden with sugar. Eating some sea fish occasionally is good as protein is important for keeping the immune system healthy. All food intolerances should be strictly avoided, whatever they may be for each patient. Wholemeal cereal products are also fine, but wheat should be eaten very occasionally if at all. Pulses are also fine if

77 *Alternative Medicine Review*, vol. 5, no. 2, p.152, 2000.

78 *J. American College of Nutrition*, vol. 18, no. 1, p.13, 1999.

79 *J. American Nutraceutical Association*, vol. 4, no. 1, p.11, 2001.

80 Patterson, RE, White, E, Kristal, AR, et al, Vitamin supplementation and cancer risk: the epidemiological evidence. *Cancer Causes Control.* 8: 786-802, 1997.

81 Rothkopf, M. Fuel utilization in neoplastic disease: implications for the use of nutritional support in cancer patients, *Nutrition*, supp, 6:4:14-16S, 1990.

soaked and cooked well. Strictly no refined products, sugar, fried foods, packaged foods, colourings and preservatives – nutrient-dense foods should always be sought.

Vitamin C and Cancer

Ascorbic acid (vitamin C, ascorbate) has a controversial history in cancer treatment.[82] Observational reports described ascorbate, given in pharmacologic doses of 10 g daily, as effective in treating some cancers and in improving patient well-being.[83,84,85]

Many practitioners use vitamin C with cancer patients based on Prof. Linus Pauling's and Dr. Cameron's research. What they do not realize is that there has been research to suggest that Vitamin C at ordinary doses (human equivalents of 1 to 5 grams/day) increased the growth rate of cancer while far larger doses (10 grams or more) suppressed the cancer growth rate. This is because vitamin C and alpha-ketoglutarate are both required to produce collagen.

The combination of producing collagen, a cellular building block, and a modest amount of additional energy could promote the growth of cancer. Larger amounts of vitamin C (10-12g daily minimum) would greatly enhance the respiratory chain and would restart the Citric Acid cycle and thus aerobic metabolism would be reinitiated. This would allow the cell to return to normal cell behaviour. In the process it would lower the concentrations of alpha-ketoglutarate and decrease the collagen producing (and vitamin C consuming) side chain.

Doctors A. Goth and I. Littmann[86] described how cancer most frequently originates in organs whose ascorbic acid (vitamin C) levels are below 4.5 mg% and rarely grows in organs containing ascorbic acid above this concentration. Research published in September of 2005 by Dr. Mark Levine et al[87] has shown that high-dose intravenous vitamin C can increase

82 Padayatty, S. J. & Levine, M. *J. Am. Coll. Nutr.* 19, 423–425, 2000.
83 Cameron, E. & Campbell, A. *Chem. Biol. Interact.* 9, 285–315, 1974.
84 Cameron, E. & Pauling, L. *Proc. Natl. Acad. Sci.* USA 73, 3685–3689, 1976.
85 Cameron, E. & Pauling, L. *Proc. Natl. Acad. Sci.* USA 75, 4538–4542, 1978.
86 Goth, A. and Littman, I. Ascorbic Acid Content in Human Cancer Tissue. *Cancer Research*, Vol. 8, 1948.
87 Chen, Q. et al. Pharmacologic ascorbic acid concentrations selectively kill cancer cells: Action as a pro-drug to deliver hydrogen peroxide to tissues. *PNAS*, 2005. (www.pnas.org/content/102/38/13604.abstract)

hydrogen peroxide (H_2O_2) levels within cancer cells and eradicate the cancer cells, without harming normal cells. As the researchers say: "It is unknown why ascorbate, using H_2O_2, killed some cancer cells but not normal cells. There was no correlation with ascorbate-induced cell death and glutathione, catalase activity, or glutathione peroxidase activity. The data here showed that ascorbate initiated H_2O_2 formation extracellularly, but H_2O_2 targets could be either intracellular or extracellular, because H_2O_2 is membrane permeable.[88,89]

For example, extracellular H_2O_2 might target membrane lipids, forming hydroperoxides or reactive intermediates that are quenched or repaired in normal cells but not in sensitive cancer cells. In sensitive but not resistant cancer cells, intracellular H_2O_2 could target DNA, DNA repair proteins, or mitochondria because of diminished superoxide dismutase activity.[90] New insights may follow from future studies of a very broad range of tumour cells or from microarray analysis of resistant and sensitive cells derived from the same genetic lineage."

They continue to say: "More than 100 patients have been described, presumably without glucose-6-phosphate dehydrogenase deficiency, who received 10 g or more of i.v. ascorbate with no reported adverse effects other than tumour lysis."[91,92,93,94] There are also many other scientific papers that have been written on the use of vitamin C for chronic diseases.[95]

Laetrile or Vitamin B17

There are a number of natural compounds that have been found to act as anti-angiogenesis factors – one of these is laetrile or vitamin B17. Laetrile (B-17) is a natural chemotherapeutic agent found in over 1,200 plants,

---

88 Chance, B., Sies, H. & Boveris, A. Physiol. Rev. 59, 527–605, 1979.

89 Antunes, F. & Cadenas, E. FEBS Lett. 475, 121–126, 2000.

90 Oberley, L. W. Antioxid. Redox. Signal. 3, 461–472, 2001.

91 Cameron, E. & Pauling, L. Proc. Natl. Acad. Sci. USA 73, 3685–3689, 1976.

92 Cameron, E. & Pauling, L. Proc. Natl. Acad. Sci. USA 75, 4538–4542, 1978.

93 Riordan, HD., Hunninghake, RB., Riordan, NH., Jackson, JJ., Meng, X., Taylor, P., Casciari, JJ., Gonzalez, MJ., Miranda-Massari, JR., Mora, EM., et al. P. R. Health Sci. J. 22, 287–290, 2003.

94 Riordan, NH., Riordan, HD., Meng, X., Li, Y. & Jackson, JA. Med. Hypotheses 44, 207–213, 1995.

95 http://www.garynull.com/Documents/vitaminc-cancer.htm

particularly in the seeds of common fruits such as apricots, peaches, plums, and apples.

The systematized study of amygdalin did not really begin until the first half of the past century when crystalline amygdalin was isolated in 1830 by two French chemists, Robiquet and Boutron. Now known as Prunus Amygdalus, of the rose family Rosaceae, amygdalin is hence appropriately named after the scientific name of the bitter almond. The chemical structure of amygdalin is well established as laevo-D-mandelonitrile-B-D-glucoside-6-B-D-glucoside.[96]

When the laetrile compound molecule comes across a cancer cell, it is broken down into 2 molecules of glucose, 1 molecule of hydrogen cyanide and 1 molecule of benzaldehyde. Initially, it was thought that the cyanide radical was the major cancer-killing radical, but now it is known that it is the benzaldehyde molecule that is responsible.

The most widespread theory ("cyanide theory") on the action of amygdalin was propounded by Ernest Krebs, Jr., in the seventies. Kreb's hypothesis is the resulting end products of the hydrolysis of amygdalin are the hydrocyanic acid (HCN) and benzaldehyde. In order to produce these products, B-glucuronidase is required. It has been demonstrated that this enzyme is present in cancerous tissue about 1,000 to 3,600 times higher than in normal tissue.

Rhodenase is an enzyme found in the liver cell and is known to be concerned with the conversion of toxic hydrocyanic acid to thiocyanate, a harmless substance.[97] Rhodenase is part of the normal detoxification process of the body. However, it was found that normal cells contain a relatively high concentration of rhodenase and low concentration of B-glucoronidase, whereas cancerous cells are high in available B-glucoronidase and low in available rhodenase.

Thus, the normal cellular protective mechanism is decreased in tumour cells and they become more sensitive to the effects of the cyanide and benzaldehyde ions. The hydrogen cyanide and benzaldehyde molecules

---

96 Viehoever, L. and Mack, N. Biochemistry of amygdalin. *Amer. J. Pharm.* 107: 397-450, 1935.
97 Manner, H. and Poletti. M. The activity of the enzyme rhodanese in normal and malignant mouse tissue. Presented at the Illinois State Academy of Science. April, 1977.

would tend to depress the enzyme functions of the cancer cell and thereby destroy it. Since normal cells contain large quantities of rhodenase and relatively low quantities of available B-glucoronidase, the available rhodenase would detoxify the cyanide ion (CN-) forming the non-toxic thiocyanate. Then according to Ernest Krebs, amygdalin's toxic effect is against the cancerous cell and not the host. Generally, therapeutic dosages of laetrile have been found to be non-toxic.[98] Laetrile has been found to be effective for some cancers, but not all types.[99,100,101,102,103,104]

Zinc is one of the most critical parts of the laetrile therapy as zinc is the transportation mechanism for laetrile and nitrilosides in the body. Biochemists and researchers have found that you can give Laetrile to a patient in large doses, but if the patient is lacking zinc then it would be difficult for the laetrile to get into the body tissues. They also found that nothing heals within the body without sufficient vitamin C, and magnesium; selenium, vitamin A,[105] and B5 all played an important part in maintaining the body's defence mechanism. This is why it's important to provide a holistic approach consisting of an optimal diet, vitamins, minerals, laetrile and pancreatic enzymes.

Rubin (1977)[106] found in their clinical investigations in Israel that amygdalin (Laetrile) was most effective against adenocarcinoma and Hodgkin's disease, somewhat less effective in certain other of the sarcomas

98 Manner, H., DiSanti, S., Michalsen, T. The non-toxicity of amygdalin to laboratory mice. *Sd. Biol. J.* 347-349. May-June. 1977.

99 DiSanti, SJ, Amygdalin, Vitamin A and Enzymes Induced Regression of Murine Mammary Adenocarcinomas, *Journal of Manipulative and Physiological Therapeutics*, Vol 1, No. 4, December 1978.

100 Moertel CG, Fleming TR, Rubin J, et al. A clinical trial of amygdalin (Laetrile) in the treatment of human cancer. *N.Engl.J.Med.* 28;306(4):201-206, Jan 1982.

101 Milazzo S, Ernst E, Lejeune S, et al. Laetrile treatment for cancer. *Cochrane Database Syst Rev* 2006.

102 Moertel CG, Fleming TR, Rubin J, et al. A clinical trial of amygdalin (Laetrile) in the treatment of human cancer. *N.Engl.J.Med.* 28;306(4):201-206, Jan 1982.

103 Moss RW. Patient perspectives: Tijuana cancer clinics in the post-NAFTA era. *Integr Cancer Ther* 4(1):65-86, Mar 2005.

104 Wodinsky, I. and Swiniarski, J. K. Antitumor activity of amygdalin MF (NSC-15780) as a single agent and with beta-glucosidase (NSC-128056) on a spectrum of transplantable rodent tumours. *Cancer Chemother Rep* 59(5):939-950, 1975.

105 Manner, HW, Michaelson, TL, and DiSanti, SJ, Amygdalin, Vitamin A and Enzymes Induced Regression of Murine Mammary Adenocarcinomas, *Journal of Manipulative and Physiological Therapeutics*, Vol 1, No. 4, December 1978.

106 Moertel, CG., Ames, MM., Kovach, JS., Moyer, TP., Rubin, JR., and Tinker, JH. A pharmacologic and toxicological study of amygdalin. *JAMA* 245(6):591-594, Feb 1981.

and melanomas, and relatively poor results were achieved with the leukemia. Similar results have been obtained by other clinicians in the United States and elsewhere. The best results with amygdalin (Laetrile) therapy have been achieved with lung, prostate, breast, lymphomas, liver and brain cancer. The chemical quality of the amygdalin (Laetrile) also has a bearing on the clinical therapeutic results.

Halting Metastasis

Over the last two decades, research into controlling or halting cancer metastasis has led to two promising new strategies. The first, anti-angiogenesis, targets the growth of new blood vessels (angiogenesis) that are required for tumour growth. Originally pioneered by noted cancer researcher Dr. Judah Folkman, anti-angiogenesis grew from his observation that tumours cannot grow without access to a constant supply of new blood vessels. Folkman theorized that cancer cells actively communicate with surrounding tissues to trigger the growth of new blood vessels (neovascularization) needed to supply nutrients and remove waste products. Once neovascularization is initiated, hundreds of new capillaries converge on the tumour site and are quickly coated with new layers of rapidly dividing tumour cells.

Shark Cartilage

Shark cartilage has gained increased popularity as an unconventional cancer treatment and in prevention of cancer. Shark cartilage was initially promoted by William Lane, Ph.D. in his book "Sharks Don't Get Cancer."[107]

Shark cartilage contains approximately 40% protein (troponin-I, tetranectin-type protein, collagenase, cartilage-derived inhibitor/CDI, tissue inhibitor of metalloproteinases) and 5-20% glycosaminoglycans (chondroitin sulfate-D, chondroitin-6-sulfate, keratan sulfate). The remainder is made up of calcium salts (up to 25% of some preparations) and glycoproteins (sphyrnastatin-1 and 2, galactosamines, glucosamine).[108,109] Shark cartilage is also a rich source of other trace

---

107 Lane, IW., Comac, L. Sharks Don't Get Cancer. Garden City, NY. Avery Publishing Group, 1992, updated 1993.
108 Talks, KL and Harris, AL. Current status of antiangiogenic factors. *Br J Haematol.* 109(3):477-489, 2000.

elements and minerals such as calcium, iron, zinc, selenium, copper, manganese, molybdenum, titanium, and strontium, but it is also a rich source of toxic metals too.

Brem, Langer, and Folkman conducted early basic science research on cartilage and angiogenesis inhibition.[110,111,112] In humans, shark cartilage supplementation reduced endothelial cell densities, an indirect measurement of angiogenesis.[113] A proposed biochemical basis of shark cartilage's antiangiogenic activity is blockade of vascular endothelial cell growth factor (VEGF) receptors, which in turn inhibits endothelial cell proliferation.[114],[115] Shark cartilage has also been found to modify the organization of focal adhesion proteins responsible for endothelial attachment[116] and to inhibit the proteolytic enzymes that break down extracellular matrix and allow tumour invasion and metastasis ("matrix metalloproteinase inhibition").[117,118,119,120,121]

---

109 Moses, MA., Wiederschain, D., Wu, I., Fernandez, CA., Ghazizadeh, V., Lane, WS., Flynn, E., Sytkowski, A., Tao, T., and Langer, R. Troponin I is present in human cartilage and inhibits angiogenesis. *Proc Natl. Acad. Sci.* 96(6):2645-2650, Mar 1999.

110 Brem, H. and Folkman, J. Inhibition of tumor angiogenesis mediated by cartilage. *J Exp. Med* 141(2):427-439, Feb 1975.

111 Langer, R., Brem, H., Falterman, K., Klein, M., and Folkman, J. Isolations of a cartilage factor that inhibits tumor neovascularization. *Science* 193(4247):70-72, Jul 1976.

112 Langer, R, Conn, H, Vacanti, J, and et al. Control of tumor growth in animals by infusion of an angiogenesis inhibitor. *Proc National Acad Sci* 77, 1980.

113 Berbari, P., Thibodeau, A., Germain, L., Saint-Cyr, M., Gaudreau, P., Elkhouri, S., Dupont, E., Garrel, D. R., and El Khouri, S. Antiangiogenic effects of the oral administration of liquid cartilage extract in humans. *J Surg Res* 87(1):108-113, 1999.

114 Beliveau, R., Gingras, D., Kruger, E. A., Lamy, S., Sirois, P., Simard, B., Sirois, M. G., Tranqui, L., Baffert, F., Beaulieu, E., Dimitriadou, V., Pepin, M. C., Courjal, F., Ricard, I., Poyet, P., Falardeau, P., Figg, W. D., and Dupont, E. The Antiangiogenic Agent Neovastat (AE-941) Inhibits Vascular Endothelial Growth Factor-mediated Biological Effects. *Clin Cancer Res* 8(4):1242-1250, 2002.

115 McGuire, TR., Kazakoff, PW., Hoie, EB., and Fienhold, MA. Antiproliferative activity of shark cartilage with and without tumor necrosis factor-alpha in human umbilical vein endothelium. *Pharmacotherapy* 16(2):237-244, 1996.

116 Chen, JS., Chang, CM., Wu, JC., and Wang, SM. Shark cartilage extract interferes with cell adhesion and induces reorganization of focal adhesions in cultured endothelial cells. *J Cell Biochem* 78(3):417-428, July 2000.

117 Langer, R., Brem, H., Falterman, K., Klein, M., and Folkman, J. Isolations of a cartilage factor that inhibits tumor neovascularization. *Science* 193(4247):70-72, July 1976.

118 Langer, R, Conn, H, Vacanti, J, and et al. Control of tumor growth in animals by infusion of an angiogenesis inhibitor. *Proc National Acad Sci* 77, 1980.

119 Sheu, JR., Fu, CC., Tsai, ML., and Chung, WJ. Effect of U-995, a potent shark cartilage-derived angiogenesis inhibitor, on anti-angiogenesis and anti-tumor activities. *Anticancer Res* 18(6A):4435-4441, 1998.

Ongoing research suggests that shark cartilage interferes with cellular adhesion.[122] Lee and Langer reported that shark cartilage extract (incorporated into pellets) implanted alongside tumours in rabbit cornea inhibited tumour neovascularisation.[123] Inhibition was 75% greater than controls, with statistical significance.

Animal studies have demonstrated that shark cartilage inhibits angiogenesis in rats[124,125,126] and exhibits activity against several mouse tumour lines in vivo in laboratory studies.[127,128,129,130,131] This has been

120 Moses, MA. A cartilage-derived inhibitor of neovascularization and metalloproteinases. *Clin Exp.Rheumatol.* 11 Suppl 8:S67-S69, 1993.

121 Gingras, D., Renaud, A., Mousseau, N., Beaulieu, E., Kachra, Z., and Beliveau, R. Matrix proteinase inhibition by AE-941, a multifunctional antiangiogenic compound. *Anticancer Res* 21(1A):145-155, 2001.

122 Chen, JS., Chang, CM., Wu, JC., and Wang, SM. Shark cartilage extract interferes with cell adhesion and induces reorganization of focal adhesions in cultured endothelial cells. *J Cell Biochem* 78(3):417-428, June 2000.

123 Lee, A. and Langer, R. Shark cartilage contains inhibitors of tumor angiogenesis. *Science* 221(4616):1185-1187, Sept 1983.

124 Davis, PF., He, Y., Furneaux, RH., Johnston, PS., Ruger, BM., and Slim, GC. Inhibition of angiogenesis by oral ingestion of powdered shark cartilage in a rat model. *Microvasc. Res* 54(2):178-182, 1997.

125 Cataldi, JM and Osborne, DL. Effects of shark cartilage on mammary tumor neovascularization in vivo and cell proliferation in vitro (meeting abstract). *FASEB Journal* 9(3):A135, 1995.

126 Gonzalez, RP., Soares, FS., Farias, RF., Pessoa, C., Leyva, A., Barros Viana, GS., and Moraes, MO. Demonstration of inhibitory effect of oral shark cartilage on basic fibroblast growth factor-induced angiogenesis in the rabbit cornea. *Biol. Pharm. Bull.* 24(2):151-154, 2001.

127 McGuire, TR., Kazakoff, PW., Hoie, EB., and Fienhold, MA. Antiproliferative activity of shark cartilage with and without tumor necrosis factor-alpha in human umbilical vein endothelium. *Pharmacotherapy* 16(2):237-244, 1996.

128 Sheu, JR., Fu, CC., Tsai, ML., and Chung, WJ. Effect of U-995, a potent shark cartilage-derived angiogenesis inhibitor, on anti-angiogenesis and anti-tumor activities. *Anticancer Res* 18(6A):4435-4441, 1998.

129 Anonymous. Angiostatic and antitumoral activity of AE-941 (neovastat-R), a molecular fraction derived from shark cartilage (meeting abstract). *Proc Annu Meet Am Assoc Cancer Res* 38:A1530, 1997.

Shimizu-Suganuma, Masum, Mwanatambwe, Milanga, Iida, Kazum, and et al. Effect of shark cartilage on tumor growth and survival time in vivo (meeting abstract). *Proc Annu Meet Am Soc Clin Oncol* 18:A1760, 1999.

130 Barber, R., Delahunt, B., Grebe, SK., Davis, PF., Thornton, A., and Slim, GC. Oral shark cartilage does not abolish carcinogenesis but delays tumor progression in a murine model. *Anticancer Res* 21(2A):1065-1069, 2001.

131 Shimizu-Suganuma, Masum, Mwanatambwe, Milanga, Iida, Kazum, and et al. Effect of shark cartilage on tumor growth and survival time in vivo (meeting abstract). *Proc Annu Meet Am Soc Clin Oncol* 18:A1760, 1999.

demonstrated in a mouse model of lung carcinoma.[132,133] Other animal anti-tumour models have been less definitive and one study showed no improvement after 25 days in SCCVII tumours implanted in the feet of mice.[134] A more recent report demonstrated regression of implanted mouse brain tumours after 43 days of shark cartilage, but no additive effect with the chemotherapy agent boronophenylalanine-mediated neutron capture therapy (BNCT).[135] Intravenous shark cartilage derivative AE-941 (500mg/kg) was given to mice using the Lewis lung carcinoma metastatic model and resulted in a statistically significant 49% reduction in lung surface metastases vs. placebo.[136] Notably, in this study cisplatin (4mg/kg) reduced metastases by 69% (with greater toxicity) and cisplatin with shark cartilage reduced metastases by 87%.

Other causes of cancer

Constipation
By far the worst predisposing factor to cancer that contributes to the deterioration of the internal milieu is constipation. It is important to remember that a regular daily bowel movement does not mean the absence of constipation; what counts is the time food residues take to transit the digestive tract. On the traditional Western diet of mainly cooked food, the transit time is about seventy-two hours, which means that "regular" or not, there are always stagnant putrefying residues occupying the colon producing carcinogenic substances, some of which provoke local problems and some of which perfuse back into the bloodstream. Sir William Arbuthnot Lane,[137] the famous British surgeon, repeatedly emphasized he

---

132 Riviere M, Alaoui-Jamali M, Falardeau P, and et al. Neovastat: an inhibitor of angiogenesis with anti-cancer activity. *Proc Amer Assoc Cancer Res* 39:46, 1998.

133 Dupont, E., Falardeau, P., Mousa, S. A., Dimitriadou, V., Pepin, M. C., Wang, T., and Alaoui-Jamali, MA. Antiangiogenic and antimetastatic properties of Neovastat (AE-941), an orally active extract derived from cartilage tissue. *Clin Exp Metastasis* 19(2):145-153, 2002.

134 Horsman, MR., Alsner, J., and Overgaard, J. The effect of shark cartilage extracts on the growth and metastatic spread of the SCCVII carcinoma. *Acta Oncol* 37(5):441-445, 1998.

135 Morris, GM., Coderre, JA., Micca, PL., Lombardo, DT., and Hopewell, JW. Boron neutron capture therapy of the rat 9L gliosarcoma: evaluation of the effects of shark cartilage. *Br J Radiol.* 73(868):429-434, 2000.

136 Jamali MA, Riviere P, Falardeau A, and et al. Effect of AE-941 (Neovastat), an angiogenesis inhibitor, in the Lewis lung carcinoma metastatic model, efficacy, toxicity prevention and survival. *Clin Invest Med* (suppl):S16, 1998.

137 Sir William Arbuthnot Lane, BART CB; Consulting Surgeon to Guys Hospital; Consulting Surgeon to The Hospital for Sick Children, London; President of The New Health Society; author of The Prevention of the Diseases Peculiar to Civilization (1929).

had never known a single case of cancer that had not been preceded by prolonged intestinal stasis.

In his surgical practice, Sir William noted that so common were diseased colons he was forced to conclude the colon to be the seat of most chronic diseases, and for some time he specialized in the removal of diseased colons. This procedure confirmed his ideas because most of his patients' chronic disorders cleared up very quickly after losing their colons, and their overall health improved. Eventually he realized that the colon was not, itself, a troublesome organ, and became diseased only because of the kind of food people ate, and that the resulting disorders were the result of what he called 'auto-intoxication'. It was at this time in his career he became converted to the concept of natural health and thereafter concentrated his efforts on educating patients rather than cutting pieces out of them.

Professor Aviles of the Biochemistry of Cancer Department, Guadalajara, Mexico reported that out of 7,715 cancer patients examined by him over a fifteen-year period, at least ninety-nine per cent had suffered from constipation and that the degree of malignancy was parallel to the degree of constipation. Doctors Dennis Burkitt and Hugh Trowell, who both spent twenty-five years working in rural Africa, agreed that in those areas where the diet of the natives consisted almost entirely of fruit and vegetables, the "transit time" of the natives was about twenty-four hours, there was no such thing as constipation and cancer was non-existent. Dr E. H. Tipper in his book The cradle of the world and cancer: a disease of civilization (1927) said:[138]

"Cancer has been suspected of being a disease of civilization. judging from my experience in general practise in London, twenty years in West Africa, and again in rural England, I am convinced that this is true. It is due to the conventionalism and bad feeding of civilization, and is an exact index of the degree to which the alimentary tract has deviated from its natural and normal state of health. In the case of cancer, constipation and excessive meat-eating should be the two suspects, when they are present cancer is rife, where absent there is none."

---

138 Tipper, EH. The cradle of the world and cancer: a disease of civilization (Unknown Binding) ASIN: B00088KECS, 142 pages.

Diseased teeth and cancer

Dr. Joseph Issels of Germany,[139] who has researched and treated cancer for fifty years, asserts that poisoning from infected teeth is one of the prime causes of cancer, and this viewpoint is supported by Dr Mulhim Hassan of Lebanon in his book *Prevention and Cure of Cancer*. Dr Max Garten, also of Germany, said in agreement with Issels: "This is one phase in the cancer treatment that requires adamant and uncompromising attention."

Root canals are a major cause of the immune system being suppressed and they are a major cause of cancer:

"Dr. Thomas Rau, who runs the Paracelsus Clinic in Switzerland[140] recently checked the records of the last 150 breast cancer patients treated in his clinic. He found that 147 of them (98%) had one or more root canal teeth on the same meridian as the original breast cancer tumor. His clinic has a biological dentist section where all cancer patients, on reporting in, have their mouth cleaned up first - especially all root canal teeth removed.

Root canal fillings were proven deadly disease agents in 1925 in a study by Dr. Weston Price and 60 prominent researchers. That study has been suppressed ever since by the ADA and the American Association of Endodontists (AAE). Read the book "Root Canal Cover-Up" by George Meinig, DDS, FACD for the full story.[141] Dr. Meinig was an endodontist for 50 years. He helped found the AAE in 1943. His book is a mea culpa (apology) to the thousands of patients whose health he ruined doing root canal fillings. He discovered the Weston Price research only after he retired in 1993. His book was published first in 1994 and he has lectured widely since then trying to alert people to this danger to their health.

In comparison to the volume contained in the accessory canals and the dentine tubules, that of the root canal is actually quite small. It is not possible to remove dead infected soft tissue from the whole tooth. When only the root canals are treated there remains a massive amount of gangrenous tissue which is infected by anaerobic microorganisms, producing lethal toxins that can be a main trigger to triggering oncogenes.

---

139 Issels, J. Immunotherapy in Progressive Metastatic Cancer, A Fifteen-Year Survival Follow-up. *Clinical Trials Journal*, London, 7, No. 3, 1970.
140 www.paracelsus.ch
141 Meinig, G. Root Canal Cover-up. USA: Bio Publishing, 2004.

Inflammation and cancer

Recent data have expanded the concept that inflammation is a critical component of tumour progression.[142] Many cancers arise from sites of infection, chronic irritation and inflammation. It is now becoming clear that the tumour microenvironment, which is largely orchestrated by inflammatory cells, is an indispensable participant in the neoplastic process, fostering proliferation, survival and migration. In addition, tumour cells have co-opted some of the signalling molecules of the innate immune system, such as selectins, chemokines and their receptors for invasion, migration and metastasis. These insights are fostering new anti-inflammatory therapeutic approaches to cancer development.

Leukocyte infiltration is a cardinal feature of almost all cancers. Chemokines are generally responsible for eliciting local accumulation of inflammatory cells and they appear to play the same role in the formation of peri- and intra-tumoural infiltrates.[143] Chronic inflammation predisposes to cancer formation and progression, and it is likely that the chemokine system contributes to this process. In part, this may be a consequence of its ability to attract mononuclear cells to cancer sites, where they provide growth or angiogenic factors that enhance cancer development.

However, accumulating evidence also points to a direct effect of chemokines on cancer cells that express chemokine receptors. In particular, some chemokines can activate anti-apoptotic pathways in these cells. By either mechanism, tumour cells that secrete and/or respond to chemokines would have a selective advantage. This provides another example of cancer's ability to co-opt host systems in order to promote tumour progression.

A very well-researched herb that has been found to be a potent anti-inflammatory is Turmeric which has been associated with the inhibition of tumor necrosis factor-α, interleukin-8, monocyte inflammatory protein-1, interleukin-1B, and monocyte chemotactic protein-1.[144] Turmeric and its constituent curcumin have been found to inhibit lipoxygenase and

---

142 Coussens LM, Werb Z. Inflammation and cancer. *Nature*. 26:420(6917):860-7, Dec 2002.
143 Rollins BJ. Inflammatory chemokines in cancer growth and progression. *Eur J Cancer*. 42(6):760-7, April 2006.
144 Abe Y, Hashimoto S, Horie T. Curcumin inhibition of inflammatory cytokine production by human peripheral blood monocytes and alveolar macrophages. *Pharmacol Res*. 39(1):41-7, Jan 1999.

cyclooxygenase in rat tissues and in vitro,[145,146,147] as well as thromboxane B2[148] and leukotriene B4 formation.[149]

Based on animal study, oral administration of curcumin may reduce expression of several cytokines, chemokines, and proteinases known to mediate aneurismal degeneration.[150] In rat macrophages, curcumin inhibits the incorporation of arachidonic acid into membrane lipids, as well as prostaglandin E2, leukotriene B4, and leukotriene C4, but does not affect the release of arachidonic acid.[151] Curcumin also inhibits the secretion of collagenase, elastase, and hyaluronidase. Inhibition of neutrophil function has been noted,[152] and in vitro research demonstrates that curcumin inhibits 5-hydroxy-eicosatetraenoic acid (5-HETE) in intact human neutrophils.[153] Turmeric has been found to block cytokine-induced transcription of leukocyte adhesion molecules ICAM-1, VCAM-1, and E-selectin,[154] and it appears to induce the production of endogenous TGF-B1

145 Flynn DL, Rafferty MF, Boctor AM. Inhibition of 5-hydroxy-eicosatetraenoic acid (5-HETE) formation in intact human neutrophils by naturally-occurring diarylheptanoids: inhibitory activities of curcuminoids and yakuchinones. *Prostaglandins Leukot Med.* 22(3):357-60, Jun 1986.

146 Rao CV, Simi B, Reddy BS. Inhibition by dietary curcumin of azoxymethane-induced ornithine decarboxylase, tyrosine protein kinase, arachidonic acid metabolism and aberrant crypt foci formation in the rat colon. *Carcinogenesis.* 14(11):2219-25, Nov 1993.

147 Ammon HP, Safayhi H, Mack T, Sabieraj J. Mechanism of antiinflammatory actions of curcumine and boswellic acids. *J Ethnopharmacol.* 38(2-3):113-9, Mar 1993.

148 Srivastava KC, Bordia A, Verma SK. Curcumin, a major component of food spice turmeric (Curcuma longa) inhibits aggregation and alters eicosanoid metabolism in human blood platelets. *Prostaglandins Leukot Essent Fatty Acids.* 52(4):223-7, Apr 1995.

149 Ammon HP, Anazodo MI, Safayhi H, Dhawan BN, Srimal RC. Curcumin: a potent inhibitor of leukotriene B4 formation in rat peritoneal polymorphonuclear neutrophils (PMNL). *Planta Med.* 58(2):226, Apr 1992.

150 Parodi FE, Mao D, Ennis TL, Pagano MB, Thompson RW. Oral administration of diferuloylmethane (curcumin) suppresses proinflammatory cytokines and destructive connective tissue remodeling in experimental abdominal aortic aneurysms. *Ann Vasc Surg.* 20(3):360-8, May 2006.

151 Joe B, Lokesh BR. Effect of curcumin and capsaicin on arachidonic acid metabolism and lysosomal enzyme secretion by rat peritoneal macrophages. *Lipids,* 32(11):1173-80, Nov 1997.

152 Mukhopadhyay A, Basu N, Ghatak N, Gujral PK. Anti-inflammatory and irritant activities of curcumin analogues in rats. *Agents Actions.* 12(4):508-15, Oct 1982.

153 Flynn DL, Rafferty MF, Boctor AM. Inhibition of 5-hydroxy-eicosatetraenoic acid (5-HETE) formation in intact human neutrophils by naturally-occurring diarylheptanoids: inhibitory activities of curcuminoids and yakuchinones. *Prostaglandins Leukot Med.* 22(3):357-60, June 1986.

154 Gupta B, Ghosh B. Curcuma longa inhibits TNF-alpha induced expression of adhesion molecules on human umbilical vein endothelial cells. *Int J Immunopharmacol.* 21(11):745-57, Nov 1999.

in animal wounds.[155] Curcumin down-regulates transcription of genes responsible for the production of chemotactic cytokines in bone marrow stromal cells.[156] Curcumin reduces liver inflammation.[157]

Formation of fibrin on the tumour cell membrane supports this adhesive process and serves as a protective barrier against tumour cell recognition by the immunological system.[158] Proteolytic enzymes inhibit both excess fibrin deposition and inflammation, thus helping to prevent the spread of tumour cells.

At the turn of the century, Dr. John Beard,[159] of the University of Edinburgh, made a series of discoveries that led him to believe pancreatic enzymes did more than just aid in digestion — they could be an effective treatment for pancreatic cancer.[160] However, his work was quickly dismissed and over the years, the claim that enzyme pills could treat serious conditions, especially cancer, has not been taken seriously. But recent evidence suggests there might be something to it. A 1993 pilot study by Dr. Nicholas Gonzalez, published in the medical journal *Nutrition and Cancer* (June 1999),[161] found that pancreatic cancer patients on enzyme therapy lived significantly longer than expected - in some cases, three times longer than the usual survival rate.

What the enzymes do to help is that they discover the receptors. Enzymes also facilitate the reaction of recognition. Another important action of the enzymes is to improve immunity, which is done by breaking the circulating immune complexes by activating the natural killer cells and the

155 Sidhu GS, Singh AK, Thaloor D, Banaudha KK, Patnaik GK, Srimal RC, Maheshwari RK. Enhancement of wound healing by curcumin in animals. *Wound Repair Regen.* 6(2):167-77, Mar-Apr 1998.
156 Xu YX, Pindolia KR, Janakiraman N, Noth CJ, Chapman RA, Gautam SC. Curcumin, a compound with anti-inflammatory and anti-oxidant properties, down-regulates chemokine expression in bone marrow stromal cells. *Exp Hematol.* 25(5):413-22, May 1997.
157 Srimal RC, Khanna NM, and Dhawan BN. A preliminary report on anti-inflammatory activity of curcumin. *Indian J Pharmacol* 3:10, 1971.
158 Rakoff-Nahoum S. Why cancer and inflammation? *Yale J Biol Med.* 79(3-4):123-30, Dec 2006.
159 Beard J. The action of trypsin upon the living cells of Jensen's mouse tumor. *Br Med J.* 4:140-141, 1906.
160 Beard J. The Enzyme Treatment of Cancer. London: Chatto and Windus, 1911.
161 Gonzalez NJ, Isaacs LL. Evaluation of pancreatic proteolytic enzyme treatment of adenocarcinoma
of the pancreas, with nutrition and detoxification support. *Nutr Cancer.* 33:117-124, 1999.

T-cells, and also by inducing mediators and cytokines, such as TNF, Tumor Necrosis Factor.

Enzymes have the ability to reduce the thick fibrin layer which is abnormally 15 times thicker than normal. By reducing this fibrin layer the stickiness of the cancer cells is also diminished, and by this means we can prevent metastasis. Proteolytic enzymes are well-absorbed from the gastrointestinal tract into the systemic circulation[162,163] to exert anti-tumour, anti-inflammatory, anti-oedematous and immuno-stimulatory actions, which are the result of different and synergistic effects, including the following:[164,165,166,167]

- ❖ Reduction in substance P production.
- ❖ Reduction in PG-E2 production.
- ❖ Dose-dependent stimulation of reactive oxygen species production and anti-cancer cytotoxicity in human neutrophils.
- ❖ A pro-differentiative effect.
- ❖ Fibrinolytic effect.
- ❖ Anti-thrombotic effect, mediated at least in part by a reduction in 2-series thromboxanes.
- ❖ Modulation of adhesion molecules.
- ❖ Modulation of cytokine balance.
- ❖ Induction of endogenous proteinase inhibitors (e.g., alpha-1-antitrypsin and alpha-2-macroglobulin).
- ❖ Reduction in circulating immune complexes.
- ❖ Possible antimicrobial effect in the gastrointestinal tract, thereby alleviating dysbiosis and reducing de novo immune complex formation.

---

162 Gotze H, Rothman SS. Enteropancreatic circulation of digestive enzymes as a conservative mechanism. *Nature* 257(5527):607-609, 1975.

163 Liebow C, Rothman SS. Enteropancreatic circulation of digestive enzymes. *Science* 189(4201): 472-474, 1975.

164 Zavadova E, Desser L, Mohr T. Stimulation of reactive oxygen species production and cytotoxicity in human neutrophils in vitro and after oral administration of a polyenzyme preparation. *Cancer Biother* 10(2):147-52, 1995.

165 Maurer HR, Hozumi M, Honma Y, Okabe-Kado J. Bromelain induces the differentiation of leukemic cells in vitro: an explanation for its cytostatic effects? *Planta Med* 54(5):377-81, Oct 1988.

166 Gaspani L, Limiroli E, Ferrario P, Bianchi M. In vivo and in vitro effects of bromelain on PGE(2) and SP concentrations in the inflammatory exudate in rats. *Pharmacology* 65(2):83-6, 2002.

167 Vellini M, Desideri D, Milanese A, Omini C, et al. Possible involvement of eicosanoids in the pharmacological action of bromelain. *Arzneimittelforschung* 36(1):110-2, 1986.

One advantage of using enzymes is that we can combine them with orthodox treatment, that is, chemotherapy and/or radioactive therapy. As a bonus, the patient will have fewer side effects by combining these natural enzymes.

Modified Citrus Pectin (MCP)

Another strategy for controlling metastasis works by intercepting migrating cancer cells before they have a chance to establish new tumours. This approach targets a family of carbohydrate-binding proteins called galactoside-binding lectins, that help cancer cells stick together to form multi-celled clusters that are believed necessary for metastasis formation. Lectins also enable cancer cells to communicate with each other, as well as with other types of cells (cell-to-cell communication) to trigger cellular transformations that assist the spread of cancer.

A number of cancer researchers have focused on galectin-3 which strongly binds with galactose. Once the cancer cell in firmly lodged in the microcapillary network, galectins on the surface of the cancer cell start to bind to galactose receptors on endothelial cells and penetrate through the blood vessel walls. The final step after invading the vessel involves the release of chemical signals that trigger new blood vessel growth (angiogenesis), and a new tumour colony is firmly established.

Modified citrus pectin (MCP) is a unique dietary fibre that is produced by processing natural citrus pectin by altering its pH and splitting the carbohydrate chains to form a low molecular-weight, water-soluble fibre that is rich in the sugar, galactose. It is this presence of particularly high amounts of galactose that led researchers to wonder if MCP might bind with proteins (lectins) on cancer cells to inhibit their ability to bind with other   tissues.

In 1992, Platt and colleagues demonstrated that MCP was effective at reducing metastases in mice injected with live melanoma cells. Seventeen days after being injected, the mice receiving untreated melanoma cells were found to have, on average, 33 new tumours (metastases) in their lungs, while the mice receiving the MCP-treated cells had virtually no lung tumours.

In several animal rat and mouse models of breast, colon, and lung cancers, oral MCP has significantly inhibited carbohydrate-mediated tumour growth, angiogenesis, and metastasis, presumably via its effects on galectin-3 function.[168,169,170,171]

Galectins (galactose-specific lectins) are a group lectins found on the surface of mammalian cells that bind to galactosides. Galectin-3 lectins may be key in mitosis and proliferation, especially as metastatic cells of specific cancers have more galectin-3 on their surface compared to healthy cells. Galactose-rich MCP is thought to saturate the galactose-binding sites on the cancer cell surface by tightly binding with galectins.[172,173,174,175] With MCP bound to the galectins, the cancer cell is unable to aggregate with other cancer cells or adhere to normal cells, thereby reducing the cancer cell's ability to metastasize. This provides a preclinical evidence for a possible mechanism of action in prostate cancer. In an in vitro study, the addition of MCP to the media of cultured androgen-independent human prostatic JCA-1 cells reduced cell growth and correspondingly [3H] thymidine incorporation into DNA.[176] This also provides preclinical evidence for a possible mechanism of action in prostate cancer.

---

168 Hayashi A, Gillen AC, Lott JR. Effects of daily oral administration of quercetin chalcone and modified citrus pectin on implanted colon-25 tumor growth in Balb-c mice. *Altern Med Rev.* 5(6):546-52, Dec 2000.
169 Hsieh TC, Wu JM. Changes in cell growth, cyclin/kinase, endogenous phosphoproteins and nm23 gene expression in human prostatic JCA-1 cells treated with modified citrus pectin. *Biochem Mol Biol Int.* 37(5):833-41, Nov 1995.
170 Nangia-Makker P, Hogan V, Honjo Y, Baccarini S, Tait L, Bresalier R, Raz A. Inhibition of human cancer cell growth and metastasis in nude mice by oral intake of modified citrus pectin. *J Natl Cancer Inst.* 18;94(24):1854-62, Dec 2002.
171 Pienta KJ, Naik H, Akhtar A, Yamazaki K, Replogle TS, Lehr J, Donat TL, Tait L, Hogan V, Raz A. Inhibition of spontaneous metastasis in a rat prostate cancer model by oral administration of modified citrus pectin. *J Natl Cancer Inst.* 1;87(5):348-53, Mar 1995.
172 Bresalier, RS., Yan, PS., Byrd, JC., Lotan, R., and Raz, A. Expression of the endogenous galactose- binding protein galectin-3 correlates with the malignant potential of tumours in the central nervous system. *Cancer* 80(4):776-787, Aug 1997.
173 Kidd, P. A new approach to metastatic cancer prevention: modified citrus pectin (MCP), a unique pectin that blocks cell surface lectins. *Altern Med Rev* 1:4-10, 1996.
174 Raz, A. and Loton, R. Endogenous galactoside-binding lectins: a new class of functional cell surface molecules related to metastasis. *Cancer Metastasis Rev* 6:433-452, 1987.
175 Strum, S., Scholz, M., McDermed, J., and et al. Modified citrus pectin slows PSA doubling time: A pilot clinical trial. Presentation: International Conference on Diet and Prevention of Cancer. May 28 - June 2, 1999.
176 Hsieh, TC. and Wu, JM. Changes in cell growth, cyclin/kinase, endogenous phosphoproteins and nm23 gene expression in human prostatic JCA-1 cells treated with modified citrus pectin. *Biochem Mol.Biol Int* 37(5):833-841, 1995.

The collagen-dissolving mechanism also plays a major role in the spread of cancer and the growth of secondary tumours in other organs or parts of the body (metastases). With the help of collagen-digesting enzymes called malignin (a sterioisomer of trypsin), a cancer cell can "eat" its way into the lumen of the small blood vessel and into the blood stream. The blood can then carry away cancer cells, by which means they can spread and invade other organs.

The DaVinci Cancer Programme

If you have read this book from the beginning, you will have seen a lot written about the importance of detoxification on many different levels of the body. When cancer patients come to the DaVinci Natural Health Centre for help, one of the first things that we recommend is the DaVinci Cancer Detoxification Programme. This involves many different detoxifying and therapeutic protocols, as will be outlined below.

In addition, based on the bespoke data for each patient obtained from the IDEL Diagnostic Programme (see Chapter 2), there will be a number of other treatments recommended such as hyperthermia, low intensity laser therapy (LILT), nutritional supplements, homeopathy, digital homeopathy, homotoxicology, herbal medicine, bioresonance, Su Jok acupuncture, psychotherapy, sex therapy, EFT, Hellinger's soul healing and more. All the levels of health are addressed, as required.

Here is an example of a typical programme that the average cancer patient would follow – you can see details of all these therapies at www.docgeorge.com or go back through the book as they have all been discussed in detail in different chapters. International patients coming in from abroad would stay a minimum of two weeks to complete the IDEL Diagnostic Programme as well as take full advantage of all the therapies offered – by the time they return to their home country to continue with their supplement programme, they are well on the way to healing:

- ❖ Ozone Sauna
- ❖ Infrared Sauna
- ❖ Matrix Regeneration Therapy (MRT)
- ❖ Orgone Accumulator
- ❖ Ionizer Foot Bath
- ❖ Colon Hydrotherapy
- ❖ Rife Technology

- ❖ PAPIMI
- ❖ Low Intensity Lazer Therapy for tooth and scar foci
- ❖ Sex therapy
- ❖ Brief psychotherapy, EFT and Hellinger's Soul Healing
- ❖ 15-day alkaline detoxification diet
- ❖ Liver and gallbladder cleanse
- ❖ Parasite Cleanse
- ❖ Heavy metal detox using the HMD® Ultimate Detox Protocol
- ❖ Optimized nutrition based on the patient's Metabolic Typing
- ❖ Bespoke supplement programme based on the IDEL Diagnostic testing
- ❖ Use of Digital Homeopathy, homeopathy and homotoxicology where appropriate
- ❖ Use of the Cesium High pH Mineral protocol, PolyMVA, MMS, DCA, Graviola, Vitamin C, ozone, bicarbonate and other protocols to reduce tumour load
- ❖ Su Jok therapy where appropriate to deal with pain conditions as well as help the body to heal
- ❖ Hyperthermia – topical
- ❖ Bioresonance Therapy
- ❖ The bespoke use of naturopathy, herbal medicine, homeopathy, clinical nutrition and many other healing modalities, based on the patient's needs.

Epilogue

It is important to realize that once upon a time a cancer cell was a normal cell sitting in your body, breathing happily and going about its work. Over time, as the body became more and more toxic, acidic and deoxygenated this happy cell had one of two choices. Either it dies and the whole body leaves with the Angels, or it switches a gene and becomes an anaerobic cell that no longer requires oxygen to survive – this is the cancer cell.

Seen in this light, the cancer cell is an adaptive response to an imbalanced internal milieu – cancer is not a disease but the symptom of the imbalance – cancer is a mechanism of survival and self-protection. It is not the enemy that should be burned, radiated, cut out or poisoned. Cancer is a desperate attempt of the body to live, not die.

Many times these can be psychological, emotional or systemic entanglements. Whatever happens in our emotional body also occurs in our physical body. Fear and suppression are two key emotions that can quickly poison your body and create the circumstances for cancer cells to develop.

Cancer may be the wake-up call to bring harmony, joy and love back into our lives – if these are missing, then the heart or fundamental soul of the person becomes paralyzed. Cancer maybe a way out of this paralysis of the heart and soul – it may trigger us to change and help us to break old patterns of guilt, shame and low self-esteem, aspects that crush the soul. This inward change is crucial to induce a cure of your cancer. Cancer's purpose is not to destroy the body but to heal what is no longer whole and holy – the disease is a reflection of our inner world, the one that needs nurturing so that we can talk from our heart openly and lovingly.

I sincerely hope that this chapter will help the layperson as well as their doctors and healers to radically alter our current thinking on cancer and its treatment. Let's stand still, listen to our body, mind and soul and ask, "Why has it developed cancer?" Once we understand the answers, then we are well on our way to heal our body on all levels, as many people have done even with metastatic cancers.

In the next chapter we will examine detailed case histories of 15 patients with "incurable" diseases, as defined by the medical profession, and how they found their way back to health using holistic medicine.

PART C

Chapter 12

Patient Case Histories

This last and final chapter is a living testimonial of 15 patients that I have seen and applied the holistic model to at the DaVinci Natural Health Centre in Larnaca, Cyprus. Pretty much all of these patients had spent years seeing a number of medical doctors and had received many different types of medical treatments but their health problems remained or got worse.

I am deeply grateful, indebted and beholden to every single one of these patients (and all other patients that I see); all, without exception placed their trust in me – sometimes the going got tough, but their trust in me, and my trust in holistic medicine helped to get through the dark patches of the tunnel where we could see light again. I also express gratitude to them for placing their trust in me when I would say: "I have never tried this before, but I think it is going to work because ……" Nearly without exception most patients agreed to experiment and we managed to move one step forward. I believe these qualities of trust, commitment, developing a healthy therapeutic relationship with a mutual respect, and a determination to get well play a very important role in the whole therapeutic process for both patient and therapist.

There are, off course, patients that simply do not have the self-discipline to persevere, experiment, be their own doctor, discuss therapeutic strategies with their therapist and are generally pessimistic about outcomes. These patients are the most difficult cases to work with, even with relatively simple problems.

Most of these are fairly recent patients that I have seen in the last couple of years or so – there are many, many others that I have seen in the past 20 years and who have seen many benefits to their health, but it was easier to take the active patients as opposed to those seen many years ago. In a busy practice like I run, it is always difficult to take meticulous notes when time is of essence and this is probably the main reason why many practitioners with equal successes do not write their cases up due to time restraints. I believe it is important, however, for more cases to be published as this is important testimonial to holistic medicine, as well as a learning tool for all.

The cases are presented in the same format throughout, as follows:

> ➤ The presenting problem
> ➤ the medical diagnosis consisting of blood tests, scans and medical reports written by medical practitioners
> ➤ the holistic diagnosis, which consists of all the testing that was conducted by myself and sometimes other natural medicine practitioners
> ➤ the holistic treatments that the patient followed as part of their healing journey, usually based on the diagnostics.
> ➤ a personal account by the patient concerning how they perceived their health problem and what this meant to them
> ➤ comments by myself about the particular case. This was taken by an independent medical doctor who would spend about an hour with each patient taking their personal account.

Finally, I just want to add that apart from the gratitude that I have towards all these brave souls who persevered with their wellness programmes, I am also in reverence to the Higher Power that guided myself and supported my patients throughout their healing journey.

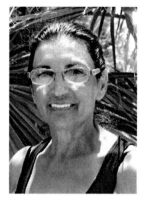

Case No. 1, Mrs. A, aged 62

Main presenting problem: Depression, asthma, hypertension, psoriasis, mitral valve prolapse, kidney cyst, hypercholesteremia, rheumatoid arthritis.

This is an interesting case as it shows the power of how a traumatic experience can lock a person into illness for many decades. This lady was on 13 different medications amounting to a total of 30 pills taken daily – when speaking to her for the first time in my office she was on a different level of consciousness and had difficulty following and partaking in the dialogue we were trying to have – it was the daughter accompanying her that did most of the talking.

Medical diagnosis

This lady presented with a clinical depression of 20-years standing, taking a variety of psychotropic drugs over the years as prescribed by the local psychiatrist. She was also asthmatic and taking various inhalers, she had psoriasis which was severe, spreading all over her body; she was hypertensive (150/95) and taking a variety of anti-hypertensive medications. She has cardiovascular problems with a mitral valve thickening, mild regurgitation, with the tricuspid and aortic valves calcified. She also has hypercholesteremia and takes Statin drugs for this. Her hepatic enzyme levels are usually high and so are her CRP and ESR levels. She also suffers from rheumatoid arthritis with deformities in her fingers of both hands, as well as other joints. She has a kidney cyst on one of her kidneys.

She had spinal surgery three years ago for a compressed vertebral disc, as well as a gallbladder removed about the same time.

Her cholesterol levels were 219mg/dl (100-200), gamma-GT hepatic enzymes were 41U/L (9-38) and her CRP was 0.69 (0.10-0.50).

Her complete cardiac report showed thickening of the mitral valve leaflets and calcified tricuspid aortic valve with mild aortic valve regurgitation.

There was also a confirmed diagnosis of rheumatoid arthritis, depression, psoriasis, kidney cysts, hypertension and hypercholestermia.

A recent MRI brain scan taken in June 2009 has shown multiple small focal hyperintensities of the subcortical white matter of both parietal lobes on T2W images compatible with a small vessel disease with an empty sella syndrome. This testing was done due to her complaining of short-term memory problems. With so much psychotropic medication taken over the years this finding may not come as a surprise.

Holistic diagnosis

The thermography scan showed a hyperthermic symmetry over the left side of the mouth which suggested dental inflammation. ART testing had shown tooth foci in the lower jaw, which was confirmed with the panoramic X-ray. There was an area of hyperthermia in the upper outer quadrants of both breasts that were compatible with fibrocystic and fibrofatty changes. There was also hyperthermia noted over T2 which suggest autonomic dysfunction and may correlate with the history of hypertension. There was hyperthermia over the base of the left lung which may be compatible with lung dysfunction and correlate with her history of asthma. There was also intense hypothermia over the epigastrium which suggests upper GI autonomic dysfunction. Hyperthermia was noted over the hepatic flexure, transverse colon and splenic flexure of the colon which may be compatible with irritation or dysfunction. There was also inflammation present over the left acromioclavicular joint which suggest arthritis.

VEGA food intolerance testing revealed a number of food intolerances such as: wheat, lactose and milk products, chicken, pork, the nightshade family of vegetables, citrus, sugar and caffeine. All these food intolerances are highly likely to lead to inflammation in the body.

Further energetic testing using VEGA and ART showed that there were a number of organs that were energetically imbalanced: brain, thyroid, heart, lungs, liver, fallopian tubes and ovaries, auditory tubes, coronary arteries, aorta, stomach, kidneys, adrenals, pancreas, jejunum and rectum. Prioritization of these organs showed that the brain was the primary organ affected.

Darkfield microscopy showed a picture of low vitality with very few protits – the integrity of the cell walls of the RBC's would diminish in less than 10 minutes (lack of antioxidants to protect cell wall), the WBC's were viable but somewhat sluggish (compromised immunity), there were signs of elliptocytes (possible liver dysfunction), with B12 and folic acid deficiency. Generally, this was a picture of very low vitality with a number of nutritional deficiencies, including antioxidants.

Iridology showed a "daisy iris" which is an indication of inherited connective tissue weaknesses, with particular weaknesses in the liver, kidney, uterus, lung and thyroid areas which had large lacuna. Stomach lining was irritated and yellow, indicating a chronic hypochlorhydria; there was a cholesterol ring which is an indication of an inherited predisposition towards hypercholestermia. The iris colour was murky with isolated psora spots of concentrated toxicity in the liver and uterus. There were cervical and lumbar subluxations.

Heart Rate Variability testing showed a decreased parasympathetic system with a moderately increased sympathetic system. The general functioning of all the physiological systems was generally reduced – score of 10 (7 is average, 1 is excellent) and the adaptation reserve which is an indicator of how she copes with stress was very low too – score of 6 (7 is the lowest, 1 is excellent).

Hair Tissue Mineral Analysis showed low levels of copper, selenium, cobalt and molybdenum, and a cocktail of heavy metals such as arsenic, mercury, aluminium with cadmium. On the first hair test dated 16th March 2009 the cadmium levels were fairly low, but on the second test dated 6th May 2009, after taking the natural chelator HMD,™ her cadmium levels had shot up to extremely high levels, indicating high storage levels in the organs and tissues – it has still not been determined where she had obtained these amounts of cadmium, even though the husband is quite a heavy smoker.

Cadmium can lead to the development of cardiovascular disease, kidney disease, arthritis and many others. One reason may be that cadmium replaces zinc in the body. Mrs. A had many of these degenerative diseases.

This case is particularly important as it shows how this lady became "got stuck" when she was 29-years old, after the death of her young 4-year old son who died in a tragic tractor accident, with the husband driving, as described in Chapter 10.

During the IDEL testing, I casually asked her when her problems had begun. She immediately answered: "when I was 29 years old." I asked her why 29 and she went on to explain that at that age when her young boy was 4 years old, he was taking a ride on her husband's tractor and fell over and was crushed by the heavy tire. She picked the child up and took him to the local hospital, but by the time they could treat the boy he had died. Since this time she has been 'locked-in' with her young boy in a delayed grieving reaction, literally lying next to the child in the grave where she felt she belonged. She saw no one, as one of her daughters bitterly complained: 'we never had a mother, ever.' This mother felt so guilty about her child's death that she stopped living herself and became loyal to her child's grave, not seeing or hearing anyone else (the representative was able to sense and channel the mother's emotions).

One of her 4 daughters came to a Hellinger Family Constellation workshop and set up a constellation about her mother not seeing her and never paying much attention to her. The representative for the young child was placed on the ground and as soon as the mother's representative saw the child in the grave she immediately went down and embraced the child very tightly, while she was crying and wailing at the top of her voice. This continued for over 20 minutes and no attempts to separate them was possible.

The lack of freedom and strength to get on with her life due to her failure to 'consent to what is' became very apparent. Through Hellinger's Family Constellation or soul healing she was able to overcome this blockage and move on with her physical healing.

Holistic treatments

Apart from the soul healing mentioned above and some brief psychotherapy, there were many other levels of healing that took place after this monumental blockage was removed.

The other level of healing was to detoxify her of the myriad of toxins that she had exposed her body to over the last 40 years – she was taking 30 pills comprising 13 different combinations of drugs when I first saw her. It was difficult to determine what symptoms were related to the side-effects of this lethal cocktail, and what true pathology was. Most of her consequent health problems had began 8-10 years of taking potent anti-depressants and anxiolytics – there was a strong cocktail of these psychotropic drugs which no doubt played a role in creating the rheumatoid arthritis, the hypertension, the heart valve defects, the hypertension, the high liver enzymes and the high cholesterol. Needless to say she received a myriad of other medications to control this syndrome of health issues.

I referred her to a medical doctor who worked with her to reduce her medication, concomitantly with her detoxification which lasted over 30 days. She first began with cutting out her food intolerances, as well as cereal products, refined foods and for the first week she ate fish, pulses, salads, steamed vegetables, fruit and fresh carrot and green juices. The second week she cut out the fish and remained with the rest. The third and fourth week she cut out the pulses and continued with the fruit and veg. This is a "compromised" DaVinci detoxification diet for chronically ill patients who would suffer if detoxification was to take place too quickly.

She was also given a number of drainage remedies from the homotoxicology range such as lymphomysot for the lymphatic system, berberis for the kidneys and nux vomica for the liver. There were other herbal remedies for helping the detoxification organs too, one was the Organic Lavage.[1]

There was a high-potency multivitamin formula added to deal with her chronic nutritional deficiencies, along with Omega 3,6 and 9 fatty acids[2,3] to help her heart, circulation and joints, glucosamine[4,5] as well as MSM for

---

1 See www.detoxmetals.com for further details

2 Martin C. Omega-3 Fatty acids: proven benefit or just a "fish story"? *Consult Pharm.* 23(3):210-21, 2008.

3 Simopoulos AP. The importance of the omega-6/omega-3 fatty acid ratio in cardiovascular disease and other chronic diseases. *Exp Biol Med* (Maywood). 233(6):674-88, 2008.

4 Herrero-Beaumont G, Ivorra JA, Del Carmen Trabado M, Blanco FJ, Benito P, Martin-Mola E, Paulino J, Marenco JL, Porto A, Laffon A, Araujo D, Figueroa M, Branco J. Glucosamine sulfate in the treatment of knee osteoarthritis symptoms: a randomized, double-blind, placebo-controlled study using acetaminophen as a side comparator. *Arthritis Rheum.* 56(2):555-67, Feb 2007.

5 Vangsness CT Jr, Spiker W, Erickson J. A review of evidence-based medicine for glucosamine and chondroitin sulfate use in knee osteoarthritis. *Arthroscopy.* 25(1):86-94, Jan 2009.

the joints, Lugol's Iodine[6] for the metabolism and thyroid functioning which was sluggish as seen on the Barne's Temperature test (35.7 degrees centigrade average).

As there were high levels of heavy metals, particularly cadmium, she was started on the HMD™ Ultimate Detox Protocol consisting of HMD, Organic Lavage and Chlorella.[7]

Tumeric[8] was also added as a general anti-inflammatory, as well as adding herbal formulas for her asthma and adrenal glands. A Salt Pipe was added to further help the respiratory system.[9] Within 3 weeks of taking the asthmatic herbs and salt pipe she was completely off the medicinal inhalers and was walking considerable distances with no breathing problems.

The DaVinci Candida Protocol (see chapter 5) was also began on the 24th April for her systemic candidiasis and this cleared in July.

Finally, Bach Flower remedies were given to suit her psychoemotional state in order to begin balancing on this level.

Patient's own account

Towards the end of last year I was a walking zombie – all I would do most of the day is lie on the couch either watching TV or sleeping. The chronic fatigue that I felt can only be explained by someone who has had this experience – I could not do the basic housework, I would begin wheezing heavily and feel asphyxiated if I walked to the shop or neighbour next door – it was like I had been running non-stop for an hour. Going to the shop I had to take my little basket on wheels as I could not carry even a kilo of fruit back with me without dropping it. My husband ran the household, shopping, cleaning and everything else that was required.

My brain was quite non-functional, I could not even remember simple things and had difficulty holding a conversation most of the time. My

---

6 The prevalence of thyroid dysfunction in a population with borderline iodine deficiency. *Clin Endocrinol* (Oxf). 51(3):361-7, Sept 1999.

7 http://www.detoxmetals.com/Toxic-Metal-Detoxification-Protocol.html
8 Molnar V, Garai J . Plant-derived anti-inflammatory compounds affect MIF tautomerase activity. *Int Immunopharmacol*. 5(5):849-56, May 2005.
9 See www.thesaltpipe.co.uk

mood was constantly depressed and many people around me commented that I never could smile, which was true. I just felt that it was pointless being with people as I was such a misery that it would make me fall into a deeper depression and it was a bit of a vicious cycle – this is why I preferred being alone most of the time. My quality of life was zero but there did not seem to be anything that I could do about it – it was like someone had 'locked me in' and I did not know how to escape.

I had 4 daughters who cherished over me but throughout their life I was never there for them and this just made me feel worse. The grandchildren too – I so much wanted to play with them but I couldn't – it was so frustrating and depressing. One of my daughters wanted me to go to see Dr. Georgiou at the DaVinci Natural Health Centre in Larnaca which was only a short drive from where we lived. Our first meeting took place on the 18th December 2008, but I really do not remember much of what took place apart from booking another appointment a couple of weeks later to see him for a fuller assessment.

On the 12th January 2009 I underwent a 5-hour rigorous testing that involved many tests – on the same day Dr. Georgiou said that for the next month I would be changing my diet drastically – the first week I had to eat a little fish, pulses, salads, steamed vegetables, fruit and vegetable juices like carrot. The second week I was to cut out the fish and stay with the rest, and the third and fourth weeks I was to 'eat like a bunny' as I remember him telling me – only vegetables and fruit with juices. I told him that this would be difficult to implement but he smiled and said that he would help me to take a step at a time and that I would be pleasantly surprised. He was so convincing that as soon as I got home I began organizing the household for the new diet.

To my surprise, and that of my husband and family, by the end of the second week I was actually doing the housework, began walking to the shops and neighbour much easier and generally finding that my mood was lifting. I was actually smiling and people around me would shout this out every time I did it.

It is now about 7 months into therapy and I am a different person, as my husband says continuously it is the difference between night and day. Dr. Georgiou sent me to a medical doctor to reduce the 13 different drugs that I was taking, including a number of different psychotropic drugs. I am now down from taking a cocktail of 30 pills to taking only 6 – most of the other ones that I have been taking for years have now been stopped. I now wake at 6 am every morning and take the bus down to the sea where I will swim for an hour and lie in the sun as this helps my psoriasis. On returning I walk about 6 kilometres to my daughter's house – another younger relative used to join me but she dropped out as she said that she could not keep up with me! I am doing most of the shopping, the cleaning, the housework and I have even gone out and began doing some gardening which I thoroughly enjoy.

All my daughters are really happy for me and I am now playing games with my grandchildren which I could only dream of. Most people now see me smiling – a really big smile as it is a marvelous gift to feel so much alive again and live a quality life – thank you so much Dr. Georgiou, your work is truly blessed!

Dr Georgiou's final comments on Mrs. A's case

Seven months have now gone by and this lady has reduced her medication from 13 different kinds to only three. She is doing all her household chores, walking to her daughter's houses (6 kms), which takes her just over an hour, as well as swimming every morning in the sea.

Her blood pressure has dropped from 150/85 to 110/65, even though she has stopped taking a number of anti-hypertensive medications. She is still taking some and this may need to be eliminated in the future as her diastolic pressure is quite low at present. Probably the elimination of the general inflammation in her body has also helped the blood pressure as inflammatory chemicals in the body can certainly cause hypertension.[10,11,12]

The pain in her joints is much better, and so is the flexibility, even though she has reduced a lot of the analgesics as well as the arthritis medication – the glucosamine, MSM, omega fatty acids as well as the multivitamin will

10 Hansson GK. Inflammation, atherosclerosis, and coronary artery disease. *N Engl J Med* 352: 1685–1695, 2005.

11 Willerson JT, Ridker PM. Inflammation as a cardiovascular risk factor. *Circulation* 109: II2–II10, 2004; Chae CU, Lee RT, Rifai N, Ridker PM. Blood pressure and inflammation in apparently healthy men. *Hypertension* 38: 399–403, 2001.

12 Chrysohoou C, Pitsavos C, Panagiotakos DB, Skoumas J, Stefanadis C. Association between prehypertension status and inflammatory markers related to atherosclerotic disease: The ATTICA Study. *Am J Hypertens* 17: 568–573, 2004.

help here. The psoriasis has more or less healed completely, even though it can reappear as soon as she gets upset over something or faces acute stress.

Her cholesterol levels taken 5th January 2009 were 219 and are now 187 on 17th June. Her gamma-GT levels were 41 and have now dropped to 19. Her CRP levels were 0.69 and have now dropped to 0.40. We are still monitoring her cadmium levels every two months as she continues with her natural chelation protocol.

It is very likely that many of her symptoms were iatrogenic or caused by the myriad of drugs that she was on – blindly given by a number of state doctors without thinking of the consequences of this polypharmacy on the body – this lady could have very easily died of kidney or heart disease due to the massive doses of drugs that she was on. I see this often and it makes absolutely no biological sense whatsoever – it certainly makes good economics for the pharmaceutical companies.

She has overcome her depression and her husband is delighted with his new-found wife, the one he so much remembered all those years ago when they married. It would have been difficult to achieve so much in so little time if she had not dealt with the suppressed trauma of her deceased child – the retrieval and healing of the Soul from the grave in this case was probably the key factor that led to her amazing recovery and this was all done in her absence by her daughter who set up the constellation. This is also one of the mysteries of the Field (see Chapter 10), that the healing effects when family members are reconstituted back into the family system can affect people who were not even present in the same room.

Case No. 2, Mr. S, 24 years old

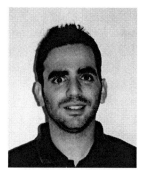

Main presenting problem: Astrocytoma stage II (Brain tumour)

Medical diagnosis

In 2006 this young, postgraduate university student was diagnosed with a diffuse WHO grade II astrocytoma (left parietal and temporal lobes) which was surgically removed in the UK – about 60% was resected. This was also confirmed by routine histology in anatomic pathology in the UK.

In September 2007 he had developed numbness in the right leg, dizziness and focal seizures with speech arrest and paresis of the right arm. An MRI scan showed a non-contrast enhancing tumour in the left insular region. The tumour reached the Broca's area with its frontal and the Wernicke's area with its dorsal circumference. The pyramid tract is medially dislocated. A German neurosurgeon performed another resection with bilingual speech monitoring and neuronavigation under awake conditions – the histology exam showed a Glioblastoma WHO Grade IV.

Holistic diagnosis:

The IDEL Diagnostic Programme brought to light a number of potential causative factors. VEGA testing for food intolerances identified the following foods: wheat, lactose and dairy products, chicken, pork, citrus and sugar (he was a 'sugarholic' in his teens). Lactose was his primary allergens that completely blocked his regulation or ANS.

Organ testing using VEGA and ART showed energetic organ imbalances in the liver, gallbladder, tonsils, adrenals, jejunum, left brain – cerebrum motor area, and right teeth quadrant, as well as the pancreas. The pancreas was the primary organ on prioritizing testing using ART – this organ is commonly found in cancer patients as it is highly significant in dissolving the sialo-glycogen coating of cancer cells (see chapter 11). He also had systemic Candidiasis, probably related to the IV antibiotics, but also his high sugar consumption.

There were also high levels of electromagnetic and mobile phone stress detected. Apparently he was quite addicted to electronic games when younger, sitting in front of the TV for many years, as well as using the mobile phone for many years – he is left-handed and used the mobile phone mainly on the left ear where the tumour was identified (exactly in the area where the mobile phone sits).

Thermography showed hyperthermic patterns encircling the buccal cavity on the left side which indicated an oral dental or periodontal pathology. There was a slight vertical type hyperthermia that may relate to the epigastric hyperthermia possibly indicating a developing GERD (this was also picked up on the iridological analysis). There was also a slight muscular type diffuse hyperthermia over the entire posterior neck region extending inferiorly to the upper back, through the right and then through the spine to the left side between the scapulas. These muscular inflammatory findings indicate a possible involvement of the trapezius, levator scapula and rhomboid muscles.

Iridological analysis showed hypochlorhydria (he had difficulty digesting protein concentrates with stomach bloating and discomfort), subclinical hypothyroidism with extremely cold hands and feet, pancreatic enzyme deficiency with bowel distension after eating, as well as considerable liver and kidney congestion. There were also indications of cervical and lumbar subluxations.

Darkfield microscopy revealed a number of parasites (there were more than 10 identified in one single drop of blood), as well as a lot of rouleau and high valence fibrinogen, indicating a very congested blood picture with an imbalanced tissue pH. There were also some colourful red symplasts that are characteristic of cancer patients taking chemotherapy such as Thelozamide that he was taking last year.

The white blood cells were viable but generally sluggish showing compromised immunity.

The Biological Terrain Analysis from saliva and urine indicated the saliva pH was very alkaline with highly acidic urine indicating an acidic tissue pH and there were malabsorption problems with mineral levels low, high free radical activity with a biological age of 53; chronological at time of testing was 23.

Hair Tissue Mineral Analysis showed high levels of heavy metals such as beryllium, mercury, arsenic and aluminium, with low levels of minerals and trace elements such as copper, manganese and cobalt.

Heart Rate Variabilty (HRV) testing a relatively healthy picture with a slightly increased sympathetic activity, but the overall HRT score on the orthotest was 6,3 which is slightly above the average found generally (perfect score is 1,1).

Holistic treatments

Bach remedies were given to help ease the anxiety and fear of the disease, as well as the despondency. He has noticed that when he is stressed, particularly during the summer when his friends from university disband, he feels a little down and some symptoms come back. He was also advised to keep away any electrical devices to the brain, including mobile phones and use the speakerphone if necessary. A whole body detoxification with fruit, vegetables and their juices, vegetable soups and steamed vegetables and salads were allowed for 2 weeks – this greatly helps to alleviate the inflammatory chemicals in the body caused by a number of toxins and imbalanced pH.

He was advised to stop using the mobile phone and only use it for a few minutes at a time with Bluetooth which uses sound waves, not microwaves. Using Tachyon energy chips in the mobile phone would also help to reduce the electromagnetic fields. Also, tachyon crystals can be used on his person and in his surroundings to neutralize the electromagnetic fields from electronic equipments and computer screens.

The HMD™ Ultimate Detox Protocol was used to eliminate the cocktail of heavy metals. Interestingly, on the initial hair tissue mineral analysis there was no heavy metals shown in circulation, but two months later, while on the HMD protocol, it showed that there were quite high levels of beryllium, mercury, arsenic and aluminium in storage sites of the body. Mr. S is now being monitored every two months using the hair test to determine whether the level of metals is dropping. On the last test it showed that the levels of toxic metals had dropped to a significantly low levels, an indication that there is probably very few metals in storage sites of the body. Removing this high load of toxic metals will greatly reduce the free radical load and facilitate health and healing.

In addition, he took a number of nutritional supplements such as a high-potency multivitamin and multimineral supplement, as well as omega 3,6 and 9 fatty acids, betaine HCl plus pepsin for stomach digestion and a pancreatic digestive enzyme to facilitate gut digestion. He was also given Essiac Tea which contains Burdock root, Turkey rhubarb, Sheep's sorrel in order to help boost immunity. He also took powdered calcium ascorbate, a buffered form of vitamin C – approximately 12-15 grams daily. He has also been taking systemic enzymes – Wobenzyme-N in order to help digest the silao-glycoprotein coating of the cancer cells and allow the WBC's access to attack.

Another important treatment that he has been doing courses of intermittently is the PAPIMI – this has helped with the loss of sensation, coordination and balance problem and general "brain fuzziness" which he developed in September 2009 on his right side and is intermittent. The PAPIMI has greatly helped to bring sensation back into the right side and clear this fuzziness and help his balance and coordination.

He is presently on an optimum diet. All cells contain special "suicide genes" - p53 - that, when activated, can kill them. Normally, this is what happens when a cell is in danger of becoming a cancer cell. More and more nutrients have been found to wake up this vital gene, including extracts of both green tea and persimmon, curcumin, apigenin, quercetin, luteolin and resveratrol. DHA, from omega-3 fats, can also activate the cancer cell's suicide genes.

As I have mentioned and explained in detail in chapter 11, inflammation is key to the development of cancer. Recent studies have shown that it also plays a major role in the growth and spread of the disease. Experiments found that when inflammation was triggered near a small cancer, it became very aggressive and spread faster. Mr. S is now very aware of this fact and takes precautions to avoid excessive inflammation -

Curcumin is a powerful anti-inflammatory comparable to the strongest drugs - minus their side effects - and has turned out to be one of the most powerful cancer inhibitors found thus far. It uses a number of mechanisms to effectively restore bone marrow cells, build muscle, heal wounds, stimulate detoxification and suppress the COX-2 enzyme.

Proanthrocyanadins (from grapes), resveratrol (grape skins), quercetin (onions, apples and teas), hesperidin (oranges), naringenin (grapefruit), aged garlic extract, vitamin E succinate, gamma-tocopherol (type of vitamin E), boswellia and bromelain have all been shown to significantly reduce inflammation and do so safely.

Optimizing diet and avoiding foods that can acidify the body and fuel cancer cells such as sugar, omega-6 fats, methionine, glutamate and aspartate, as well as making it more prone to inflammation. Recent findings have shown that glutamate is a powerful stimulant of cancer growth and invasion has caused great concern. In fact, drugs that block glutamate were proven to significantly slow the growth of cancers and remarkably enhance the effectiveness of cancer chemotherapy agents. Most sensitive were malignant brain tumors, as well as cancer of the breasts, colon and lungs. It's a shame that most oncologists are not aware of this as they can use it for the best benefit of the patient.

All of this becomes very important when you realize that the modern American diet is loaded with glutamate in the form of MSG (monosodium glutamate), hydrolyzed proteins, caseinate, soy products and natural flavourings. Our obsession with soy is ludicrous when you realize that soybeans have one of the highest glutamate levels in the plant kingdom. Mushrooms, especially portobello mushrooms, also have high levels.

One of the most concise studies on the ability of fruits and vegetables to prevent cancer used the best of over 200 human and 22 animal studies available. The conclusion was that eating five servings of fruits and vegetables daily reduced cancer incidence by fifty percent. For some cancers, the reduction was seventy-five percent. On the other side of the coin, deficiencies in certain nutrients have been shown to increase cancer risk anywhere from 200 to 1,600 percent. Mr. S very rarely ate fruit and vegetables during childhood and teenage years.

Further things on his "to do" list include: detoxifying every 6 months, removing heavy metals, taking a constant supply of the anti-inflammatory nutrients as well as those that that keep the p53 gene switched on and more.

Patient's own account

It was a beautiful Sunday morning 2006, when I woke up and I felt the whole of the right side of my body going numb. I couldn't feel anything. Even the same side of my head was numb. I was a university student at that time in Greece. I went to the hospital with my room-mate for blood tests and the results showed nothing pathological and we went home. On the following Wednesday, I felt this paresthesia again on the same side of my body and I also had an epileptic crisis and they took me immediately to the hospital. They conducted a CT scan and an MRI scan of my brain and the diagnosis was a brain tumour in the left side of my brain. They suggested to leave the country immediately, go to UK and have the tumor removed, because they did not perform such kind of operations there.

I quit my studies in the middle of the year and in June 2006 my parents arranged the hospital in UK which I would be operated. I had 60% of the tumour removed. The doctors told me that the biopsy showed that it was low grade astrocytoma and that I shouldn't worry, because most probably it would not grow again or metastasize. So I left England and the same story with epileptic crisis went on. I started antiepileptic drugs but no change at all.

In July 2007, I had an MRI scan again and unfortunately, I had bad news again. The rest of the tumour which could not be removed started to grow again. I was 26 years old at that time and my stress levels were really going through the roof having to cope with all this. It was overwhelming because I never had to deal with any health problems before. We did a lot of searching with my parents and we found out that in Germany there is one of the best neurosurgeons dealing with brain tumors. So in the middle of September 2007 I had the operation in Germany which took 12 hours!

This time, 95% of the tumour was removed. They did a biopsy again and this time thy told me that it is a Stage IV malignant glioma and I needed radiotherapy and chemotherapy. The doctor was very positive about my situation and very encouraging. When I arrived in Cyprus in October, I started chemotherapy and I had nine sessions. I felt terrible! These were indeed the worst days of my life. I had nausea and vomiting all the time, felt very weak, my energy levels were extremely low, I was lethargic and I could hardly walk from one room to the other of the house.

After the operation in Germany though, I felt better. I started being more positive despite the chemotherapy. I also had radiotherapy for about 6 weeks. I still had this right-sided paresis, sometimes with dizziness and speech arrest but not so often now. I tried to stay positive despite the continuation of my problems even though the tumour was removed.

During my stay in Germany, I met a woman from Cyprus and she told me about the DaVinci Natural Health Center, here in Larnaca, She insisted that I visit the Centre as soon as I returned and see Dr. Georgiou in person.

In August 2008 I called and spoke to Dr. Georgiou and arranged to be seen the same month. I had an extensive series of tests called the IDEL Diagnostic Program, designed to identify and eliminate all the possible causative factors of my health problems. It took Dr. Georgiou just over 5 hours to complete all the testing and he explained things on the way. After collecting all the health data from these tests I began a treatment programme that made me feel so much better. At the same time I learned a lot of things which I was ignorant of.

I began to realize how terrible my eating habits were and as long as I can remember I was always playing electronic games for many hours a day, watching TV, using the mobile phone as if it was going out of fashion – I was heavily laden with electromagnetic and mobile phone stress – this was a highly likely cause that harmed my brain.

After the first two weeks of the treatment protocol at the DaVinci Centre I felt so much more energetic. My progression is very interesting as I feel I have myself back again, my legs are feeling a lot stronger to climb up the stairs and this right-sided paresthesia doesn't happen so often anymore. I live a healthy life without making my body toxic with chemotherapies and different kinds of food that harm my body.

I am thankful to the lady that insisted that I visit the DaVinci Natural Health Center as well as to Dr. Georgiou himself for all the support that he has given me even in my more desperate moments.

I feel an 80% improvement in all my symptoms and my energy levels are really quite optimal, something that is helping me to complete my MSc and keep up to speed with everyone else, even though I have part of my brain missing.

Last months MRI scan (May 2009) showed that there was no change as far as the 5% of the remaining tumour is concerned. I am really heartened that the DaVinci Centre is just around the corner and I will continue to have follow-up treatments, including the PAPIMI which has greatly helped the paresthesia and balance issues. I am now much more optimistic about my prognosis as one of the things that Dr. Georgiou has helped me to understand are the causative factors of my illness, and I have made concerted efforts to change my life-style dramatically to one that is a lot more healthy.

Dr Georgiou's final comments

It is heartening to see that Mr. S's MRI scans have shown stability since I first met him in November 2007. Specifically, his latest MRI scan a few months ago read: "There have been no changes in the appearance of the post operative changes in the left parietal and temporal lobe in comparison with the previous scan dated 14.4.08. There is no evidence of abnormal enhancement in the surgical bed to indicate recurrent or residual tumour. There have been no changes in the gliosis surrounding the post operative cavity."

It is difficult to be certain what causes such brain tumours at such a young age – probably the high use of the electromagnetic equipment and mobile phone was one major factor, along with the very poor diet with its high sugar content and no fruit and vegetables, that helped to keep his body in a state of inflammation and acidic pH – again factors that facilitate oxygen levels to drop in the body which would trigger oncogenes and begin the cascade of cancer cell proliferation. Heavy metals, low levels of mineral, systemic candidiasis and poor digestion will add to the load and make things worse.

There is now considerable research that has shown the link between mobile phone use and brain tumours,[13,14,15] specifically the research has shown that mobile phone use leads to:

---

13 Schüz, et al., Cellular phones, cordless phones, and the risks of glioma and meningioma (Interphone Study Group, Germany), *Am. J. Epidemiol.* 163 (6) 512–520, Mar 2006.
14 Hansson Mild, et al., Pooled analysis of two Swedish case–control studies on the use of mobile and cordless telephones and the risk of brain tumours diagnosed during 1997–2003, *Int. J. Occup. Safety Ergon.* (JOSE) 13 (1) 63–71, 2007.

❖ a statistically significant doubling of brain cancer risk[16],[17]
❖ a statistically significant dose-response[18] risk of acoustic neuroma with more than 6 years of cellphone use[19]
❖ findings of genetic damage in human blood when exposed to cellphone radiation.

There is no doubt that microwaves and RF from mobile phones can penetrate the brain causing harm.[20]

Eating a lot of sweets and carbohydrates could also cause brain damage for three reasons:

1. Sugar dramatically increases metabolism, and high rates of metabolism are the major source of free radicals. In fact, 95 percent of all free radicals come from metabolism.

2. Second, high levels of sugar in the body cause the sugar to react with various critical proteins, including enzymes that repair DNA damage caused by free radicals.

3. When high levels of sugar are combined with high fat levels over a long period of time, cells cannot absorb the sugar needed to produce energy.

Finally, consumption of large amounts of excitotoxins can seriously damage the brain. Excitotoxins found in many fast foods, sweets with colourings and other processed foods dramatically increase free radical generation for a prolonged period after a single exposure. Heavy metals such as aluminium and mercury have a natural affinity for the brain and can cause serious free radical damage.

---

15 Morgan LL. Estimating the risk of brain tumours from cellphone use: Published case–control studies. *Pathophysiology*, Apr 2009.

16 Christensen, et al., Cellular telephones and risk for brain tumors. A population-based, incident case–control study, *Neurology* 64, 1189–1195, 2005.

17 Hepworth, et al., Mobile phone use and risk of glioma in adults: case–control study, *BMJ* 332, 883–887, April 2006.

18 Lönn, et al., Output power levels from mobile phones in different geographical areas; Implications for exposure assessment, *Occup. Environ. Med.* 61 (2004) 769–772.

19 Lönn, et al., Mobile phone use and the risk of acoustic neuroma, *Epidemiology* 15, Nov 2004.

20 Cardis, et al., Distribution of RF energy emitted by mobile phones in anatomical structures of the brain, *Phys. Med. Biol.* 53, 2771–2783, 2008.

Mr. S is still young and has many years ahead of him – he is presently in remission and it is predicted that he will stay this way for a long time to come if he is careful with his lifestyle. He has a lot to achieve as he is completing his Master's degree presently at the University of Cyprus and is considered a good scholar. Let's all bow to Mr. S for his courage, determination and struggle to keep ahead when faced with such a life-threatening illness at such a tender age.

Case No. 3, Mrs. K, Age 30

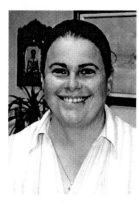

Main presenting problem: Acute Gallbladder Colic due to stone obstruction

Medical diagnosis:

This patient presented with acute pains in the liver area which reached the shoulder area. An ultrasound scan taken 8.9.08, showed: "the gallbladder is distended, with a length of 8.5 cm and a transverse diameter of 5.3 cm. There are no large gallstones evident, but there are echogenic contents in the dependent part of the gallbladder, suggestive of bile sludge (on a previous examination, small calculi were identified within the gallbladder). There is mild dilation of the common bile duct, which measures 9mm in diameter, down to the level of the ampulla of vater. The features are in keeping with a partial obstruction to the distal gallbladder, probably as a result of microlithiasis, or bile sludge."

In addition, she presented with blood analysis taken 4.9.08 showing the following elevated enzymes:

ALT - (alanine aminotransferase) - was previously called SGPT is more specific for liver damage. The ALT is an enzyme that is produced in the liver cells (hepatocytes) therefore it is more specific for liver disease than some of the other enzymes. It is generally increased in situations where there is damage to the liver cell membranes. All types of liver inflammation can cause raised ALT. Her levels of ALT were 400 U/l which are extremely high as they should be below 32 U/l.

GTT - (gamma glutamyl transpeptidase) is often elevated in those who use alcohol or other liver toxic substances to excess. An enzyme produced in many tissues as well as the liver. It may be elevated in the serum of patients with bile duct diseases. Her GGT levels were 323 U/l which again were very high as the acceptable parameters are between 5 and 36;

AST - (aspartate aminotransferase) which was previously called SGOT. This is a mitochondrial enzyme that is also present in heart, muscle, kidney and brain therefore it is less specific for liver disease. In many cases of liver inflammation, the ALT and AST activities are elevated roughly in a

1:1 ratio. Her levels were again very elevated at 188 U/l when acceptable parameters should be below 32 U/l.

Bilirubin is the major breakdown product that results from the destruction of old red blood cells (as well as some other sources). It is removed from the blood by the liver, chemically modified by a process call conjugation, secreted into the bile, passed into the intestine and to some extent reabsorbed from the intestine. It is basically the pigment that gives faeces its brown colour. Her levels of Total bilirubin were very high at 4.7 mg/dl when acceptable parameters should be below 1 and her direct bilirubin (see explanation below) was 2.7 when acceptable parameters are closer to zero (0.0 – 0.2).

Elevated levels of bilirubin can mean:

a) Bilirubin concentrations are elevated in the blood either by increased production, decreased uptake by the liver, decreased conjugation (modification to make it water soluble), decreased secretion from the liver or blockage of the bile ducts.

b) In cases of increased production, decreased liver uptake or decreased conjugation, the unconjugated or so-called indirect bilirubin will be primarily elevated.

c) In cases of decreased secretion from the liver or bile duct obstruction, the conjugated or so-called direct bilirubin will be primarily elevated.

AP - (alkaline phosphatase) is elevated in many types of liver disease but also in non-liver related diseases. Alkaline phosphatase is an enzyme, or more precisely a family of related enzymes, that is produced in the bile ducts and sinusoidal membranes of the liver but is also present in many other tissues. An elevation in the level of serum alkaline phosphatase is raised in bile duct blockage from any cause. Her levels were elevated at 137 U/l were acceptable parameters are 35 to 104.

Given that all the blood parameters were pointing to a blockage of the gallbladder duct by calculi, she was strongly advised to remove the gallbladder immediately (cholecystectomy) the same day. She had suffered from gallbladder problems back in 2005 - this was the first time that I saw her and we managed to deal with this using a natural gallbladder flush that cleared all the stones from her gallbladder and her symptoms disappeared.

Based on this past experience, she was now adamant to repeat the gallbladder flush again and avoid the cholecystectomy, even though her situation now was a little more pressing than before!

Holistic diagnosis:

Given the time constraints with the current medical and biochemical diagnosis, there were not many tests that were run apart from the Hair Tissue Mineral Analysis. This showed extremely low levels of many minerals including calcium, magnesium, potassium, manganese and cobalt with heavy metals such as mercury, arsenic, cadmium and aluminium appearing in circulation.

Holistic treatments:

As I pointed out to Mrs. K on initial consultation, her situation was a little more critical than previously as there was now an obstruction in the gallbladder ducts that had led to the high hepatic enzymes and the stress on the liver. She was also in acute pain with intense pain in the upper and middle abdomen that would radiate to the right shoulder blade. Pain would be worse after eating and could last a few hours and become very intense at times to the point of feeling nausea. It was an indication of the disruption of bile flow with the bile duct muscles contracting to try to force the bile though the ducts.

There was little time to undergo a series of tests, so I told her that we should begin working on clearing the obstruction using a gallbladder flush[21] that she had done in the past, helping the flow of bile using herbs and neutraceuticals, as well as working towards softening the stones with magnesium malate and plenty of apple juice, which contains malic acid. We would monitor the situation closely with the help of the medical doctor who could do further ultrasound scans and blood tests. If all else failed she would go in for surgery, even though she was very determined to avoid it at all costs.

She began a 15-day alkaline detoxification diet with fresh fruit, steamed vegetables, salads, freshly made carrot and green juice and herbal teas on the 8.9.09. She was given a number of nutritional supplements such as a high-potency multivitamin formula, omega 3, 6 and 9 fatty acids to help

---

21 www.docgeorge.com/20080521179/GallBladder-Flush.html

with the inflammation. Globe artichoke (Cynara scolymus) has been found to increase bile secretion in perfused rat liver and liver cell cultures[22,23] and has been reported in one small double-blind, placebo controlled trial and several case series to increase choleresis (secretion of bile).[24]

A herbal formula that contained vitamin B1, B6, B12, folic acid (all required for the P-450 Cytochrome detoxication pathways of the liver), N-Acetyl-Cysteine, Trimethylglycine, Scutellaria baicalensis root extract, Milk thistle, Artichoke and Lipoic Acid (a universal fat and water soluble antioxidant to protect the liver against damage). Moreover, she took Aloe Vera juice and vitamin C as calcium ascorbate powder – 2 grams, three times daily to help further in the dissolution of the stones.

Scutellaria baicalensis is a botanical commonly used in Traditional Chinese Medicine. Research has indicated it has many interesting effects on the liver. A number of in vitro and animal studies indicate that Scutellaria baicalensis can improve liver health. A recent cell culture study tested three active flavonoid components of the root of Scutellaria baicalensis on a human liver cancer cell line. The results indicated that the components of Scutellaria baicalensis inhibited the oxidation of protein in the liver and the decrease of cell viability that had occurred in the cancer cells prior to exposure to the botanical compounds. The Scutellaria baicalensis component baicalin had the strongest inhibitory effect. The researchers concluded that all three components of Scutellaria baicalensis could inhibit liver injury in a dose dependent manner.[25]

This same protective effect was seen in a study investigating the use of the Scutellaria baicalensis component baicalin in rats given high doses of acetaminophen. When acetaminophen is given at high doses it is extremely toxic to the liver. In this study, however, when rats were given baicalin a half hour after acetaminophen administration, it significantly prevented many of the toxic effects observed in rats given acetaminophen without baicalin. Furthermore, none of the rats given baicalin with acetaminophen

---

[22] Kraft K. Artichoke leaf extract - Recent findings reflecting effects on lipid metabolism, liver and gastrointestinal tracts. *Phytomedicine* 4(4):369-378, 1997.

[23] Matuschowski P. Testing of Cynara scolymus in the isolated perfused rat liver. 43rd *Ann Congr Soc Med Plant Res* 3-7, 1996.

[24] Kirchhoff R, Beckers CH, Kirchhoff GM, and et al. Increase in choleresis by means of artichoke extract. *Phytomedicine* 1:107-115, 1994.

25 Zhao Y, Li H, Gao Z, Gong Y, Xu H. Effects of flavonoids extracted from Scutellaria baicalensis Georgi on hemin-nitrite-H2O2 induced liver injury. *Eur J Pharmacol.* 24;536(1-2):192-9, Apr 2006.

died, whereas 43 percent of the rats given only acetaminophen died. Baicalin also prevented the acetaminophen-related drop in levels of glutathione, a critical antioxidant mentioned below.[26]

N-Acetyl-Cysteine (NAC) is a powerful antioxidant, which increases the production of the critical antioxidant glutathione. Glutathione is the chief chemical used by the liver exerting a variety of protective effects, including detoxification and intracellular defense against oxidative stress. NAC is even used by conventional medicine to treat life threatening acetaminophen poisoning.[27]

Milk Thistle seeds contain a bioflavonoid complex known as silymarin, responsible for the health benefits of the plant. Today, laboratory and clinical tests confirm milk thistle's significant liver-protective effects. A potent antioxidant in its own right, silymarin is particularly remarkable for its beneficial effects on glutathione. Researchers have found that silymarin increases levels of glutathione by up to 35 percent. Silymarin has also been shown to regenerate injured liver cells. In addition, silymarin has the ability to block fibrosis, a process that contributes to the eventual development of cirrhosis.[28]

On 30.9.09, twenty five days after beginning her holistic treatments she had another blood test that showed that her hepatic enzymes had began to reduce; gamma-GT from 324 to 164 (still high); SGOT from 188 to 22 (now in normal range); SGPT from 400 to 60 (still high) – the clinical chemist and medical doctor commented that this was an extremely rapid decline, indicating that the liver was beginning to regain functioning again.

This test was performed 5 days after she had done her first gallbladder flush which removed a number of stones and 25 days into the holistic treatment programme. The blood results were encouraging as all pathological parameters were normalizing and this greatly encouraged her to continue. Besides, she was now feeling a lot better and the pain in the

---

26 Jang SI, Kim HJ, Hwang KM, Jekal SJ, Pae HO, Choi BM, Yun YG, Kwon TO, Chung HT, Kim YC. Hepatoprotective effect of baicalin, a major flavone from Scutellaria radix, on acetaminophen-induced liver injury in mice. *Immunopharmacol Immunotoxicol.* 25(4):585-94, Nov 2003.

27 Ellenhorn MJ, et al. Ellenhorn's Medical Toxicology: Diagnoses and Treatment of Human Poisoning. 2nd edition. Baltimore, MD. Williams & Wilkins, 1997.

28 Ferenci P, Dragosics B, Dittrich H, et al. Randomized controlled trial of silymarin treatment in patients with cirrhosis of the liver. *J Hepatol.* 9:105-13, 1989.

gallbladder region had reduced considerably and she was no longer getting shooting pains into her right shoulder.

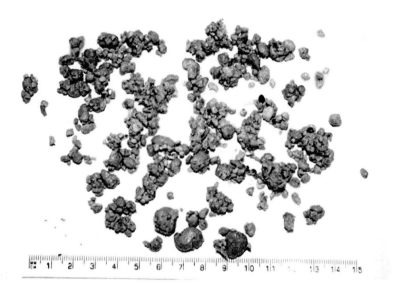

Gallstones flushed the first time

During the gallbladder flush apple juice is taken which is high in malic acid, which is thought to act as a solvent to weaken adhesions between solid globules. Epsom salts (magnesium sulphate) are used because it's believed it relaxes smooth muscle and will relax and dilate the bile duct to enable larger solid particles (like gallstones) to exit the gallbladder. Unrefined olive oil is used to stimulate the gallbladder and bile duct to contract and expel gallstones. The image above shows the number of stones flushed from the gallbladder the first time around.

About 14 days after beginning her holistic treatment protocol she had another ultrasound scan which read: "the gallbladder is not as distended as on the previous examination, but there is now marked thickening of the gallbladder wall with an oedematous ring, indicating inflammation of the gallbladder wall. There is a large cluster of small calculi noted within the gallbladder, which is more clearly evident on today's examination. There are no features of pancreatitis sonographically. The features are suggestive of less obstruction on todays examination, but there is a complication of associated cholecystitis."

The medical doctors again strongly encouraged her to go in for gallbladder surgery but she was adamant and managed to stall them further. When the gallbladder empties, as had occurred on the first flush, the stones left in the liver ducts will slowly make their way down into the gallbladder again. This can fill with stones AGAIN, and therefore more flushes are required – sometimes as many as 5-6 flushes are required to completely clear all the stones from the liver and gallbladder – this is why the scan showed more stones a couple of weeks after the initial flush. Had the scan been taken only a couple of days after the flush, then the chances are that it would have shown no stones, or very few.

She continued her supplements and towards the end of October 2008 she did another gallbladder flush and removed more smallish stones. Another blood analysis on the 21.10.09 which was a few days after her second gallbladder flush showed a marked decrease in hepatic enzymes back to normal levels: gamma-GT fell from 164 on last count to 36 (now about normal); AST from 188 to 18 (now normal) and ALT from 66 to 23 (now normal). These results had occurred within 6 weeks of beginning her holistic protocol.

Moreover, all the pain had disappeared completely and she had no further problems after eating. In fact, she had lost considerable weight and her energy levels had greatly increased, her bowel distension was gone and generally she was feeling very well.

Patient's own account:

I have been doing gallbladder flushes for some time, ever since I visited Dr. Georgiou in 2005. However, due to excessive stresses at work and at home, with a hectic lifestyle, I failed to look after myself over the last two to three years, eating anything but an optimum diet, not drinking enough water and generally putting on excess weight. This was not the advice that I received from Dr. Georgiou who mentioned doing a general body detox every 6 months with fruit and vegetables, as well as flushing the gallbladder at least once per year based on my previous history of gallstones.

When I returned to Dr. Georgiou early September 2008 I was in a real state. I had lots of pain in the gut area that kept shooting up to my upper back, I was bloated most of the day and I was afraid to eat as the pain would get worse. I was also feeling tired and run down, so I went to see a medical doctor first to see whether it was what I suspected, gallstones again. Indeed, the ultrasound scan confirmed this, as did the blood tests where all my liver enzymes were sky high! When the doctor had completed his examination he was determined to get me into surgery the same day and actually called the surgeon there and then to book me an appointment that afternoon.

Even though I was worried as I knew that this was serious, I always had faith in natural medicine as I and my family had relied on it for many years and I really did not want my gallbladder whipped out. Over the years I have developed a sort of "allergy" towards medical doctors due to many of the mistakes and consequences that I have seen in other friends and family members.

I therefore called Dr. Georgiou who is normally very busy and puts you on a waiting list, but as soon as he heard my voice he recognized me and luckily he had a cancellation the same day. I did not hesitate and got my husband to drive me to Larnaca where we met. He looked at the results with a worried frown and said after a few minutes, well it looks like you are really close to surgery – why are you here? How can I help?

I told him quite categorically that I had no intention of being put under the knife and that I wanted to do another gallbladder flush under his supervision. He continued to tell me that my liver was under considerable stress as the liver enzymes had shot up, possibly because of an obstruction of the gallbladder ducts. However, he said that if we moved quickly and monitored the situation with the help of the medical doctor, we would see. He said that he had a similar case and they had succeeded, but each case has its own individual qualities. He said that the reassuring thing was that he knew me from previous consultations and that I was a good and well-behaved patient.

He immediately put me on an alkaline detoxification diet with supplements to help reduce my liver enzymes, as well as others to soften the gallbladder stones and asked to see me in a weeks time. By that time I began to feel better, so we decided to implement the first gallbladder cleanse which went well with no pain or complications. A few days later the blood tests had confirmed that my liver was improving by leaps and bounds and this was really encouraging. Dr. Georgiou advised that I continue the supplements and plan for another gallbladder flush soon.

By the time I completed the second flush at the end of October I was a new woman – all the pains had gone, as well as the bloating – I was eating normally now but within a more optimal diet (I got my knuckles wrapped by Dr. Georgiou on this), my energy and stamina had much increased and so had my overall moods which were much happier. My blood tests also showed that my liver enzymes were pretty normal, which relieved me considerably as this was very worrying. Dr. Georgiou was also again smiling!

I was elated and very happy to have saved myself the ordeal and expense of gallbladder surgery. I am also grateful to Dr. Georgiou for his faith in natural medicine and the results that it can bring to many patients like me. He really is a most caring and committed practitioner that finds amazing ways of getting people well, even with critical cases like mine.

Dr. Georgiou's final comments on Mrs. K:

This was a most interesting case where natural medicine showed its power by healing the liver and gallbladder in a very short period of time. Even though I have personally supervised hundreds of gallbladder flushes, this one was a little "on the edge" due to the high liver enzymes and the possible blockage. However, with a positive attitude, a healthy optimism and a systematic approach, having faith in the power of natural healing remedies, as well as the innate healing forces of the body, it is amazing how healing miracles are performed.

It is important to state here that patients facing similar crises should not simply take their treatments into their own hands without the supervision of an experienced holistic practitioner, who will work with other medical specialists to carefully monitor the patient every step of the way.

Case No. 4, Mrs. A, Age 38.

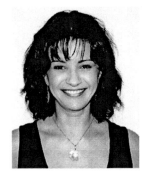

Main presenting problem: Crohn's Disease, pericarditis

Crohn's disease, a type of inflammatory bowel disease (IBD), is a condition in which the lining of the digestive tract becomes inflamed, causing severe diarrhoea and abdominal pain. The inflammation often spreads deep into the layers of affected tissue. Like ulcerative colitis, another common IBD, Crohn's disease can be both painful and debilitating and sometimes may lead to life-threatening complications. While there's no known medical cure for Crohn's disease, therapies can greatly reduce the signs and symptoms of the disease and even bring about a long-term remission. Two-thirds of people with Crohn's usually require surgical resection of a part of the intestine.

Medical diagnosis

A biopsy from the colon in 2004 reported the following: "Histopathology examination done in July 2004 from the caecum, ascending, descending, transverse and sigmoid colon showed colon mucosa heavily infiltrated by lymphoplasmocytes and eosinophils, with features of cryptitis and isolated crypt destruction with intraluminal abscesses. There was also evidence of epitheliod granuloma formation. The appearances are those of crypts destructive colitis with features compatible with idiopathic (unknown cause) disease and history very much suggestive of Crohn's Disease".

Blood ESR was 17, indicating an active inflammation in the body.

In addition to the Crohn's disease, the patient had a history of recurrent pericarditis (inflammation of the sac surrounding the heart) beginning in August 2004 which required pericardial effusions with methyprednisone therapy (tapering course of oral steroids) – this would appear approximately two times per year, every Christmas and Easter.

Holistic diagnosis

The first time I examined Mrs. A, a petite, charming and pleasant lady, I thought she was at least 6 months pregnant; such was the distention in her gut. She said that most evenings she would be in this very uncomfortable and painful condition. She had all the classic symptoms of Crohn's disease such as Diarrhoea, abdominal bloating, cramp-like abdominal pain, awaking in the night to defecate, occasional blood in the stool, vomiting, nausea and itchiness or pain around the anus.

During the initial consultation, it was agreed to dig deeper and discover the potential causative factors to these symptoms that had been labeled Crohn's Disease. The label unfortunately had not helped cure the disease as the aetiological factors remained hidden. She was a little skeptical at first as many gastroenterologists in Cyprus and Germany had told her that her disease was incurable and that she would have to live with it all her life.

The IDEL Diagnostic Programme identified a number of causative factors that were not identified in the 7 years of medical tests that she had in her thick file.

VEGA testing identified food intolerances to all gluten grains such as wheat, oats, rye and barley (possible coeliac), lactose and all dairy products, nightshade family of vegetables such as potatoes, tomatoes, peppers and aubergines, all citrus fruits such as oranges, lemons, mandarins and grapefruit, sugar and caffeine-related products – food intolerances are well known for causing the production of cytokinines and cox-2 inflammatory chemicals in the gut[29,30] and there has been research on food intolerances and Crohn's disease spanning more than 25 years (surprising that gastroenterologists in Cyprus do not read this literature).[31,32,33,34]

29 Brostoff, J., and Gamlin, L. The Complete Guide to Food Allergy and Intolerance, 3rd Ed, Bloomsbury Publishing Plc, 1998.
30 Pearson, M., Teahon, K., Levi, AJ and Bjarnason, I. Food intolerance and Crohn's disease. *Gut*. 34(6): 783–787, June 1993.
31 Workman EM, Alun-Jones V, Wilson AJ, Hunter JO. Diet in the management of Crohn's disease. Human Nutrition *Applied Nutrition* 38: 469-73, 1984.
32 Alun-Jones V, Workman E, Freeman AH, Dickinson RJ, Wilson AJ, Hunter JO. Crohn's disease: maintenance of remission by diet. *Lancet* i: 177-80, 1985.
33 Giaffer MH, Cann P, Holdsworth CD. Long-term effects of elemental and exclusion diets for Crohn's disease. *Aliment Pharmacology and Therapeuties* 5: 115-25, 1991.
34 Riordan AM, Hunter JO. Multicentre controlled trial of diet in the treatment of active Crohn's disease. *Gastroenterology* 102: A612, 1992.

Organ imbalances as tested using VEGA and ART included: uterus, thyroid, stomach, ascending, descending and transverse colon, ileum, adrenals, lymph nodes, myocardium, endocardium, pericardium, kidneys and pancreas. During ART testing the gluten was blocking autonomic nervous system regulation which was a critical factor. On further VEGA testing there were vitamin, mineral and trace element deficiencies detected, hormonal imbalances, tooth and scar foci, dysbiosis of the gut, systemic Candidiasis.

Mercury levels were high on the Hair Tissue Mineral Analysis, as well as arsenic and lead, which also confirmed low levels of minerals and trace elements. Vaccination stress, bacterial infection with Borrelia[35] and viral infection with Cytomegalovirus (CMV) were also detected on the VEGA.

Iris analysis showed chronic hypochlorhydria (low hydrochloric acid production), pancreatic enzyme deficiency, irritation marks on the thyroid, liver, kidneys and lungs, with cervical and lumbar spinal subluxations.

The Heart Rate Variability (HRV) test showed a sympathetic dominance with decreased parasympathetic activity with the level of functioning of the physiological systems being at 11 (1 is best and 13 is worst) and the adaptability scale – being able to adapt to changes in the environment being at 6 (1 is best and 7 is worst). This profile corresponded well with her poor physiological functioning and low adaptation reserves, not surprising given the number of causative factors she was carrying.

Thermography showed focal dental lesions, thyroid dysfunction, cervical joint disease, fibrocystic activity of the breasts, myofascial inflammation in the trapezius, rhomboids and paraspinous musculature, as well as the upper lumbar spine with some degree of scoliosis, concave towards the left. There was some hyperthermia in the colon and small intestine.

The Biological Terrain Analysis, taken from urine, saliva and blood is a measure of the pH, oxidation-reduction potential (amount of electron potential that exists in a tested solution) and resistivity (relative concentration of electrically conductive ions in solution) of all these body fluids. The results showed a lack of adequate and normal mineral concentration or malabsorption with indications of a leaky gut, an extremely increased saliva pH is an indication of increased sympathetic

---

35 This bacterium causes the well known Lyme's Disease.

nervous system activity, liver and lymphatic congestion and poor pancreatic enzyme efficiency. The urine pH was low (acidic) and the blood pH was high (alkaline) – this usually indicates that the kidney is not removing acids efficiently and the blood makes a compensatory shift to a more alkaline state. Viral loads and heavy metal toxicity were other factors present.

Live Blood Analysis showed a very congestive picture throughout with high valence rouleau (very sticky red blood cells), poikilocytosis (iron deficiency anaemia), many microcytes (impaired haemoglobin synthesis – haemoglobin levels were low on medical blood tests), high valance spicules or fibrinogen (related to liver toxicity), sluggish white blood cells with many lyzing prematurely, and undigested fat. Generally the blood picture was one of imbalanced pH, toxicity, iron, folic acid and B12 deficiencies, and possible free radical damage.

Psychosomatically, there were a number of unresolved psychoemotional issues relating to family matters that had systemic entanglement issues attached to them. There was also an element of fear with her Crohn's, whether she would ever be able to function normally again, as well as an underlying depression that the disease had caused the last few years.

Holistic treatments

Mrs. A's holistic treatments began by simply avoiding the foods that were causing the inflammation in the gut; these food intolerances were later treated using bioresonance therapy. Supplemental Betaine HCl, Pepsin and pancreatic enzymes were utilized to improve her digestion, absorption and assimilation of nutrients.

Amazingly, within the first five days her symptoms overall had improved by 60% (her estimation), while specifically constipation and bloating declined by 80%. She also underwent a course of PAPIMI and hyperthermia treatments of the gut region which also helped considerably with the inflammation.

Her systemic Candidiasis was then treated using the DaVinci Candida Protocol (see chapter 5). She also received a series of digital homeopathic treatments for her vaccination stress, CMV and Borrelia, as well as dietary supplements including a high potency multivitamin and multimineral, omega 3, 6 and 9 fatty acids for the inflammation, acidophilus and bifidobacteria species to repopulate the bowel flora, A-Lipoic acid, a water and fat soluble antioxidant capable of penetrating deep into the tissue, vitamin B12, Aloe vera for healing the mucous membranes of the gut, chlorella, HMD® and Organic Lavage to remove the toxic metals (see chapter 7). Additional selenium was given based on indications from her hair tests. Coenzyme Q10 was given for the intermittent pericarditis and to increase ATP production in cells, as well as vitamin E for her fibrocystic breast disease and heart.

In addition to these treatments, Mrs. A also began prioritizing life's issues and clearing out old, unwanted patterns of behaviour that were burdening her psyche. There were many systemic entanglements that surfaced during these Soul Healing constellations and there was a dramatic improvement in her symptoms within days of this workshop. Bach Flower remedies also helped with her high anxiety levels and depressed state and generally helped to balance her psychoemotional state.

Patient's own account

I have always remembered myself since adolescence with stomach pains, feeling of fullness, with periods of either constipation or diarrhea. Everybody knew that I was always the sensitive, stressed girl and as a consequence of this, my stomach was always hurting me. I used to take anxiolytics from time to time. My symptoms were mild until the age of 31, around the time when I got pregnant.

I had an unforgettably difficult pregnancy 7 years ago. I remember that from the beginning until the end of my pregnancy, I constantly felt nausea and I was vomiting almost every day. I felt a bloating sensation, discomfort and had diarrhea every day. I was living a nightmare - I could not go out with my husband or socialize, because of my multiple diarrheas.

After giving birth to a beautiful boy, my situation got worse; my nausea, abdominal pain, vomiting, and the diarrhea got worse. Even though I was very happy to be a mother, at the same time I felt so sick that I could not offer much - this made me feel depressed and helpless.

I went back to work after my pregnancy and I was literally struggling to find the energy to get through the day. I couldn't feel my knees, I suffered from dyspnoea, I felt weak and almost fainted many times, but I tried to hide my pain by not complaining to anyone. I started having headaches, I was lethargic and my abdominal pains got worse. Every time I went to the toilet I was in so much pain that I was sweating and having chills. I felt like I was giving birth every day.

I finally visited a doctor and I had a gastrointestinal endoscopy and colonoscopy. I was diagnosed with Crohn's disease, a chronic inflammatory gastrointestinal disease that can affect any part of the gut. I was also diagnosed with Helicobacter pylori bacteria in the stomach, that could cause peptic ulcer and I took medicine for that.

In the meantime, before I found out about the DaVinci Natural Health Centre, my doctor told me that treatment was palliative, which actually meant 'incurable' and this made me feel very depressed so I began a course of antidepressant pills for this reason. After trying a variety of drugs that were supposed to help Crohn's, I decided to visit a clinic in Germany that confirmed the diagnosis of Crohn's disease; even worse it reaffirmed that there was no cure.

As my illness progressed, I also developed a heart problem, pericarditis, which appeared about 4 years ago. Doctors drained the fluid from the pericardium the first time, but this occurred again three more times – every time I was given large doses of cortisone to help the problem.

Looking back in retrospect, with what I know now, my diet was atrocious – I hardly ate any fruits and vegetables which was reinforced by my gastroenterologists. I then decided to visit a nutritionist and I felt quite relieved with the specific diet she gave me. Still my symptoms were persistent and I was still feeling depressed.

Fortunately, one day while my mother was watching a programme on television, she heard Dr. Georgiou talking about various health issues. I decided to call him and ask his opinion – to my surprise he said that he had quite a few cases of Crohn's and did not see it as a major problem, assuming we could identify the causes. The initial appointment lasted a total of 5 hours and there were many tests conducted.

In early July 2008 I began a bespoke treatment programme based upon the diagnostic information that was gathered by Dr. Georgiou. Honestly, I have to admit that my life changed completely. I feel like I was born again! Since the treatment, my symptoms have pretty much vanished and I now live a normal life. No more diarrhoeas, no abdominal pain and I often feel positive and happy, with a desire to devour life. On a psychological and emotional level I am a different person with so much more confidence and I am no longer the "yes lady" that I used to be – no doubt some people around me are unhappy because of this. I can also enjoy being a mother without worrying that I cannot hold my baby in my arms because of my abdominal pains.

I truly thank Dr. Georgiou for his wisdom, patience, caring attitude (I used to call him numerous times with various questions) and his healthy respect towards myself, his work, his belief in holistic medicine and more.

Dr. Georgiou's final comments on Mrs. A's case

There were many factors that were important triggers in the development of the bowel inflammation, labeled Crohn's disease. Systemic Candidiasis[36] is an important issue as this fungus that infiltrates the gut can cause considerable inflammation. Ironically, the inflammation caused by Candida, is then treated by gastroenterologists with the powerful anti-inflammatory cortisone. The resulting introduction of corticosteroid to the gut results in a dramatic increase in the Candida colonies. While the corticosteroid then masks the increasing inflammation, it continues to assist in the colony growth, making the symptomatic disease become both chronic and incurable – a true vicious cycle. Numerous research sources report a direct fact: In every case of corticosteroid use, the patient has demonstrated a severe increase in Candida pathogenic colonization. In short, the use of cortisone for more than a few weeks, results in Candida overgrowth and pathology, with an exacerbation of the inflammation.

The food intolerances were another major issue as these specific foods that the person is intolerant too, such as the gluten grains that she was eating daily, will cause severe inflammation by provoking inflammatory cytokinines and Cox-2 chemicals. Identifying and eliminating these food intolerances is crucial to the removal of these inflammatory markers, not simply pulling out a ready-made diet sheet that is standard to all patients, as every patient will inevitably have different food intolerances. Interestingly, this patient was told to eat white bread, but not brown as well as to avoid life-giving fruits and vegetables as the fibre content will apparently be abrasive to the gut, something that has never been proven scientifically.

---

36 Standaert-Vitse, A. et al. Candida albicans colonization and ASCA in familial Crohn's disease. *American Journal of Gastroenterology*, 2009.

Digestive issues such as hypochlorhydria and pancreatic enzyme deficiency will increase the putrefactive and fermentative processes in the gut, releasing more inflammatory chemicals, therefore increasing the symptoms. Addressing the digestive issues is crucial to the success of the therapy. Concomitantly, it is also very important to replace the minerals and vitamins that are deficient to provide the raw materials required by the body to produce these acids and enzymes for digestion, while helping to repair and rebuild the body – this is the essence of orthomolecular nutrition.

It is clear from Mrs. A's case that there are a myriad of causative factors that are responsible for Crohn's disease – in A's case she had more than 20 causative factors that were incorporated into her bespoke treatment programme and gradually offloaded. Once these issues were addressed, then slowly over time – within 6 months of treatment – she had regained her health with no symptoms of Crohn's noticeable any more.

The Hellinger Soul Healing has also helped to eliminate the yearly pericarditis that she used to be hospitalized for twice a year, every new year's eve and during the summer holidays. This was clearly a psychosomatic and deeper Soul connection that has now been broken forever – her soul and heart and gut are now at peace and fully functional to the point where she is eating ice-cream, crepes and bread with no symptoms! It is truly heartening to see an "incurable" case such as Crohn's Disease now completely cured and their quality of life significantly increased.

Case No. 5, Miss S, Age 32

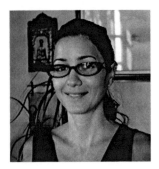

Main presenting problem: Polycyctic ovaries, irregular periods, chronic constipation, migraines, hypothyroidism,

Medical diagnosis:

Pelvic sonography showed enlarged polycystic ovaries – the report reads: "the uterus appeared normal, regular endometrium 4.8mm thick, no endometrial abnormality could be detected. Both ovaries were enlarged and polycystic - right ovary 28 x 46 mm and the left ovary 30 x 51 mm. Conclusions: Enlarged polycystic ovaries."

These clinical signs are accompanied by irregular periods approximately every 45 days, with 3 days of bleeding. There are also symptoms of Premenstrual Syndrome (PMS) accompanied by sweet cravings. There is a weight gain of about 10 kilos in a two year period.

There is a history of chronic constipation, bowel distension and flatulence. Migraines are also quite frequent. Thyroid function tests show a hypothyroid picture and has been prescribed 50 mcg thyroxine – this seems to run in the mother's family.

Blood test showed low levels of Glucose-6-phosphate dehydrogenase (G6PD) = 0.45 U/GHB (7.0-20.5). This is an X-linked recessive hereditary disease characterized by abnormally low levels of G6PD, a metabolic enzyme involved in the pentose phosphate pathway, especially important in red blood cell metabolism. Individuals with the disease may exhibit non-immune hemolytic anemia in response to a number of causes, most commonly infection or exposure to certain medications or chemicals. G6PD deficiency is closely linked to favism, a disorder characterized by a hemolytic reaction to consumption of broad beans.

Hepatic enzymes were somewhat elevated GGT = 32 U/L (7-32); GOT = 35 (<32); GPT = 40 (<31). Progesterone levels were also low at 1.08 (5.3-86). TSH was low at 0.28 μIU/ml (0.4-4) but T4 and T3 were within the normal range. This may be an early sign of Hashimoto's thyroiditis. Iron and serum ferritin levels are also low and ESR levels at 27 indicate an active inflammation.

Holistic diagnosis:

VEGA testing for food intolerances found wheat, rice, milk products and lactose, eggs, chicken, nightshade family of vegetables, peas, citrus fruits and bananas. Lactose is her primary intolerance as ART testing shows that this completely blocks regulation.

ART testing has shown tooth foci on teeth 16 (stomach meridian), 25, 36 and 47 (all large intestine meridian). There were also three scar foci detected on the right leg, scars on both breasts and a small scar on the chin. In addition, there were organ weaknesses such as spleen, pituitary, adrenals, ascending and descending colon and lymphatics. Ascending colon was her primary organ that was causing blocked regulation. She is also resonating with Ascaris and Oxyuren parasites.

Thermography screening showed the following: slight area of local hyperthermia over the left side of the mouth which may indicate either dental or periodontal infection. There were slight areas of hyperthermia in the upper right quadrants of both breasts that do not appear suspicious and there are no neovascularities, but should be monitored for change.

Iris analysis showed a very toxic, dark area around the large intestine, liver irritation, a genetic predisposition towards pancreatic weakness (exocrine), thyroid markings – has been diagnosed with hypothyroidism. There was also a cervical subluxation indicated with lacunas (weak areas) in the adrenal glands.

Hair Tissue Mineral Analysis indicated low levels of copper which is a critical mineral for building and repairing connective tissue, including the hair and nails, to produce energy (required for the final steps of the Kreb's cycle in the electron transport system), immune system, the thyroid and adrenal glands, it is closely related to oestrogen metabolism and can be one of the causes of ovarian cysts, and it is also required for the stimulation of neurotransmitter substances such as epinephrine, norepinephrine and dopamine, as well as serotonin production (required for monomine oxidase enzyme). Deficiencies can cause depression, anxiety and memory loss.

Manganese and molybdenum were also low - Manganese is an essential trace nutrient in all forms of life.[37] It is important for the production of a number of enzymes such as oxidoreductases, transferases, hydrolases, lyases, isomerases, ligases, lectins, and integrins. The best known manganese-containing polypeptides may be arginase and Mn-containing superoxide dismutase (Mn-SOD),[38] present in all mitochondria.

Molybdenum is present in approximately 20 enzymes in the body, including aldehyde oxidase, sulfite oxidase and xanthine oxidase.[39] In some animals, the oxidation of xanthine to uric acid, a process of purine catabolism, is catalyzed by xanthine oxidase, a molybdenum-containing enzyme. The activity of xanthine oxidase is directly proportional to the amount of molybdenum in the body. So, low levels of manganese can lead to high uric acid levels.

There were also elevated levels of circulating mercury found in the hair analysis – this is probably related to amalgam removal some years ago.

Darkfield microscopy of a live blood sample indicated an acidic milieu with a protit veil and very sluggish WBC's – there were also signs of a pancreatic weakness as there were undigested fat globules in the fasting blood sample that was examined. There were also indications of iron, folic acid and vitamin B12 deficiency.

Holistic treatments:

There were many reasons why Miss S. had endocrine imbalances and polycystic ovaries. Progesterone is the primary raw material for producing cortisol. When the glands are in overdrive, the body will divert progesterone to the adrenals to support cortisol production. With reduced progesterone, the body may experience estrogen dominance, i.e. PMS, fibroids, polycystic ovaries, heavy bleeding, breast tenderness, weight gain, etc. Excessive cortisol also blocks progesterone receptors, further

---

37 Emsley, John (2001). "Manganese". Nature's Building Blocks: An A-Z Guide to the Elements. Oxford, UK: Oxford University Press. pp. 249–253.
38 Law, N. Manganese Redox Enzymes and Model Systems: Properties, Structures, and Reactivity. 46. pp. 305, 1998.
39 Emsley, J. Nature's Building Blocks. Oxford: Oxford University Press. pp. 262–266, 2001.

contributing to low progesterone.[40] These two imbalances are the primary reasons why adrenal exhaustion leads to estrogen dominance.

The thyroid, which regulates metabolism, may turn down its hormonal activity in an attempt to reverse adrenal overdrive. Some symptoms of hypothyroidism include fatigue, weight gain, fibroids, endometriosis, ovarian cysts, heavy bleeding, fibrocystic breast disease, depression, PMS, migraines, lack of concentration, cold hands and feet, menopausal symptoms, miscarriage and infertility.

Hypothalamus-Pituitary-Adrenal axis activation due to stress causes decreased production of thyroid-stimulating hormone (TSH), and blocks inactive thyroxin's conversion to the biologically active triiodothyronine. (T3), which has the greatest effect on the body.

Her holistic treatment programme was therefore designed to eliminate these underlying causes and regain balance. She detoxified on many levels including a 15-day alkaline detoxification diet, liver and gallbladder cleanse, parasite cleanses using the Hulda Clark protocol.[41] She also underwent a series of ozone saunas and Matrix Regeneration Therapy[42] for deep tissue cleansing, which also cleared a large proportion of cellulite.

Her supplement programme consisted of building the adrenals and thyroid which are two major endocrine organs underlying menstrual imbalances and polycystic ovaries. She began taking taking a high-potency multivitamin formula, omega 3,6 and 9 fatty acids, a formula consisting of B vitamins (especially B5), vitamin C, magnesium, manganese, zinc, adaptagenic herbs, adrenal extracts and the amino acids tyrosine as well as iodine taken as Lugol's solution for the thyroid gland. Milk thistle was also added for the raised hepatic enzymes. She was also given the natural chelator HMD™ Ultimate Detox protocol[43] for her high mercury levels. The DaVinci Candida protocol was also followed (see Chapter 5).

A herbal formula consisting of Agnus castus (Vitex/Chastetree berry) was also given - this herb stimulates and normalizes the function of the

---

40 John Lee, MD, What Your Doctor May Not Tell You About Premenopause, Warner Wellness, p 133, Jan 1999.
41 This consists of taking Walnut tincture, Wormwood and Cloves for a period of 14 days in gradually increasing dosages.
42 http://www.docgeorge.com/Matrix-Regeneration-Therapy.html
43 www.detoxmetals.com

pituitary gland which in turn helps to balance hormone output from the ovaries and to stimulate ovulation. Agnus castus is also useful when there is an excess of prolactin which can be suppressing ovulation. Natural progesterone was also used, which is nearly identical to what the body produces and is manufactured in scientific laboratories from wild yams and soy beans.

It is applied on the skin transdermally, and once it reaches a saturation level in the underlying skin tissue, it diffuses into the capillaries, then passes into the general blood circulation for use by the body. Some women feel effects in less than a week of usage. For those who are especially deficient in progesterone, it may take two to three months to restore optimum levels.[44]

Further treatments included Su Jok therapy and Su Jok acupuncture[45] was used quite extensively, along with bioresonance programmes on the BICOM bioresonance device for hormonal balancing and within a short period of time using the basic correspondence system of the hand and foot her migraines disappeared completely. Constipation had also much improved. The tooth and scar foci were also repolarized using Low Intensity Lazer Therapy.[46] Hyperthermia was also applied on the abdominal and pelvic areas.

Within two months she was seeing regular periods on a 28-day cycle with no pains or symptoms of PMS. Within 4 months a further pelvic sonography showed NO FURTHER cysts on either the right or the left ovary – the radiologist did the scan very thoroughly twice to be absolutely certain. The volume of the ovaries had also returned back to normal.

Her thyroid function tests were now back to normal – TSH = 1.46 (0.4-4.0); Free T4 = 13.58 (10.3-24.4) and Free T3 = 2.94 (1.45-4.20) and she was now off thyroxine completely.

Patient's own account:

I tend to be quite an anxious person, always running around concerned about everyone's welfare – it really does take it out of me sometimes. I

---

44 Lee, J.R. What Your Doctor May Not Tell You About Menopause. Warner Books, May, 1996.
45 http://www.su-jok.eu
46 http://www.docgeorge.com/2008040474/Low-Intensity-Lazer-Therapy-LILT.html

remember suffering from constipation, migraines, irregular periods and the diagnosed ovarian cysts for a long time. As I am not the person to rush to medical doctors as most of my family have been following natural medicine treatments for a long time, it was only natural that I landed on Dr. Georgiou's doorstep as I have known him for a long time, given that he was the primary care practitioner for most of my family.

It was not long after he took my latest history that he suggested that we do some thorough testing to determine the underlying causes of all these health issues – so we began the 5-hour testing protocol called the IDEL Diagnostic Programme. This was a most interesting experience and one really learns a lot about their health on a very deep level. Many things came up when the results were collated – hormonal issues, systemic Candida, food intolerances, parasites, tooth and scar foci – many, many factors that orthodox medicine does not even look for – all they wanted to do was suppress these problems using hormonal drugs.

We immediately got to work to offload these factors and after 4 months it was incredible, I really felt like a new person – my ovarian cysts were gone, completely disappeared even though the radiologist really looked hard to find them before saying: "this is very unusual to see ovarian cysts disappear, have you been taking natural remedies as this is the only explanation?" I admittedly said "yes" and he nodded his head. My periods had regulated with no further pains and PMS, my constipation was gone, so was my bloating, and a big surprise was that my intractable cellulite was also gone, thanks to all the detoxifying regimes including the ozone sauna and the MRT.

I am obviously thrilled about my newfound health, even though it is a struggle to keep the balance as stress plays such an important role in our health that it is a juggling act trying to keep the balance.

Dr Georgiou's final comments on Miss S:

This is an interesting case were we can trace the pathogenesis of disease back to stress related to the hypothalamus-pituitary-adrenal-thyroid axis and the relationship between these organs. There are also other obvious factors that can upset this balance including nutritional deficiencies, heavy metals being antagonistic to the essential minerals, upsetting the endocrine balance further, constipation causing autointoxication which further aggravates the sensitive endocrine balance, tooth and scar foci that can deregulate the autonomic nervous system and cause various imbalances to the sensitive electromagnetic balance of the body, as well as unbalancing acupuncture meridians.

A few simple symptoms with a myriad of causes, but it is always heartening to be able to identify and eliminate these causative factors and help the body repair and rebuild using various natural healing methods where you are doing to the body the least harm.

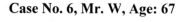

Case No. 6, Mr. W, Age: 67

Main presenting problem: Stomach and bowel distension of 35 years standing, pains in feet, tinnitus, hypercholestermia

Medical diagnosis:

Mr. W has seen many doctors over a 35-year period for stomach pains, bloating, constant burping and reflux. He has excessive belching after eating any type of food. He has undergone many types of tests including ultrasound scans, blood tests, numerous gastroscopy and rectoscopy tests, which showed Helicobacter pylori. This was treated with antibiotics, but the stomach distension and pain still remain to this day.

He was operated for a herniated disc at level L6 in 2002.

Recent blood tests showed elevated triglyceride levels but nothing else of significance.

Holistic diagnosis:

The main point in conducting the IDEL Diagnostic Programme was to determine what the causative factors of his chronic problems were – clearly there were unresolved issues with the stomach that spanned over 35 years with numerous consultations to many medical and naturopathic physicians, but no complete resolution yet of his symptoms.

VEGA food intolerance testing identified a number of food intolerances – wheat, lactose and all dairy products, eggs, beef, chicken, crustacean fish family and caffeine. All these food intolerances can cause inflammation in organs and tissues of the body.[47] Wheat was his primary intolerance that would block his regulation or ANS completely.

There was also systemic Candidiasis detected, along with oxyuren vermicularis, otherwise known as the common pinworm on energetic, resonance testing.

---

47 Brostoff, J and Gamblin, L. Food Allergies and Food Intolerance. Rochester: Inner Traditionals International, p.119, 2000.

Testing his organs energetically using Autonomic Response Testing (ART) as well as VEGA showed that there were a number of imbalances such as stomach, pancreas, liver, teeth, larynx, auditory ossicles, diaphragm, duodenum, ileum and prostate. In addition, there was a scar focus identified on the right foot that appeared significant as this was the primary deregulating factor of the ANS – meaning that this was the primary factor of all the organs identified that was keeping his autonomic nervous system from functioning correctly. Scar foci can become impulse generators, disturbing the subtle electromagnetic fields of the body, with resulting symptoms (see chapter 9).

There was also one tooth focus identified with ART testing, number 13 which is attached to the Large Intestine meridian that was detected on resonance testing.[48] However, a panoramic X-ray showed that there were 8 tooth implants and 5 root canal fillings which may require further investigation.

There was also considerable electromagnetic stress detected, probably as a result of using computers for long hours.

Thermography[49] showed focal mild hyperthermia at the right side of the mouth that may relate to focal, oral or dental inflammation. There were hyperthermic patterns in the right mandibular and digastric regions which may indicate increased lymph gland activity. No other significant findings.

Investigation of the iris in iridology showed a severe case of hypochlorhydria (low secretion of hydrochloric acid) which was probably the primary pathogenesis of his stomach issues can include: diarrhoea, steatorrhea, macrocytic anemia, weight loss, protein-losing enteropathy, abdominal discomfort or bloating and reflux. Deficiencies in certain nutrients may result in limb weakness, memory or mood changes, circulatory weaknesses in the capillary network leading to tinnitus, numbness and tingling in the limbs and other symptoms. Many researchers now believe that hypochlorhydria is present in about 80% of the population and is often wrongly diagnosed for hyperchlorhydria (excess secretion of HCl) and treated with hydrogen proton inhibitors or antacids which only aggravate the problem further.

---

48 See Chapter 8 for more details on tooth foci.
49 www.meditherm.com

The body tissues were quite acidic and inflamed, and so was the stomach lining, probably as a result of the hypochlorhydria that causes food to remain in the stomach for much longer periods of time. There was a cholesterol ring which is an indication of an inherited predisposition to hypercholestermia.

Darkfield microscopy of living blood showed a high level of congestion with stickiness in the red blood cells (rouleau) with high valence fibrinogen causing cells to tear and be destroyed. There was poikilocytosis, an indication of low iron, folic acid and vitamin B12 levels. The white blood cells were viable with good movement, indicating an active immune system. There was also considerable fermentation in the blood picture, probably a result of the systemic Candidiasis.

Biological Terrain Analysis (BTA),[50] a test conducted using urine and saliva, indicated an inability of the body to detoxify the cellular waste, which results in fluid congestion and stagnation. There was also a lack of available minerals in the body, most notably the blood. The kidneys were not cleaning the blood adequately and that the remaining detoxification organs of the body are unable to compensate. There was also a depletion of minerals that may be due to an imbalance in normal dietary factors, or intestinal malabsorption.

It is recommended that lymphatic drainage be improved, also kidney function, support liver function and rule out dehydration (he was drinking about 2 glasses of water per day at this stage which was increased to 8-10 glasses daily).

Hair Tissue Mineral Analysis has shown that the levels of iron and manganese are relatively low and levels of molybdenum are non-existent. Manganese is an essential trace nutrient in all forms of life.[51] It is important for the production of a number of enzymes such as oxidoreductases, transferases, hydrolases, lyases, isomerases, ligases, lectins, and integrins. The best known manganese-containing polypeptides

---

50 Correlative Urinalysis: The Body Knows Best, Morter, MT Jr., BEST Research Inc., Rogers, Arkansas, 1987.
51 Emsley, J. Manganese: Nature's Building Blocks: An A-Z Guide to the Elements. Oxford, UK: Oxford University Press. pp. 249–253, 2001.

may be arginase and Mn-containing superoxide dismutase (Mn-SOD),[52] present in all mitochondria.

Molybdenum is present in approximately 20 enzymes in the body, including aldehyde oxidase, sulfite oxidase and xanthine oxidase.[53] In some animals, the oxidation of xanthine to uric acid, a process of purine catabolism, is catalyzed by xanthine oxidase, a molybdenum-containing enzyme. The activity of xanthine oxidase is directly proportional to the amount of molybdenum in the body. So, low levels of manganese can lead to high uric acid levels leading to pains in the joints of the feet.

The hair analysis also showed a number of circulating toxic metals such as arsenic, mercury (he had 6 amalgams removed some time ago), lead and aluminium (probably from the antacids taken over the years which contain aluminium). Most of these toxic metals create free radicals which will cause further inflammation and degeneration of body tissues and organs.

Holistic treatments:

First, Mr. W began with an alkaline detoxification diet for 15 days with fruit, steamed vegetables, salads, vegetable juices and herbal teas. He also did the Hulda Clark parasite cleanse with Walnut tincture, wormwood and cloves during the alkaline detoxification diet.

He was also given nutritional supplements such as a high-potency multivitamin, a multimineral, omega 3, 6 and 9 fatty acids for the inflammation, betaine HCl and pepsin to improve the stomach digestion and eliminate the hypochlorhydria, as well as pancreatic enzymes to help improve the gut digestion. In addition, he was given homotoxicological glucosamine sulphate (2,000 mg daily), calcium with magnesium, drainage remedies for the kidneys (Berberis), the liver (Nux Vomica) and the lymphatic system (Lymphomyosot), aloe vera juice and a herbal drainage formula called Organic Lavage which addresses all the detoxification

---

52 Law, N. Manganese Redox Enzymes and Model Systems: Properties, Structures, and Reactivity. 46. pp. 305, 1998.
53 Emsley, J. Nature's Building Blocks. Oxford: Oxford University Press. pp. 262–266, 2001.

organs. In addition, he was given a ginkgo biloba[54] based formula to help alleviate the tinnitus and increase capillary circulation.

In addition, the HMD™ Ultmate Detoxifaction Protocol[55] was added to the supplemental regime to mobilize and eliminate the toxic metals. For the pain in the feet, he was checked and found to have a Rothbart's foot or a Primus Metatarsus Supinatus[56] foot type which can greatly aggravate the spine and misalign the body posture,[57] also putting pressure on the knees.[58] He was fitted with 6mm proprioreceptor insoles[59] in order to adjust the Rothbart's foot.

The tooth and scar foci were also repolarized using Low Intensity Lazer Therapy.[60] The belching of the stomach and distension had improved by about 40-50% within a couple of weeks of adding the HCl, even though he was on a reduced dosage due to the gastritis which we did not want to aggravate. At this point he also reported that his eyesight had improved a little, the tinnitus was much improved and so had his back improved considerably. The hot feeling in the feet and itchiness had more or less disappeared.

Six months into the treatment his health has improved overall – he has at least an 80% improvement in his stomach belching which he has had since he was 33 years old. He is very pleased at the fact that he can more or less eat what he likes. We believe that the stomach will improve completely as soon as he has completed the Candida treatment which he has not done to date due to his busy travelling schedule. He also still eats some of the foods that he is intolerant to which causes further aggravations on

---

54 Blumenthal M, Busse WR, Goldberg A, Gruenwald J, Hall T, Riggins CW, et al, eds. The complete German commission E monographs: therapeutic guide to herbal medicines. Austin, TX: American Botanical Council, 1998.
55 www.detoxmetals.com
56 Rothbart BA, Medial Column Foot Systems: An Innovative Tool for Improving Posture. *Journal of Bodywork and Movement Therapies* (6)1:37-46, 2002.
57 Rothbart BA, Liley P, Hansen, el al. Resolving Chronic Low Back Pain. The Foot Connection. *The Pain Practitioner* (formerly American Journal of Pain Management) 5(3): 84-89, 2002.
58 Rothbart BA, Yerratt M. An Innovative Mechanical Approach to Treating Chronic Knee Pain: A BioImplosion Model. *The Pain Practitioner* (formerly American Journal of Pain Management) 4(3): 13-18, 1994.
59 Rothbart BA. Proprioceptive Insoles. From a Podiatric Point of View. Health and Healing Wisdom (*Price-Pottinger Nutrition Foundation Journal*) Vol 29(3):11, 2005.
60 http://www.docgeorge.com/2008040474/Low-Intensity-Lazer-Therapy-LILT.html

occasions. The eyesight, hearing and tinnitus are stable with very negligible symptoms on occasions. His posture has much improved with the help of the proprioreceptor insoles and this has greatly helped his low back pain as well as the pain in his feet.

Patient's own account:

I have suffered for many years from bad digestion, with excessive belching, particularly after eating. It seems to me that my food is not digesting properly and perhaps coming up from the intestine back into the stomach as my belching often smells bad as though the food has not been digested properly. I have had this for some 35 years and have been treated by many doctors without success.

I have also had an operation for a herniated disc about 7 years ago, and still have a small herniated disk, which causes some discomfort from time to time. I also developed a recent foot pain which stopped me jogging, something that I have loved doing for years now.

I was really getting quite concerned about my deteriorating health as I am an active traveler and wanted to continue enjoying my travels and active lifestyle. Even though I have been seeing a Naturopathy abroad for over 25 years and his treatments have helped me to improve the quality of my life, no-one had got to the bottom of my stomach problems which was the most chronic and worse problem for me as it made it difficult for me to enjoy social eating.

While I was staying in Cyprus for a while, I found Dr. Georgiou's DaVinci Centre in Larnaca and thought that it was appropriate to pay him a visit to see if he could help me. After an initial assessment interview we booked for more extensive testing – the IDEL Diagnostic Programme which took a complete morning of about 5 hours to complete. This gave a lot of new information that had not been discovered before – all the causative factors to my underlying health problems – the most critical was the fact that my stomach was not producing enough hydrochloric acid and protein digestion was very strained and this was the primary cause of the belching, distension, pain and reflux.

There were many other factors identified such as food intolerances, mineral deficiencies, toxic metals, dehydration (no-one had told me ever to drink enough water), stagnated toxins due to compromised detoxification organs and a congested lymphatic system. Even my blood picture that I saw on the screen while Dr. Georgiou was conducting the live blood analysis was congested with all the red cells stuck together and torn apart by lots of fibrinogen – I was told that this was because my body getting enough oxygen and nutrients, nor was it eliminating the toxins.

Even my feet where causing a misalignment in my body posture that was putting pressure on my spine, knees, and neck – this was simply rectified by wearing special insoles that made such a difference, and so quickly.

I was very impressed with Dr. Georgiou's approach and the health problems that I have lived with for decades started to disappear in just a few months. I realized that this was beyond coincidence – there must be something to what Dr. Georgiou now calls Holistic Medicine.

I have learnt during my visits to Dr. Georgiou, that the premise of this wonderful medicine is that first you need to identify the causes of the problem, not simply put a label on it. Then you have to offload the causative factors – preferably as many as possible in the shortest period of time – then use natural remedies to repair and heal the body. This is exactly what Dr. Georgiou did, but each patient is obviously different and this type of medicine does not appear to be one that can be applied generally to all people in the same manner – each person needs to go through the testing to determine their causative factors.

I am truly grateful to Dr. Georgiou and his approach, as I never thought that I would be rid of the unpleasant health problems that I have had for over 3 decades, even though I have seen many medical doctors as well as natural medicine practitioners. Now that I know better, the missing element in all these other doctors that I had seen, was that they did not identify the true underlying causes to my illness, that made my life difficult up until today.

I did not expect to regain quality of life at my age, particularly after having been treated by so many doctors, some of whom even suggested that my problems could be psychosomatic.. The global population at large needs to learn more about this form of healing, as there are far to many people like myself whose quality of life could be improved so much if they had access to the method that Dr Georgiou uses in diagnosing and treating patients.

Dr Georgiou's final comments on Mr. W:

This is really quite a typical case where a critical underlying digestive issue can cause so many other health issues over time. The digestive system is indeed the most important system of the body as it gives all the raw materials such as minerals, vitamins, trace elements and more to all the other organs. If the digestive system is out of sync, then you can bet that the rest of the body will suffer as a consequence.

The issue of hypochlorhydria or deficient hydrochloric acid production is one that is under-diagnosed by many medical doctors, and particularly gastroenterologists. Indeed, often it is misdiagnosed as the opposite problem, too much acid and treated with various drugs that block the hydrochloric acid production. This simply perpetuates the problem further and the patient enters into a degenerative downward spiral that becomes more difficult to reverse over time.

My advice to all other practitioners entering into the field of Holistic Medicine is first check the functioning of the digestive system before looking elsewhere! The problem with gastroenterologists is that they check the structure of the digestive system while ignoring its function – we need to concentrate our efforts on combing the two for the benefit of the patient.

Case No. 7, Mrs. D, Age: 40

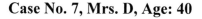

Main presenting problem: Asthma, recurrent urinary tract infections, irregular periods, GERD (reflux), spots on face that are permanent, constipation, knee pains, depression.

Medical diagnosis:

Mrs. D was diagnosed with asthma when she was 5 years old and has been taking cortisone inhalers for many years, along with anti-histamines. She was also diagnosed with Helicobacter pylori and attempts were made to eradicate this with high-doses of antibiotics over a 3-year period. She has also had a number of courses of antibiotics for recurring urinary tract infections. More courses of antibiotics followed recently when red, pussy spots appeared on her face that became permanent.

She has a history of GERD, diagnosed by a gastroenterologist and was given hydrogen-proton inhibitors that decrease the production of hydrochloric acid in the stomach and relieve symptoms.

Knee pains appeared a couple of years ago and she has been taking anti-inflammatories for this symptom too.

A histopathology examination of cervical tissue showed obvious minimal dysplasia of the superficial layer with hyperchromatic cells with no mitoses and little underlying inflammation and fibrosis. The diagnosis was: "the appearances are those of koilocytosis of the superficial squamous epithelial cells with minimal nuclear atypicalities compatible with HPV infection."

A DEXA Bone Densitometry report for femur and AP spine diagnosed osteopenia.

She was also diagnosed as suffering from depression and given anti-depressants as well as anxiolytics for recurring panic attacks related to hyperventilation. She always carried a brown bag in her car for dealing with these panic attacks.

Holistic diagnosis:

This was a young lady who had chronic health issues whose underlying aetiology had not been identified. The IDEL Diagnostic Programme was therefore conducted which consists of a series of tests to identify underlying causative factors.

The VEGA food intolerance test showed that she was intolerant to a number of foods such as: wheat, rye, barley and oats (these are all the gluten grains), lactose and milk products, eggs, citrus fruit, chicken, pork, nightshade family of vegetables (potatoes, tomatoes, peppers, aubergines), sugar and caffeine. Further regulation testing using Autonomic Response Testing (ART) showed that gluten was her primary food intolerance that would block her ANS.

Further ART testing of organ functioning showed an energetic imbalance in the following organ systems: thyroid, teeth, heart, ascending colon, adrenals, liver, stomach, breasts, kidneys, pancreas, ovaries and vagina. There has been a long history of irregular periods whose menstrual cycle ranges between 25-35 days, accompanied by pain and PMS symptoms.

On prioritization testing it was found that the primary organ that was causing the imbalance of the other organ systems was the ascending colon.

There was also two tooth foci identified at numbers 15 (stomach meridian) and 18 (Large Intestine meridian). There was also a vaccination scar that was blocking her ANS on the left arm. These foci can cause a myriad of health problems in other parts of the body.

Mrs. D. was also examined with Digital Infrared Thermal Imaging (DITI) or Thermography to determine if asymmetrical thermal findings indicate abnormal physiology. DITI findings were: "a hyperthermic pattern over the frontal region that correlates with a discrete bilateral hyperthermia over the ethmoid sinuses indicating a developing sinusitis.

Hyperthermic patterns encircling the buccal cavity possibly indicate an oral (dental or periodontal) pathology. At the inferior border of both lateral neck regions, diffuse hyperthermia (high temperature) is recorded suggesting an increased musclar tension over the platysma (neck area), but a developing vascular inflammation of the platysma should not be excluded. There is an intense muscular type diffuse hyperthermia over the entire posterior neck region extending inferiorly to the upper back toward the deltoids and posterior to the right side mainly over the scapula. These muscular inflammatory findings indicate a possible involvement of the deltoids, trapezius, right levator scapula and rhomboid muscles.

Central type hyperthermia observed over the thyroid region may suggest a thyroid dysfunction.

There are areas of hyperthermia in the upper quadrants of both breasts and most significantly there is a focal hyperthermia of the right breast and a hemilunar type hyperthermia on the left breast surrounding a focal hyperthermic area indicating an increased tissue density. These thermal patterns should be closely monitored for any future changes. Bilateral diffuse hyperthermia over the axillas may indicate increased lymphatic activity.

There is slight hyperthermia recorded over both lower lateral abdominal regions, mainly in the right side extending inferiorly to the inguinal region that may indicate a visceral involvement of the colon but a probable renal organ involvement shouldn't be excluded. The characteristic hyperthermic patterns recorded on the epigastrium and right hypochondrium could relate to the already reported GERD and to a developing gallbladder inflammatory involvement."

Iridology indicated pancreatic weaknesses of the exocrine system resulting in a deficiency of pancreatic enzymes resulting in bowel distension. There was also another digestive problem whereby the stomach was not producing enough hydrochloric acid (hypochlorhydria); there was kidney and liver irritation with accompanied toxicity, spinal subluxations at the level of the cervical, thoracic and lumbar regions, and lung irritation.

Darkfield examination using live blood showed a low vitality with very few protits, protein linkage indicating an acidity of the tissues and organs, undigested fat which is an indication of weak pancreatic enzymes, poikilocytosis indicating low iron, folic acid and vitamin B12 levels, viable WBC's but with a lot of lyzing indicating a weakened immune system (she is very prone to colds and flus).

Biological Terrain Analysis (BTA) using urine and saliva indicated a lowered ability to produce high-energy cellular fuel such as ATP due to mitochondrial dysfunction. There was also an increased cellular acidity probably related to the inability to adequately digest foods such as carbohydrates. There was also a diminished concentration of minerals caused by malabsorption, which restricts the minerals from being absorbed properly, as well as adrenal exhaustion which is also paramount in the regulation of specific minerals. Additionally, there were indications of a chronic, long-standing digestive condition, with possible manifesting yeast or fungal infection. Therapy aimed at the normalization of the digestive system and re-introduction of minerals was therefore essential, as well as strengthening the adrenal glands and investigation into the possibility of a systemic fungal issue.

Heart Rate Variability (HRV) testing is a test measuring the overall level of functioning of all the physiological systems of the body. The HRV test showed that this level was above average, but the level of the adaptation reserve or the ability to adapt to stress was moderately reduced below the average level. Here score was 5,5 where the average is 7,4 and perfection is 1,1. This was a good indication showing that most of her health issue are probably functional and not degenerative – she has a lot of potential to respond positively to the correct therapeutic programme.

Hair Tissue Mineral Analysis showed relatively low levels of a number of minerals such as copper, zinc, manganese, selenium and molybdenum. There was also circulating levels of mercury (she had had 10 amalgam fillings removed in the past), along with traces of uranium, arsenic and cadmium.

On a psychoemotional level there were unresolved family issues with siblings as well as the death of her beloved father about 2 years previously which have resulted in depressed moods, anxiety and a general feeling or apprehension and irritability.

Holistic treatments:

Mrs. D's holistic treatments began by her undergoing a 15-day alkaline detoxification protocol, with the Hulda Clark parasite cleanse and gallbladder flush running concomitantly. She also avoided the food intolerances identified; the identified food intolerances - these were later treated using bioresonance therapy.

She began an extensive detoxification protocol with ozone sauna, Matrix Regeneration Therapy (MRT), Infrared sauna, lymphatic drainage, bioresonace therapy, PAPIMI and an ionizing footbath for the removal of toxins.

Certain neutraceuticals and supplements were used to help the stomach digestion such as Betaine HCl and Pepsin, as well as pancreatic enzymes to help gut digestion and the assimilation of nutrients. A good quality multivitamin and multimineral were added to replenish her nutrient deficiencies, as well as omega 3,6 and 9, the HMD™ Ultimate Detox Protocol for the removal of heavy metals, a herbal formula to help rebuild the adrenal glands which also contains vitamin B5 and glandulars, coenzyme Q10 to facilitate energy levels at the mitochondrial level, vitamin E to help with the possible fibrocystic processes in the breasts, as well as supplemental selenium that was generally at a very low level.

In addition, digital homeopathic remedies were specifically made at the potency that resonated with her body to help rebuild and strengthen a number of organ systems such as the thyroid, heart, liver, kidneys, adrenals, pancreas, ovaries, small intestine, lungs, breast and colon.

She also began using a Salt Pipe for her respiratory issues on a daily basis. Salt pipes using mineral salt have been shown in scientific research to help clear the respiratory tract.

Within one month of beginning the holistic treatments she was generally feeling much better with improved moods and a lifting of her depressive tendencies – indeed, her family, colleagues and friends are now commenting on these improved moods and how much more she is laughing these days. This is one of her most significant improvements as she used to cry daily, thinking that no-one really cared for her, slept many hours, had no energy to enjoy a quality life and had put on considerable weight during this depressive period.

She also reports being more calm, has not had a panic attack since she began treatment and has not had to use her emergency brown bag that she keeps in the car to calm her down. She has also stopped taking all her medication including the anti-depressants, the anxiolytics, the anti-inflammatories, the hydrogen-proton inhibitors for her stomach, the cortisone inhalers for her asthma and the anti-histamines.

Most of the symptoms she presented with have now disappeared, such as her stomach reflux and bowel distention, her asthma (she has only had one need to use the cortisone inhaler once at the beginning of treatment when the weather was very damp and dusty – she used to use this every day for years). Her knee pains have disappeared, the spots on her face have cleared, as has her constipation – she is now regular every day as opposed to every 3 days – and her periods are beginning to regulate between 25-30 days as opposed to 25-35 days. She has also stopped taking the six Ponstan a day every month for period pains as she no longer needs them.

Her energy levels and stamina have greatly increased – she can now handle all the housework, she works a full day in a stressful job, and still has additional energy to enjoy life – not long ago she used to struggle to get through the day, would cover the basic housework and sleep many hours per day due to chronic fatigue. Her relationships with people around her have greatly improved as she is now much more positive, more patient and a lot happier.

She has also lost 9 kilos or about 22 lbs as well as dropped by two sizes – everyone is commenting on this which greatly pleases her, and her husband is showing renewed interest - although complaining that his expenses have increased this year as he needs to buy her a completely new wardrobe!

Patient's own account:

I am 40-years old but I feel 50 or more! I am a real mess and really don't know what to do to get out of the vicious cycle that I have put myself in. Every year some new symptom pops up, I go to the doctor and I come back with yet another pill to take – often with the message that I need to be popping these for the rest of my life – this is ridiculous!

I have been suffering from asthma since I was 5-years old and began taking inhalers from a very young age. I was also quite a sickly child, always coming down with colds and flus and taking antibiotics to combat this.

In early adulthood I had stomach problems that never seemed to go away – I was relieved when 3 years ago my gastroenterologist doctor diagnosed a bacteria in my stomach, Helicobacter, that he said was the main reason why I had reflux, pain and bloating – we spent nearly three years trying to treat this with a cocktail of antibiotics and other drugs but the reflux and heaviness in the stomach did not appear to go away, if anything it was getting worse.

I felt every year that my energy levels were draining from me and I was getting more and more depressed and anxious, often over nothing significant, there just seemed to be a constant apprehension that was difficult to explain. My symptoms seemed to be getting worse and knee pains appeared, I put on so much weight I was embarrassed to go out, my asthma got worse and I was taking inhalers every day, I began developing recurrent urinary tract infections, I suffered from irregular and very painful periods that required taking 6 antispasmodic painkillers a day to cope with this, not to mention the PMS which was so bad sometimes that I felt I could kill someone.

Generally, I was not seeing the light at the end of the tunnel until one day someone told me to visit Dr. Georgiou who happened to be living and working in the same town just round the corner from my house. I booked an appointment on the 29.5.09 and went to see him. When he heard my history and recorded everything, he suggested that it was time to take a deeper look to see what the causes of all these symptoms were. We scheduled the IDEL Diagnostic Programme and I spent an interesting 5 hours with Dr. Georgiou as he slowly traced out the chain of my diseases and symptoms – he found digestive problems in my stomach and gut, mineral deficiencies, heavy metals, problems with teeth, scars, food intolerances, weakened organs, inflammation in different parts of my body, spinal problems, Candida and a whole lot more. It was amazing how much information was revealed in a relatively short period of time.

We immediately began working on removing all these causative factors, and just a little more than 2 months into the treatment protocols I feel like a new woman and everyone around seems to agree, judging by the comments I hear. My energy levels have increased, my moods have changed drastically and I no longer feel anxious or depressed, my knee pains have gone, my stomach and gut have all improved and there is no more pain or bloating and the most significant thing is that I have stopped all the drugs that I was taking and only take natural supplements now which I am very happy with. Even my long-standing asthma that I have had for 35-years has disappeared, and so have the inhalers with it!

I only wish I had known that I could regain my health a lot sooner, but I am really pleased that I am now on the right road to regaining my health and learning how to maintain it and optimize it.'

Dr Georgiou's final comments on Mrs. D:

This is a classic case of ignoring the pathogenesis of disease and chasing the symptoms – this lady at the age of 40 was taking 7 different drugs in order to control her symptoms. By the age of 50 she certainly would have been on 10 different types with all the consequences of their serious side-effects. There is not a scientist in this world who truly understands the accumulative side effects of combining 7 or 10 different drugs – this is certainly not evidence-based medicine, but pure 'guesswork-medicate-and-lets-hope-for-the-best.'

One of the consequences of this polypharmacology is that there is a tremendous amount of free radicals created in the body which lead to inflammation and this can explain most of Mrs. D's symptomatology. One characteristic of inflammation is the high level of free radicals, mostly generated by the immune system, that are released into the tissues and blood. It has also been shown that free radicals and lipid peroxidation (the chemical breakdown by free radicals of fats, or lipids, in cell membranes), can cause many degenerative changes in the body.

One of the ways that can greatly reduce this inflammation is detoxification – generally when my patients discuss detoxification with their medical doctors they look at them as if they are from another planet or tell them that only the liver has the ability to detoxify and there is nothing one can do to help it – they are probably referring to there being no drugs that can do this.

What most people do not understand is that when two or more toxins are introduced into the body, the total toxicity may be equal to adding the toxicity of each together, or 'additive toxicity.' For instance, let's say mercury has a toxic value of 4 and aluminium a value of 5. The additive effect is 9, but if they react synergistically the total might be 29. We call this 'synergistic toxicity,' and it is exactly what was happening in Mrs. D's body. One symptom that Mrs. D had that is characteristic of excessive toxicity is hyperidrosis or excessive sweating - when we are sick with a virus or bacterial infection we build up a great number of internally created toxins that must be removed through sweating. Excessive toxins in the body can create an imbalance in the autonomic nervous system causing hyperidrosis.

The cells lining the gastrointestinal tract (GI) contain a great number of powerful detoxification systems, so the detoxification process can begin even before a toxin is absorbed. In addition, the GI tract contains the most elaborate portion of the immune system, which acts as a gate that guards the blood from harmful chemicals.

It is estimated that the average person consumes 25 tons of food in a lifetime. This includes the toxins naturally found in all foods. When the GI tract is not functioning correctly this further increases the number of toxins due to the putrefaction of food – add to this constipation which is a 'toxin factory' in itself and you have all the correct ingredients for making the body extremely toxic in a short period of time.

There is another very important factor involved in keeping the GI tract from auto-intoxicating itself – the friendly bacteria present in the GI tract – this normal "good" bacteria in the colon also plays an important role in detoxification, especially for removing dangerous products of oestrogen metabolism. If allowed to stay in the system and recirculate, these oestrogen toxins (called 16-alpha hydroxyestrone) can generate a number of cancers in both males and females.

This may explain why women who use antibiotics often have a higher incidence of breast cancer, since the antibiotics kill the good bacteria (probiotics). In Mrs. D's case, these friendly bacteria were eradicated by the large number of courses of antibiotics that she took in her lifetime - these antibiotics do not only kill the pathogenic bacteria but also the good bacteria too. This normally opens the door to the normal unicellular Candida species that is present in everyone's gut transforming into a pathogenic, mycelial form that will begin penetrating the gut wall and into other tissues of the body. Systemic Candidiasis, with the 79 mycotoxins that it produces is an underlying cause of many of Mrs. D's symptoms.

Mrs. D is still continuing her treatments and is, at the time of writing, about one month into her Candida protocol – she has another two months to complete this. We will also be looking at reversing the osteopenia using natural progesterone cream made from the Wild Yam, as well as other supplements. She has now learned the power of optimal nutrition and detoxification and will be repeating some of her cleanses every 6 months, as well as maintaining an optimal diet.

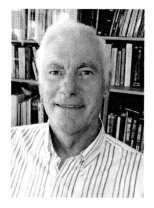

Case No. 8, Dr. H, Age: 62

Main presenting problem: IBS, Chronic Fatigue Syndrome, Myastenia Gravis, severe muscle pains, severe headaches, angina, complete fatigue resulting in 40-hour sleep episodes.

Medical diagnosis: Systemic Lupus Erythromatosus (SLE), Myesthenia Gravis, Myalgic encephalomyelitis, angina, IBS.

Mr. H. has been to many doctors and hospitals in the UK, Cyprus and other countries. There have been a variety of diagnoses that have been written up and investigated – these include Systemic Lupus Erythromatosus (SLE), a chronic, inflammatory autoimmune disorder. One report by a medical doctor that diagnosed this mentioned the "typical butterfly syndrome" with light sensitivity, chronic fatigue and more.

At one point Dr. H was admitted to the Larnaca hospital in Cyprus complaining of malaise, dizziness and diarrhoea lasting for 14 days and a 10 kilogram loss in weight during this period. Many blood tests and other examinations followed but they found "nothing pathological."

On another occasion during the same year, he presented to a medical neurologist with diplopia – provoked by fatigue and sunshine, mild ptosis of both sides, weakness of the neck muscles, stiffness and vague pain in the neck and lumbar region, general weakness, difficulty in speaking. The neurological examination showed an increase of diplopia and ptosis by provocation testing, reduction of the muscle power of the upper and low limbs by provocation testing, muscle atrophies in the limbs. EEG showed no signs of polyneuropathy or myopathy. The final conclusion was that the history and findings were indicative of a myasthenic syndrome.

A later CT scan picked up no abnormalities or lesions in the brain.

One surgeon that saw him confirmed a myasthenic syndrome and recommended a thymectomy (removal of the thymus gland) which Mr. H. kindly refused.

Holistic diagnosis:

Due to the fleeting visit of Dr. H in Cyprus, it was only possible to perform a few of the extensive tests that would normally be conducted during the IDEL Diagnostic Programme.

VEGA food intolerance testing identified a number of food intolerances – wheat, lactose and all dairy products, pork, and caffeine. He was also found to be reacting to house dust and the house dust mite. All these food intolerances can cause inflammation in organs and tissues of the body.[61] Wheat was his primary intolerance that would block his regulation or Autonomic Nervous System completely, as measured using Autonomic Response Testing (ART). Dr. H. loved bread and would often eat it on a regular basis.

There was also systemic Candidiasis detected, along with oxyuren vermicularis, otherwise known as the common pinworm on energetic, resonance testing.

Testing his organs energetically using Autonomic Response Testing (ART) as well as VEGA showed that there were a number of imbalances such as stomach, pancreas, liver, teeth, duodenum, jejunum, ileum, colon and prostate.

There was also considerable electromagnetic stress detected, probably as a result of using computers for long hours. He was also in the military responsible for radar and powerful electromagnetic equipment – this caused electromagnetic stress and a hypersensitivity to the point where he will now come up in red skin rashes when he is near Wi-Fi, computers and mobile phones.

Investigation of the iris in iridology showed pancreatic enzyme deficiency which was accompanied with considerable bloating after eating. The body tissues were quite acidic and inflamed.

The weak and dysfunctional digestive system is key to many inflammatory symptoms. The intestinal wall can allow endotoxins to invade the bloodstream causing a biochemical cascade of inflammatory conditions

---

61 Brostoff, J and Gamblin, L. Food Allergies and Food Intolerance. Rochester: Inner Traditionals International, p.119, 2000.

due to gluten sensitivity, food intolerances, and Candida overgrowth. When this occurs, there is an accompanying dysbiosis of the intestinal tract (an imbalance between the good and bad bacteria, where the bad bacteria overwhelm the good) as caused by prolonged or repeated antibiotic treatment. Commonly this is combined with a malfunctioning ileocecal valve (he often had pain in this area), which normally prevents bacteria from the large intestines to invade the small intestines.

A relevant observation is the presence of acetylcholine receptors in various bacteria, especially in E. coli, the most common type of bacteria in the large intestines. If the intestinal wall is weak, bacterial proteins or endotoxins can pass from the intestines into the bloodstream and cause antibodies to develop against any bacterial receptors. These antibodies, originally formed against E. coli receptors may, in turn, initiate the attack on thymus receptors in the presence of manganese deficiency. A surplus of antibodies spills over into the bloodstream and will then attack healthy muscle receptors.

Hair Tissue Mineral Analysis confirmed a number of mineral deficiencies such as: sodium, potassium, iron, manganese, selenium and boron. Manganese is an essential trace nutrient in all forms of life.[62] It is important for the production of a number of enzymes such as oxidoreductases, transferases, hydrolases, lyases, isomerases, ligases, lectins, and integrins. The best known manganese-containing polypeptides may be arginase and Mn-containing superoxide dismutase (Mn-SOD),[63] present in all mitochondria required for energy production.

Manganese deficiency causes defective growth, muscular weakness, lack of coordination and balance, reproductive abnormalities and disorders of the central nervous system. Manganese is required for a healthy immune system and it is also involved in the synthesis of acetylcholine.

The hair analysis did not show any circulating toxic metals on the first test, but after taking the HMD detoxification protocol for two months and retesting his level of mercury had increased tremendously. This was an indication that he had high levels of mercury stored in his organs and tissues and needed to be chelated. Mercury will create free radicals which

---

62 Emsley, J. Manganese. Nature's Building Blocks: An A-Z Guide to the Elements. Oxford, UK: Oxford University Press. pp. 249–253, 2001.
63 Law, N. Manganese Redox Enzymes and Model Systems: Properties, Structures, and Reactivity. 46. pp. 305, 1998.

will cause further inflammation and degeneration of body tissues and organs.

Myasthenia gravis has been shown to be an autoimmune disease. This means that the immune system attacks some of its own body proteins. Specifically, the transmission of signals from the nerve endings to the muscle receptors is partly blocked by antibodies. The messenger chemical or neurotransmitter released as signal from nerve endings to muscles is acetylcholine. Acetylcholine molecules travel the short distance in the gap between nerve ending and muscle to find a receptor on the motor end plate. When a sufficient number of acetylcholine molecules are attached to muscle receptors, there is an electric discharge of the normal membrane potential and the muscle fibre can contract.

In myasthenia gravis many or most of the receptors are already occupied by antibodies, therefore, not enough acetylcholine molecules find receptors to trigger this discharge and subsequent muscle contraction. Normally, the acetylcholine is split by an enzyme acetylcholinesterase and with this, removed from the receptor in a fraction of a second. Using drugs, which hinder this enzyme, acetylcholine molecules have more time to find receptors with an increased chance to lead to a discharge.

However, if too much of this enzyme antagonist is present, the cells remain discharged for too long and the muscles become more or less paralysed. This is a 'cholinergic crisis' in which heart and breathing may stop. This may have been happening to Dr. H. when he used to arrive at the hospital in a collapsed crisis state.

Research has shown that myasthenia gravis can manifest after exposure to crop sprays with chemicals as well as heavy metals which have an antagonistic effect on acetylcholinesterase. Dr. H. was full of these toxic metals.

Holistic treatments:

First, Dr. H began with an alkaline detoxification diet for 15 days with fruit, steamed vegetables, salads, vegetable juices and herbal teas. He also did the Hulda Clark parasite cleanse with Walnut tincture, wormwood and cloves during the alkaline detoxification diet. The gallbladder flush was done at the end of the alkaline detoxification diet.

As Dr. H had a history of reacting adversely to any type of detoxification programme that he had tried in the past, we decided to add plenty of homeopathic and herbal drainage remedies to facilitate the detoxification process. Specifically, he was given Berberis for the kidneys, Nux vomica for the liver and Lymphomyosot for the lymphatic system. Aloe vera was added along with a herbal drainage remedy consisting of milk thistle, dandelion, burdock, red clover, tumeric, hydrangea and uva ursi – all provided in one formula called Organic Lavage.[64]

He was also given nutritional supplements such as a high-potency multivitamin, a multimineral, omega 3, 6 and 9 fatty acids for the inflammation, betaine HCl and pepsin to improve the stomach digestion and eliminate the hypochlorhydria, as well as pancreatic enzymes to help improve the gut digestion.

In addition, the HMD™ Ultmate Detoxification Protocol[65] was added to the supplemental regime to mobilize and eliminate the toxic metals. His body posture was misaligned – upon further testing he was found to have a Rothbart's foot or a Primus Metatarsus Supinatus[66] foot type which can greatly aggravate the spine and misalign the body posture,[67] also putting pressure on the knees.[68] He was fitted with 6mm proprioreceptor insoles[69] in order to adjust the Rothbart's foot.

Shortly after completing the detoxification treatment he began the DaVinci Candida Protocol to completely eradicate the systemic Candidiasis[70,71] – there is a relationship between Candida and autoimmune diseases. If

64 www.detoxmetals.com
65 www.detoxmetals.com
66 Rothbart BA, Medial Column Foot Systems: An Innovative Tool for Improving Posture. *Journal of Bodywork and Movement Therapies* (6)1:37-46, 2002.
67 Rothbart BA, Liley P, Hansen, el al. Resolving Chronic Low Back Pain. The Foot Connection. *The Pain Practitioner* (formerly American Journal of Pain Management) 5(3): 84-89, 1995.
68 Rothbart BA, Yerratt M. An Innovative Mechanical Approach to Treating Chronic Knee Pain: A BioImplosion Model. *The Pain Practitioner* (formerly American Journal of Pain Management) 4(3): 13-18, 1994.
69 Rothbart BA. Proprioceptive Insoles. From a Podiatric Point of View. Health and Healing Wisdom (*Price-Pottinger Nutrition Foundation Journal*) Vol 29(3):11, 2005.
70 Georgiou, GJ. Scurge of the 21st Century: Systemic Candidiasis. *British Naturopathic Journal*, Vol. 25, No. 1, 2008.
71 Georgiou, GJ. Treatment of Systemic Candidiasis. *British Naturopathic Journal*, Vol. 25, No. 2, 2008.

candida escapes outside the gut it can put out receptors on its cell surface which are similar to human receptors for connective tissue affected in rheumatoid arthritis and the immune system in general affected in lupus. As the body attacks the Candida it may also attack anything which looks like the Candida - because of the connective tissue receptors on Candida, the body's immune system may attack other cells in the body which have these receptors.

Many tissues such as the joints have connective tissue receptors and as the body attacks the Candida, the body may also attack these cells. The result may be painful joints as in rheumatoid arthritis or other inflamed tissues as in lupus and other autoimmune diseases.

Patient's own account:

Back in the 1970's I was a very fit and active member of the Royal Navy, participating in many sailing sports and a member of the Field Gun racing crew which required a very high standard of fitness.

All this changed when in 1974 I was in Puerto Rico and suddenly developed flu like symptoms some hours following an injection for yellow fever.

Chronic symptoms which developed over the next few months and which lasted for over 30 years included:

- ❖ Severe headaches
- ❖ Migraines
- ❖ Hypersensitivity to light, sound and touch
- ❖ Irritable Bowel Syndrome (IBS)
- ❖ Severe muscle pains – fibromyalgia
- ❖ Chronic fatigue – a total lack of energy to perform even simple tasks
- ❖ Sleeping up to 18 hours per day and still feeling tired
- ❖ At times, unable to walk more than a few steps without needing to rest.

I was hospitalised many times in an attempt to discover the reasons for my ill-health and to form a diagnosis. Tests included barium meal, barium enema fluoroscopy examinations, crosby capsule duodenum biopsy, muscle biopsy and many psychiatric tests to establish to what extent – if any – the symptoms were psychologically related. Although there were many symptoms none added up to a specific diagnosis. Other tests done were gastrointestinal endoscopy and colonoscopy. No specific diagnosis was agreed.

Finally, in 1978 I was discharged on medical grounds even though no precise diagnosis had been found. Symptoms continued, but since I was self-employed, I was able to rest and sleep as necessary, so was able to manage symptoms.

This continued until a total collapse and hospitalisation in 1988. One hospital confirmed myasthenia gravis and MS, but tests at another hospital did not agree. Finally I was referred to Guys Hospital and the professor of neurology, following some very confusing test results, diagnosed a severe case of Myalgic Encephalomyelitis. I was informed that there was no cure and that because I had been ill for so long, it was not going to get any better. Symptom management was the only way and I would have to live with it.

It was a relief to get a diagnosis but I refused to give up on finding a cure.

I was living in Cyprus at the time and because of my inability to do anything physical, purchased a laptop computer and began to further my studies in psychology. I got to know Dr. George Georgiou, who was teaching psychology at a local college in Larnaca. We became great friends and I realised that he could help me. He had not at that time developed the protocol to cure my ill health but I came to understand much more about ME and how to handle it.

I purchased a compound microscope and became competent in live blood analysis and darkfield microscopy all in an attempt to find out more about my condition. In January of 2006, I was invited to attend seminars on cancer treatment using natural therapies in Cyprus. Following this conference, Dr. Georgiou took me back to the DaVinci Natural Health Centre and ran a gamut of tests including VEGA testing, ART, Iridology and a Hair Tissue Mineral Analysis. We established several things. I had Systemic Candida, high levels of mercury and intolerances to wheat, dairy and other foods.

I began a strict diet eliminating the foods that displayed an intolerance, all forms of sugar and, most significantly, began the heavy metal detox protocol to eliminate mercury from my system.

Following a few days of feeling very near deaths door, even having to delay a flight out of Cyprus, I began to feel changes taking place. Within three months, by the time I had completed the Sanum remedies to deal with the Candida, I was feeling fitter than I had done in over 30 years. The healing continued over the next few months, as the mercury detox continued. The severe joint pains left me, I no longer had daily headaches – in fact, I have been free of all headaches for over 3 years now! My energy levels increased and my general health was like I had not experienced since my days in the Royal Navy.

My bowels began to function normally and I found, to my amazement, that I was completely in charge of my bowels – rather than the other way round - and could defecate whenever I wanted! I had not realised this was even possible previously and could not remember ever being so healthy.

About a year later a friend was visiting from the USA who liked to walk. I decided to take him up a steep hill, at the top of which was my old house. He was puffing a bit by the time we got to the top, and I was not feeling the strain at all. It was not until we reached the bottom again, that I suddenly realised that I had no signs of the angina, which previously I had been prescribed a drug to control. When I owned the house on the hill, I could not even manage the top tier when walking the dog without severe chest and arm pain. Now, I could walk the entire hill at a good pace with absolutely no pain whatsoever. All my friends are still astounded at the new me!

Dr Georgiou's final comments on Dr. H:

Here is an interesting case which had received many diagnostic labels ranging from myalgic encephalomyelitis, to myastenia gravis to Systemic Lupus Erythromatosus (SLE), angina, Irritable Bowel Syndrome and more. These are serious auto-immune diseases that were diagnosed based on medical tests – the only problem was that no-one could cure them because no-one could identify the causative factors.

A number of studies have suggested that environmental exposure such as inhalation or ingestion of contaminants is related to the development of lupus.[72,73,74] In lupus and other autoimmune diseases, the immune system loses its ability to differentiate between foreign substances and its own cells and tissues, causing the body to attack itself.[75] Literature suggests an overall mortality rate in lupus patients that is greater than two times the rate in the general population, a serious implication.[76,77]

Metals reported to be associated with autoimmune disease include gold, cadmium, mercury (xenobiotic that is widely present in the environment), and pristine. The hypothesized mechanisms of the effects of both chemical factors and metals in the development of lupus are mainly based on animal and in vitro studies, and include activating and inhibiting immune response, apoptosis, and activation of inflammatory cytokines.[78]

Animal studies suggest that pristane and mercury may be environmental triggers for SLE.[79,80] Cooper's epidemiologic study of human exposure to mercury among dental workers reveals increased rates of immunologic disease.[81]

---

72 Balluz, L., Philen, R., Ortega, L., Rosales, C., Brock, J., Barr, D., et al. Investigation of Systemic Lupus Erythematosus in Nogales, Arizona. *American Journal of Epidemiology*, 154(11), 1029-1036, 2001.

73 Kardestuncer, T., & Frumkin, H. Systemic Lupus Erythematosus in relation to environmental pollution: an investigation in an African-American community in North Georgia. *Archives of Environmental Health*, 52(2), 85-90, 1997.

74 Mongey, AB., & Hess, E. Chapter 3 - The Role of Environment in Systemic Lupus Erythematosus and Associated Disorders. In D. a. H. Wallace, BH (Ed.), Dubois' Lupus Erythematosus (6 ed.), 2002.

75 Grossman, J. & Kalunian, K. Chapter 2 - Definition, classification, activity, and damage indices. In D. Wallace & B. Hahn (Eds.), Dubois' Lupus Erythematosus (6 ed.), 2002.

76 Bernatsky, S., Boivin, JF., Joseph, L., Manzi, S., Ginzler, E., Gladman, D., et al. Mortality in systemic lupus erythematosus. *Arthritis & Rheumatism*, 54(8), 2550-2557, 2002.

77 Krishnan, E., & Hubert, H. Ethnicity and mortality from systemic lupus erythematosus in the USA. *Annals of the Rheumatic Diseases*, 65(11), 1500-1504, 2006.

78 Mongey, AB., & Hess, E. Chapter 3 - The Role of Environment in Systemic Lupus Erythematosus and Associated Disorders. In D. a. H. Wallace, BH (Ed.), Dubois' Lupus Erythematosus (6 ed.), 2002.

79 Bagenstose L, Salgame P, Monestier M: Murine Mercury-Induced Autoimmunity. *Immunol Res* 20:67-78, 1999.

80 Mayes MD: Epidemiologic Studies of Environmental Agentsand Systemic Autoimmune Diseases. *Environ Health Perspect* 107:743-748, 1999.

81 Cooper GS, Parks CG, Treadwell EL, St Clair EW, Gilkeson GS, Dooley MA: Occupational risk factors for the development of systemic lupus erythematosus. *J Rheumatol* 31(10):1928-1933, 2004.

There were a number of potential causative factors that were identified and treated during the IDEL Diagnostic Programme that were very probably related to these auto-immune symptoms that Dr. H had:

1. Food intolerances

2. Mercury and chemical toxicity

3. Vitamin and mineral deficiencies

4. Parasites

5. Systemic Candidiasis, accompanied with severe dysbiosis

6. Electromagnetic pollution and radiation in home and workplace.

Once these factors were identified and eliminated Dr. H gained full functioning of all his physiological systems and all auto-immune symptoms disappeared. The SLE, or MG or ME was not the disease, but only the symptoms – the causes of these syndromes is the real disease, and it is these that need to be addressed. After 30-years of suffering with horrific symptoms Dr. H is now fully functional and enjoying his sailing, sports, fully active life, publishing books and the like at the age of 62.

Case No. 9; Mr. P, Age: 80

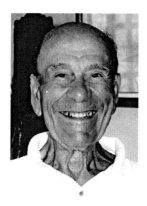

Main presenting problems:

Cancer of the oesophagus, chronic osteoarthritis of knee and shoulders, recurring urine infections, intermittent diarrhoea, bowel distention.

Medical diagnosis:

Oesophageal carcinoma – the report written by the Professor of Gastrointestinal Medicine in the UK said: "he presented with progressive dysphagia over two months with progressive weight loss - after examination it was revealed that he had oesophageal adenocarcinoma beginning at 35 cm and extending for 8 cm across the gastro oesophageal junction. EUS demonstrates that the tumour involves the right pleura, making it T4, with involved peri-oesophageal lymph nodes (N1), but no distant metastases. I have recommended neo-adjuvant chemotherapy with three cycles of ECCap. This provides a slightly prolonged course of treatment, with more opportunity for tumour shrinkage, and also limits the cisplatin dose to avoid toxicity, compared with the standard OE02 schedule."

In August 2006 he had an Ivor Lewis partial oesopagogastrectomy where part of the stomach and oesophagus was removed.

In the UK where he lived, he was also diagnosed with osteoarthritic changes in both knee and patello femoral joints. He was given Diclomax anti-inflammatories which he has been taking for 20 years to control the acute pain. Also hypercholestermia with cholesterol levels around 270.

His medical history contains information from 1982 when he developed a serious lung infection that was probably mycoplasma pneumonia. There was also an epididymal cyst which had swelling for many months. In the early 1990's he developed episodic palpitations – he was a heavy smoker but stopped in the mid 1980's. In the mid 90's he developed moderate bilateral sensori-neural loss, but he was working in a noisy environment for at least 20 years, owning his own restaurant with noisy kitchen fans.

Holistic diagnosis:

Mr. P was referred to the Davinci Natural Health Centre by his daughter who was also a patient of ours. She was concerned with a variety of symptoms that her father had which had not been alleviated by orthodox medicine. She was also concerned that he should take precautions after his initial diagnosis of oesophageal cancer in order to prevent any further metastases – prognosis for oesophageal cancer is generally not good in the elderly with less than 8% surviving for 5 years after diagnosis.[82] Mr. P went through the IDEL Diagnostic Programme to determine hidden underlying causes to his illness.

VEGA allergy testing revealed a number of food intolerances such as wheat, milk and lactose, pork, chicken, onions, garlic, leeks and caffeine. Further testing of the organ systems using VEGA and ART showed imbalances in the lymph nodes, colon, prostate, thyroid, tuba auditiva, lungs, liver, gallbladder, stomach and pancreas. The primary organ in the pathogenesis of disease was the pancreas as on ART testing this was blocking his ANS regulation completely.

Further VEGA testing indicated toxic metal burden with lead, aluminium and mercury which was later confirmed using other tests.

ART testing for scar foci indicated a scar on the right side of the head that he had incurred after a fall in the garden while he was on chemotherapy.

Iridology had shown hypochlorhydria or a deficiency in the production of hydrochloric acid, lacunas on the pancreas indicating a hereditary predisposition to pancreatic enzyme insufficiency, an arcus senilus indicating poor circulation to the brain and parts of the head, irritation of the right ear (he had considerable hearing loss in this ear) and thyroid gland. There were psora spots in the kidney and liver regions with considerable lymphatic congestion.

---

[82]Gilbert FJ, Thompson, A.M., (eds), Scottish Audit of Gastric and Oesophageal Cancer. Report 1997-2000. A prospective audit. *Scottish Audit of Gastric and Oesophageal Cancer Steering Group*: Edinburgh, 2002.

Darkfield microscopy examining living blood showed a considerable number of uric acid crystals, fibrinogen which is usually an indication of liver congestion and toxicity, rouleau of the erythrocytes indicating poor circulation and oxygenation and a fermentation of cells that was probably related to the systemic Candidiasis overgrowth.

Heart Rate Variability (HRV) testing was impressive for a 78 years old man as it showed that the functioning of the physiological systems were quite close to the average level with a score of 8 (1 is the best possible; 13 the worse). His adaptation reserve, or his ability to adapt to stress was quite low with a score of 6 (1 is best possible; 7 is worst possible). Recent testing (September 2009) has shown a dramatic improvement in his HRV – risen from 8,6 to 5,4 – there are many much younger people that do not have such a score!

Biological Terrain Analysis testing using urine and saliva showed that ATP energy production was compromised in the mitochondria, probably as a result of heavy metals and other xenobiotics. There was also a considerable depletion of minerals and a lack of available minerals in the body – this is probably related to poor stomach digestion due to the hypochlorhydria and pancreatic enzyme deficiencies that would result in poor digestion of foods and malabsorption problems. There were also indications of poor kidney drainage due to congestion and toxicity of the kidney that can also be related to minerals not being available to the body.

Tissue Hair Mineral Analysis (THMA) has shown that there was a serious zinc deficiency, which he may have had for years as this may have been the reason for him developing pneumonia.[83] Zinc is an essential co-factor in a variety of cellular processes including DNA synthesis, behavioural responses, reproduction, bone formation, growth and wound healing.[84]

Zinc is necessary for the free-radical quenching activity of superoxide dismutase (SOD), a powerful antioxidant enzyme which breaks down the

---

83 Meydani, SN., Barnett, JB., Dallal, GE., Fine, BC., Jacques, PF., Leka, LS., Hamer, DH. Serum zinc and pneumonia in nursing home elderly. *American Journal of Clinical Nutrition*, October 2007.
84 Barceloux DG. Zinc. *J Toxicol Clin Toxicol* 37:279-92, 1999.

free-radical superoxide to form hydrogen peroxide.[85] Zinc is also required for the proper function of T-lymphocytes.[86]

We know that zinc combats oxidative damage from free radicals, it plays a role in DNA repair, and that it has important anti-inflammatory properties. It also helps to shut off proliferation of mutant cells. Zinc deficiency seems to be an important factor in the pathogenesis of chronic diseases, including cancer.

Going back to Mr. P's hair analysis, there were also a number of heavy metals shown to be actively circulating including lead, aluminium and arsenic. All these metals have been implicated in the pathogenesis of cancer. These metals can also inhibit the absorption and utilization of calcium, zinc, manganese, copper, and iron, causing serious deficiencies.

We have already discussed in Chapter 11 the destruction of important cytochrome enzymes by heavy metals and xenobiotics which destroy cardiolipine, a lipid contained in the inner mitochondrial membrane, to which the cytochrome enzymes of the respiratory chain are attached. When the cardiolipine is destroyed by these pernicious agents, the oxidative processes are adversely affected[87] therefore increasing the probability of aerobic cells converting to anaerobic cancer cells.

Thermography showed: "hyperthermia over the upper border of the frontal region (L>R) that correlates with a discrete bilateral hyperthermia over the ethmoid sinuses. These thermal findings can also explain the patient's complaints of headaches. Hyperthermic patterns on the left side of the buccal cavity possibly indicate an oral (dental or periodontal) pathology. At the inferior border of both lateral neck regions, diffuse hyperthermia is recorded suggesting an increased muscular tension over the platysma mainly on the left side, but a developing vascular inflammation of the carotid artery should not be excluded (right side). Central type hyperthermia observed over the thyroid region may also suggest a thyroid dysfunction."

---

85 Diamond WJ, et al. An alternative medicine definitive guide to cancer. Tiburon: Future Medicine Publishing, Inc., 793, 1997.
86 Boik J. Cancer and natural medicine: a textbook of basic science and clinical research. Oregon: Medical Press 147, 1995.
87 Green, DR., & Kroemer, G. The Pathophysiology of Mitochondrial Cell Death. *Science* Vol. 305. no. 5684, pp. 626 – 629, July 2004.

"There is an intense muscular type diffuse hyperthermia over the entire posterior neck region extending inferiorly to the upper back, between the scapulas. These muscular inflammatory findings indicate a possible involvement of the trapezius, levarors scapula and rhomboid muscles."

"There are no significant thermal asymmetries or temperature differentials seen in the chest. There are no suspicious thermal patterns on the left side of the hemithorax suggesting any cardiovascular involvement. The only significant thermal pattern is the central hyperthermia observed on the lower level of the sternum relating to the oesophageal pathology. Slight diffuse hyperthermia is also seen on both deltoid regions suggesting a developing inflammatory involvement."

"There are no significant thermal asymmetries seen in the abdomen. There is a central type periumbilical hypothermia (R>L) that may indicate a developing visceral involvement of the colon. There are no recorded thermal patterns from the epigastrium."

Holistic treatments:

There were a number of treatments that Mr. P undertook to bring his body biochemistry back to normal – first, he began with an alkaline detoxification programme eating only fruit, salads, steamed vegetables, vegetable juices and herbal teas for two weeks. Concomitantly, he began a parasite cleanse using three herbs, walnut tincture, wormwood and cloves, which lasted two weeks. At the end of the two weeks he did a gallbladder flush, flushing out a number of gallstones.

He also began taking a number of supplements including a high-potency multivitamin formula, betaine HCl and pepsin to help stomach digestion, pancreatic enzymes to help gut digestion, HMD,® Organic Lavage and Chlorella to help eliminate the burden of heavy metals,[88] Essiac Tea,[89,90] Milk thistle[91,92] to help the liver, glucosamine to help strengthen cartilage

---

5 http://www.detoxmetals.com/Toxic-Metal-Detoxification-Protocol.html

89 Tai, J., Cheung, S., Wong, S., and Lowe, C. In vitro comparison of Essiac and Flor-Essence on human tumour cell lines. *Oncol.Rep.* 11(2):471-476, 2004.

90 Tamayo, C., Richardson, M. A., Diamond, S., and Skoda, I. The chemistry and biological activity of herbs used in Flor-Essence herbal tonic and Essiac. *Phytother Res* 14(1):1-14, 2000.

[91] Ladas EJ, Kelly KM. Milk thistle: is there a role for its use as an adjunct therapy in patients with cancer? *J Altern Complement Med* 9(3):411-416, 2003.

and aid in glycosaminoglycan synthesis, therefore helping the osteoarthritis.[93,94] He also took systemic enzymes such as Wobenzyme-N for helping to dissolve the sialo-glycoprotein coat around cancer cells which disguise them from recognition by the immune system and stimulate various components of the immune system such as Natural Killer cells, T-cells and Tumor Necrosis factor. Mr. P was also given PolyMVA, a Palladium lipoic acid complex (LAPd).

LAPd appears to be the first potential therapeutic agent developed to target and inactivate the altered pyruvate dehydrogenase (PDH) complex that is crucial to the energy metabolism of tumour cells. Through this mechanism of action, LAPd appears to stop the growth, replication, and long-term function of tumour cells.[95]

Another action of LAPd is in the reduction of electrons within DNA, which has the effect of mediating DNA synthesis, clinically applicable in restricting tumour growth or virus replication (see Bingham, reference 13 below).

Within about three weeks of beginning the detoxification protocols his diarrhoea had stopped completely and he was feeling well with good energy levels. About six weeks into the treatment protocol he was feeling and looking very well – he was working for an hour per day in the garden, he was eating well and his weight was stable. He has also stopped taking all medicinal drugs, including the painkillers and anti-inflammatories that he was taking for many years – he was quite pain-free in all joints, even though he had difficulty walking a couple of years ago.

A further tissue hair mineral analysis revealed that his aluminium levels after chelating with the natural chelator HMD® had greatly increased from 52 ppm to 73 ppm. This is an indication that he had a considerable amount of aluminium stored in his body tissues and organs, probably related to

[92] Zuber R, Modriansky M, Dvorak Z, et al. Effect of silybin and its congeners on human liver microsomal cytochrome P450 activities. *Phytother Res* 16(7):632-638, 2002.

[93] Clegg DO, Reda DJ, Harris CL, et al. Glucosamine, chondroitin sulfate, and the two in combination for painful knee osteoarthritis. *N Engl J Med* 23;354(8):795-808, Feb 2006.

[94] Herrero-Beaumont G, Ivorra JA, Del Carmen Trabado M, et al. Glucosamine sulfate in the treatment of knee osteoarthritis symptoms: a randomized, double-blind, placebo-controlled study using acetaminophen as a side comparator. *Arthritis Rheum* 56(2):555-67, Feb 2007.

95 Bingham, P, A Progress Report on the Analysis of Tumour-Cell Specific Killing by the Garnett McKeen Laboratory lipoic acid/palladium complex.

Chapter 12 – The Patient Histories

antacids that he used to take for many years which contain aluminium as a preservative. Hair mineral analysis is a good tool to use to determine whether there are toxic metals stored in the body.[96] Further hair testing have recently showed that the level of aluminium, lead and other toxic metals had began to reduce considerably with the help of the HMD.®

By the time Mr. P had completed his Candida protocol[97,98] he was feeling extremely well – he was full of joy at not having any pain in his body, he had plenty of energy to do 2-3 hours of non-stop gardening, spend a few hours fishing in the early morning hours, as well as swim in the sea regularly. He has stopped all medicinal drugs, including the anti-inflammatories that he we was taking for 25 years for the osteoarthritis of the knee and may have been one of the key factors that triggered the oesophageal cancer. He has no further arthritic pains and the difficult urine infection has cleared up, probably caused by the systemic Candida and his chronic hypochlorhydria and other digestive problems have gone completely and he is basically eating within a healthy, optimal diet.

Recent blood tests have shown that his iron levels have risen to the normal level, probably as a result of his stomach now being able to absorb the iron, vitamin B12 and intrinsic factor due to the increased production of hydrochloric acid. His liver and kidney function tests such as SGOT, SGPT, ALP, urea and creatinine are all within normal levels, and so are all his mineral levels, including zinc.

It is also worth reiterating that his Heart Rate Variability (HRV) score had improved in about one year from 8,6 to 5,4 – this is a dramatic improvement in the functioning of all the physiological systems, as well as his adaptation reserve or his ability to cope with stressful situations. This is reflected by the fact that he is capable of 2-3 hours of gardening, getting up at dawn to go fishing, as well as swimming in the sea for an hour or so.

Patient's own account:

My favourite hobby is fishing. I am 79 years old and I still enjoy waking up very early in the morning and go for fishing. One day, in April 2006,

---

[96] http://www.detoxmetals.com/THMA.html
97 Georgiou, GJ. Scourge of the 21st Century: Systemic Candidiasis. *British Naturopathic Journal*, Vol. 25, No. 1, 2008.
98 Georgiou, GJ. Treating Systemic Candidiasis. *British Naturopathic Journal*, Vol. 25, No. 2, 2008.

while I was fishing I ate some cheese cake and all of a sudden it was very painful. This pain was getting worse for the next 2-3 months.

So, I planned an endoscopy in Cyprus and I was diagnosed with gastro-oesophageal reflux and oesophageal adenocarcinoma. I decided to have the surgery done in the following August of that year in U.K. I have to say, that I had a pre-operative chemotherapy before the resection of the tumour. It was a locally advanced tumour which had spread through the wall of the oesophagus with local lymph node involvement. Fortunately, it was an early stage tumour blocking my oesophagus while eating, without any significant perforation.

Even though I felt much better after the surgery, intermittent diarrhoeas accompanied me after the surgery, urinary tract infections and urinary frequency. Most of the times when I urinated, it was very painful. I took antibiotics and there was no improvement. In fact I got worse!

Despite the fact that I am a very active, energetic person and above all very positive, these symptoms made me feel weak, tired, lethargic and made me feel very sad for losing my energy. Added to this, I have osteoarthritis problem in one knee, which can be very painful, so I used to take so many anti-inflammatory pills and as a consequence I injured my stomach and it started getting painful too. My diarrhoeas went on without finding a solution and my daughter insisted to visit the DaVinci Natural Health Center while I was next in Cyprus.

We booked an appointment and I began a bespoke treatment protocol based on the diagnostic information that was gathered by Dr. Georgiou. I started with a detox diet – to my pleasant surprise my diarrhoeas disappeared shortly thereafter! I couldn't believe that this nightmare had finally come to an end. My diet has been improved dramatically and I am also taking natural products for osteoarthritis. My knee hurts very slightly now (in 2008), and my stomach doesn't hurt anymore. I feel so much better, I gained back my energy levels and I started doing things again like before the surgery. I have to say that I had a dramatic improvement of my quality of life up to 75%.

Now in 2009, I can honestly say that most of my symptoms have gone completely – I feel full of energy, my stomach and gut are relaxed and I can eat most things with no problems, the painful knees and joints have gone and I have also stopped taking all the anti-inflammatories that I was taking for over 25 years – I think this is where my cancer came from initially with all these drugs eating away my stomach. I am thoroughly enjoying life to the full and doing all the things that I ever wanted to do such as fishing, gardening and swimming in the beautiful Mediterranean Sea on the island of Aphrodite.

Dr Georgiou's final comments on Mr. P:

Mr. P is truly a charming man who has a lot of charisma and a joyous, positive attitude to life – this spiritual state may be one of the primary reasons why he is still with us. Even at the age of 80 he was able to follow treatment protocols to a tee and never complained about anything, always trying to see the positive side of things.

Many a true scientist has commented from way back that the digestive system is the culprit for the development of many chronic diseases. Here is a case where a man was taking anti-inflammatories (NSAIDS) – the last one that he was taking was Diclomax. One of the side effects of most NSAIDS is: "NSAIDs can occasionally cause serious side effects on the gut, such as ulceration, bleeding or perforation of the stomach or intestinal lining. This type of side effect is more likely to occur in elderly people."[99]

This constant irritation of the stomach lining by these drugs will adversely affect the stomach to produce sufficient amounts of hydrochloric acid – this is called hypochlorhydria (deficiency of hydrochloric acid production). This continued over many years which did not allow the proper digestion of protein concentrates or the absorption of essential minerals and vitamins such as iron, vitamin B12, calcium and intrinsic factor.

Over many years, the hypochlorhydria will develop Gastroesophageal reflux disease (GERD), also called acid reflux disease, which occurs when liquid from the stomach backs up (regurgitates) into the oesophagus – the need for the stomach to keep food for much longer periods in its attempt to digest it will cause fermentation and gaseous production which will place stress on the sphincter muscles at the entrance and exit to the stomach. This liquid may contain stomach acids and bile. In some cases, the regurgitated stomach liquid can cause inflammation (oesophagitis), irritation, and damage to the oesophagus.[100] This inflammation and

---

99 British National Formulary: https://www.medicinescomplete.com
100 Marshall RE, Anggiansah A, Owen WA, et al. The relationship between acid and bile reflux and symptoms in gastro-oesophageal reflux disease. *Gut.* 40(2):182-7, Feb 1997.

damage to the lining of the oesophagus sets up the conditions required for cancer cells to proliferate.

To add insult to injury, he was also taking many antacids and H-proton inhibitors for stomach problem which only help to minimize the production of stomach acids, or neutralize them, making the patient feel better but greatly aggravating the hypochlorhydria driving it into achlorhydria. The antacids usually contain lots of toxic aluminium which is a further cause of cancer cells proliferating. According to a Swedish study, people with long term acid reflux are at least 5 times more likely to develop adenocarcinoma of the oesophagus than average, whether they have Barrett's oesophagus or not.

Removing a part of the oesophagus and stomach because of the cancer did not really address the underlying causes – now that the hypochlorhydria has been eradicated, as well as many of the heavy metals, and his body is nourished with the correct nutrients that it requires he is functioning symptom-free and enjoying life at the ripe age of 80. I bow to Mr. P for his determination to get to the bottom of things, his self-discipline to complete his treatment protocols and above all his joyous outlook to life and his willingness to live life to the full.

Case 10, Mrs. P, age 48

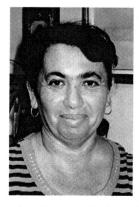

Main presenting problem: Sterility

Medical diagnosis:

Mrs. P had suffered from gynaecological problems for longer than 22 years, and headaches for more than 10 years.

She had seen a total of 5 gynaecologists who tried contraceptive pills, IV hormonal injections to stimulate ovulation, benign, fibrotic endometrial atrophic polyp with fibrosis, which was surgically removed in 2000 with the suggestion that she have a total hysterectomy that she refused. Six months later she had a D & C with histopathological analysis that found nothing abnormal. Blood hormonal assays showed high levels of testosterone that was probably responsible for her hirsuitism on arms and legs.

Polycystic ovaries were diagnosed by ultrasound scan in 1999 but no treatment was given for this. The sonography report read: "both ovaries have multiple (at least 15 on each side) small follicular cysts with diameters not exceeding 5 mm.

Her periods were very irregular with cycles ranging from 40-60 days.

She also suffered from frequent migraines and chronic fatigue.

Holistic diagnosis:

Mrs. P came to me not so much for the sterility problem as she was already 45 years old and as they had been trying for over 25 years to have more children, she had given up on any chance of getting pregnant.

She was more concerned about her increasing weight, her hisuitism and headaches that were getting worse and were more and more frequent.

Therefore, only a few tests were ran and the IDEL Diagnostic Programme was not implemented in its entirety. The VEGA food intolerance test showed a number of food intolerances such as wheat, caffeine, potatoes, tomatoes, peppers and aubergines, eggs, bananas and sugar.

VEGA testing also showed systemic mycelial, pathogenic Candidiasis.

Iridology indicated cervical and lumbar subluxations (there was pain in both these areas), a dark solaris line running through the hypothalamus-pituitary axis indicating disturbance in this important endocrine organ, irritation marks on the thyroid, liver and ovaries, as well as a pterygium on the sclera indicating fat metabolism problems related to liver stress.

Her underarm temperature readings, taken for 10-minutes every morning (Barne's Temperature Test) indicated low reading averaging about 36° C (normal range between 36.5 – 37). This indicated subclinical hypothyroidism with low metabolic rate.

Mrs. P was a very anxious, impatient, worrying-type person who felt that she should always be on the go.

Holistic treatments:
The main focus of her holistic treatment was to help balance the endocrine system. This was achieved by using Su Jok acupuncture on the basic correspondence system of the hand on the corresponding points of the ovaries, uterus, pituitary, hypothalamus and adrenals – there were 5 treatments in one month using micro needles and magnet stars and seeds in the evening (see chapter 9).

In addition, she undertook a 15-day alkaline detoxification diet with fruits and vegetables, freshly made vegetable juices, herbal teas and plenty of mineral water (see chapter 4). She also abstained from eating foods that she was intolerant to.

As soon as the detoxification was complete she began the DaVinci Candidia protocol (see chapter 5).

About two months after completing the DaVinic Candida Protocol her husband phoned me at the Centre elated at the fact that his wife was now pregnant, confirmed by urine tests at the gynaecologist. She went through a trouble-free pregnancy and a natural birth with no complications whatsoever.

Patient's own account:
My husband was an old patient of Dr. Georgiou and the DaVinci Natural Health Centre, so when he saw me suffering with headaches and worrying about my weight, he suggested that we go see Dr. Georgiou.

After a few initial tests he put me on a detoxification diet with fruits and vegetables, including freshly made carrot juices. This lasted 15 days and I began to feel very well as a lot of the bloating I had began to diminish. I also felt a lot more energetic and had a renewed interest in my house and family.

After the detoxification diet I began a treatment to clear up the candida problem that I was diagnosed with. This lasted 3 months and meant keeping off sugar and yeast products throughout this time. During this treatment I noticed that the hair on my arms and legs began getting lighter and thinner and slowly began falling away. I was really amazed as I had this problem for over a decade and it was embarrassing as the hair was very dark and thick.

Given that I was seeing the results of this treatment, I persevered and reached the end – I also felt very good, lost a considerable amount of weight, my energy levels were excellent and generally people were commenting on how good I looked.

What I was not expecting was to get pregnant at the age of 45 years old, after trying to get pregnant for more than 25 years! This was such a pleasant surprise that I remember wanting to call Dr. Georgiou from the gynaecologists office, such was my elation! I am absolutely certain that Dr. Georgiou's treatments were responsible for me getting pregnant as I had seen 5 gynaecologists over the 25 years of trying and had received so many different treatments, but nothing seemed to help.

We now have a beautiful 4-year old son who is our pride and joy and has changed our lives miraculously. May Dr. Georgiou's work be blessed forever, and may he help other women in my predicament.

Dr Georgiou's final comments on Mr. A:

This is again another interesting case where the causative factors were not investigated, but only the symptoms were suppressed by surgery or drugs. When one is faced with a uterine polyp, one needs to ask the question what caused it? The same question needs to be asked of the hormonal system – why was it so imbalanced?

In my clinical experience, seeing a number of women with fertility issues, there is not one case that I have seen that did not have systemic, pathogenic Candidiasis. This is probably not a coincidence as candida can be very virulent causing a wide array of symptoms and syndromes.[101]

Candida produces 79 different toxins[102,103] known to wreak havoc with the immune system.[104] A long list of potential symptoms associated with candida overgrowth include depression, anxiety attacks, mood swings, lack of concentration, drowsiness, poor memory, headaches, insomnia, fatigue, bloating, constipation, bladder infections, menstrual cramps, vaginal itching, muscle and joint swelling, pain, hypothyroidism, and skin problems.[105] She had a number of these symptoms.

However, it is rarely understood that candida also contributes to hormonal problems. A candida waste product produces a false estrogen, which tricks the body into thinking it has produced adequate levels, signaling a reduction of its own estrogen.[106] Similar messages can also be sent to the thyroid, reducing thyroxin production and initiating or worsening a hypothyroid problem.

Elevated estrogen levels also increase vaginal candidiasis incidence.[107,108] Estrogen will literally feed candida growth, which is why birth control pills and estrogen replacement therapy put women at a greater risk of

101 Vartivarian SE. Virulence properties and nonimmune pathogenic mechanisms of fungi. *Clin Infect Dis* 14(suppl 1) :30–36, 1992.
102 Georgiou, GJ. Scourge of the 21st Century: Systemic Candidiasis. *British Naturopathic Journal*, Vol. 25, No. 1, 2008.
103 Georgiou, GJ. Treatment of Systemic Candidiasis. *British Naturopathic Journal*, Vol. 25, No.2, 2008.
104 Iwata, K., and Yamamota, Y. Glycoprotein Toxins Produced by Candida Albicans. Proceedings of the Fourth international Conference on the Mycoses, June, 1977, PAHO Scientific Publication #356. and Iwata, K., Recent Advances in Medical and Veterinary Mycology, University of Tokyo Press, 1977.
105 Crandall M. The pathogenetic significance of intestinal Candida colonization. *Int J Hyg Environ Health* 207; 79-81, 2004.
106 Zhao, X., Malloy, PJ, Ardies, CM and Feldman, D. Oestrogen-binding protein in Candida albicans: antibody development and cellular localization by electron immunocytochemistry. *Microbiology*, 141:2685-2692, 1995.
107 Cheng G, Yeater KM, Hoyer LL. Cellular and Molecular Biology of Candida albicans Estrogen Response. *Eukaryotic Cell.* 5(1) :180-191, Jan 2006.
108 Zhang X, Essmann M, Burt ET, Larsen B. Estrogen effects on Candida albicans: a potential virulence-regulating mechanism. *J Infect Dis.* 181(4):1441-6, Apr 2000.

developing candida.[109] This woman had taken many different hormonal treatments over a number of years.

It is always heartening to see a woman at this age – 45 years old – give birth to a healthy and intelligent young boy after 25 years of trying.

109 Crook WG. The Yeast Connection and the Woman . 3 rd ed. Jackson TN: Professional Books; 1995.

Case No. 11, Mrs. P, age 42

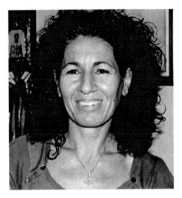

Main presenting problem: Psoriasis, vaginal discharge, constipation.

Medical diagnosis:

Mrs. P had been to 3 different dermatologists for her chronic psoriasis and all had confirmed the diagnosis of psoriasis. They had all said that this was incurable and that only cortisone creams would keep it under control.

Blood tests had shown an ESR of 17 (<20) which is borderline high for inflammation in the body. Her blood glucose was 107 mg/dl (65-100), which was borderline high. Total cholesterol levels were 231 mg/dl (<200 desirable), which was borderline high. LDL cholesterol was 148 mg/dl (<130).

Holistic diagnosis:

I have seen many cases of psoriasis in clinical practice but I can honestly say that this case was one of the worst that I have ever seen – there was heavy blotches of psoriasis on the face, forehead, back, front, legs and arms – literally the whole body was covered with a lot of pruritis.

VEGA food intolerance testing showed that she was intolerant to wheat, milk and lactose, chicken, pork, potatoes, tomatoes, aubergines and peppers, caffeine and the cruciferous vegetables. A blood analysis test of food intolerances had confirmed many of these, but also identified other foods that she never ate such as cola nuts, cashew nuts, soya beans, pineapple, as well as identifying yeast.

VEGA and ART testing confirmed the presence of pathogenic, mycelial systemic Candidiasis – it is highly probable that she had been infested with this candida for many years as she had recurrent vaginal discharge and thrush over many years. She had also taken a number of antibiotics and cortisone over the years.

Iris analysis showed a very murky iris which is an indication of chronic toxicity over the years – the fact that she was also dehydrated only helped to exacerbate this and maintained her constipation which further added to the toxicity. All the detoxification organs were irritated and toxic – kidneys, liver, gut, lymphatics – there were irritation marks on the thyroid and lungs. There were also spinal subluxations identified at the cervical and lumbar levels, with corresponding pain in these areas.

Hair Tissue Mineral Analysis had shown that she had a poor mineral profile with low levels of potassium, copper, zinc, manganese, selenium, cobalt and molybdenum. There were also traces of circulating uranium-238, arsenic, mercury and cadmium.

She was also extremely dehydrated, only drinking 2-3 glasses per day in temperatures of 40 degrees centrigrade with lots of sweating in her daily work.

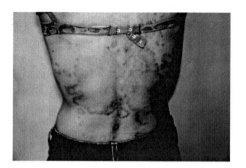 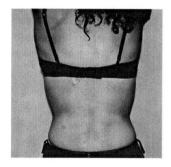

Psoriasis – before treatment (left) and after treatment (right)

Holistic treatments:

The first thing that was implemented with Mrs. P was a 15-day alkaline detoxification protocol to help balance her internal milieu and flush out a number of toxins. She also also completed a parasite cleanse for 14 days, as part of her job was to handle meat from different animals and the likelihood of having parasites were high – oxyuren had appeared on resonance testing.

By the time she had completed this cleanse she reported a 50% improvement of her psoriasis on all parts of her body, but particularly on her face. She began the Davinci Candida Protocol immediately after the detoxification (see chapter 5).

She was also given a multivitamin formula, omega 3,6 and 9 fatty acids, antioxidants, multimineral formula, zinc and a herbal formula to help the drainage of toxins through the detoxification organs.

Two weeks into the Candida protocol her vaginal discharge had much improved and her psoriasis was getting noticeably better by the day. Just over a month into the Candida protocol she reported that her psoriasis had improved by 70%.

By the time she had completed her Candida protocol over a 3-month period, her psoriasis had cleared completely from her face and body, with only very small spots visible. Her vaginal discharge had also disappeared, even though this was a daily occurrence.

Patient's own account:
I found the Davinci Centre through a sister at the hospital that I knew – she saw how desperate I was one day while visiting the dermatologist and understood the severity of my problem. I told her that I was very desperate and near suicidal with the spreading psoriasis that was disrupting my life on all levels as I no longer wanted to go out and socialize any more.

I had suffered with the psoriasis now for over 4 years and it seemed to be spreading all over my body, but the fact that it was all over my face was the worst as I could not cover this in any way.

I took the sisters advice and went to see Dr. Georgiou – he carefully took my history and immediately asked how much water I was drinking. I told him about 2-3 glasses per day. His eyes lit up and said: "you are losing 9-10 glasses of water per day and drinking two. You do not need to be a mathematician to realize that your body is in desperate need of water. Your major detoxification organs are having a tough time detoxifying and all those toxins are now showing on your skin."

I thought that he made a lot of sense and wondered why the other doctors had not told me something similar – no other doctor had asked me how much water I was drinking.

After confirming this through the iridology he did, as well as finding various foods that I was allergic to, as well as candida, he said that we had a lot of work to do over the next three months or so.

He suggested that I begin cleaning my body immediately by eating "like a bunny rabbit" was his exact words. Even though I liked my sweets and biscuits, I was so intrigued that I followed his instructions to a tee. It was not long before I noticed the psoriasis drying on my skin and flaking off –

every day there was an improvement. I was encouraged to continue with the candida treatment.

By the time I had completed the candida treatment which took 3 months, I found that my skin had cleared completely, there was literally not a spot to be found, accept a couple of very small ones behind my ears which flare up a little when I am stressed.

I am ever so grateful to this form of healing that uses gentle remedies and really works as I am a living testimonial to this. I have already began to attract attention from people that see me now completely cured and wonder how I managed it, given that I used to tell them that I was a victim of the disease and that it was incurable.

Dr Georgiou's final comments on Mrs. P:

All symptoms have underlying causes, including psoriasis. This was probably one of the worst psoriasis cases that I have seen – when investigated, it was found that she had a severe underlying systemic Candidiasis, multiple mineral deficiencies, heavy metal toxicity, food intolerances causing inflammation in the body, constipation related to dehydration and poor eating habits that made her even more toxic, overloading and congesting the liver and causing the skin to actively take over the detoxification function.

Once all these causative factors were cleared up her skin cleared and the psoriasis went into remission. She has maintained her good health for over a year now without any further psoriasis or other health issues.

Case No. 12, Mr. P, aged 36

Main presenting problem: Multiple sclerosis

Medical diagnosis:

Multiple sclerosis diagnosed in 1998 with three separate episodes – the last was in March 2007. This last crisis (myalgic symptoms of left hand) was a couple of months after removing 9 amalgams with no chelation protocol or protection taken during the amalgam removal. During attacks he receives Medrol (cortisone) I.V. as well as orally.

MRI of brain (6.11.04) showed multiple foci of high signal intensity on the FLAIR and T2W images in the subcortical and deep white matter of both cerebral hemispheres. There are also multiple similar lesions within the corpus collosum. Slight subtle focus within the right optic nerve just before the optic chiasma. The conclusion was demyelinating disease with further neurological assessment recommended.

A further MRI (12.4.07) showed on both sides, periventricular, in the corpus collosum, and mainly on the right side in the subcortical white matter, different sized (from 2mm to 8mm) hyperintense lesions. The conclusion was that these findings suggest inactive multiple sclerosis.

He had a history of allergic rhinitis, irritable bowel syndrome, acid reflux and headaches. He has been receiving the flu vaccine once yearly.

Serum magnesium levels low when had the last attack at 1.9 mg/dl (1.9-2.5).

Holistic diagnosis:

The IDEL Diagnostic Programme came up with a number of findings, such as:

VEGA testing and ART showed organ imbalances in the cerebrum, maxillary sinuses, teeth (right side), thyroid, myocardium, adrenals, spleen, pancreas, jejunum, colon and prostate. Prioritization testing showed the pancreas to be the primary organ blocking the autonomic nervous system. There were two scar foci detected – one on the left palm and the other on the lower hair line, due to hair transplant operation. There was also a tooth focus detected on the large intestine meridian. Panoramic

X-ray showed one root canal filling, but no obvious signs of cysts or abscesses.

VEGA also showed food intolerances such as wheat, lactose and milk products, pork, chicken, citrus fruits, sugar, caffeine, onions, garlic and leeks. Wheat was a major food blocking regulation or the ANS.

He also tested positive for geopathic stress, electromagnetic stress (uses computer for 8 hours per day at work), vaccination stress, viruses (coxsackie and HBV), Systemic Candidiasis, vitamin, mineral, trace element and enzyme deficiencies.

Iridology showed hypochlorhydria with an irritated stomach lining, thyroid, pancreas, with lacunas indicating an inherited weakness on the left kidney, heart and exocrine part of the pancreas. There were also subluxations at the cervical and lumbar levels (he has pains in both these areas with diagnosed osteophytes. There was also a general level of toxicity.

Darkfield microscopy study of live blood showed a non-congested picture with viable WBC's, some fermentation and some free chondroits. There was nothing remarkable about his blood as he had already began to take supplements and change his diet before seeing him.

A urine pre-post provocation test using the natural chelator HMD™ as the provocation agent, showed high levels of circulating mercury which increased further upon provocation - 8.59 ug/g (<3 ug/l). Hair Tissue Mineral Analysis at a later stage showed a cocktail of heavy metals such as uranium, arsenic, mercury, cadmium and aluminium in circulating blood. There were also low levels of copper, manganese and cobalt.

Heart Rate Variability (HRV) testing showed increased sympathetic activity over parasympathetic with moderately reduced physiological functioning and adaptation reserves – his score was 10.5 whereas a perfect score would be 1.1.

Holistic treatments:
He began a 15-day alkaline detoxification diet with fruit, vegetables and juices, followed by a gallbladder and liver flush and a parasite cleanse using black walnut tincture, wormwood and cloves. He also began taking the HMD™ Ultimate Detox protocol immediately, with the Organic

Lavage and Chlorella, in order to begin chelating the heavy metals (see chapter 7).

He also began the DaVinci Candida Protocol on 14th October 2007 and completed this successfully by the following January (see chapter 5).

Supplements given included Omega 3, 6 and 9, the Dr. Klenner protocol[110] using high doses of vitamin B-complex, vitamin B6, B1, B2, B3, B5, magnesium, and coenzyme Q10.

PAPIMI has helped his crises on a number of occasions.

Patient's own account

During the year 1998, I woke up one morning and I was really shocked that I could not see anything from the right eye. I had a complete loss of vision of my right eye. I visited a doctor and I was diagnosed with optic neuritis at the age of 25. I had an MRI scan and a fluid sample of my cerebrospinal fluid using a lumbar puncture that was sent to England for testing. They could not diagnose 100% whether this was Multiple Sclerosis or not. Soon I began a treatment with corticosteroids for three consecutive days. I used in total 3000 mg corticosteroids these three days. Fortunately, I could see again, but the same situation occurred again 10 months later and I used corticosteroids again.

Until the year 2004, I had no other intense symptoms and my life went on normally. I experienced headaches, my energy levels were very low and my eating habits were very bad. By then, I was 31 and unfortunately this year I had a relapse with optic neuritis in my right eye again. I used for the third time the treatment with corticosteroids, in order to be able to see again. I decided to repeat the MRI scan this year and it was then, when I was diagnosed with Multiple Sclerosis with certainty since plaques clearly appeared in my brain tissue.

My neurologist suggested no other treatment by that time, since he said to me that my disease is incurable and I just had to live with it. From then and onwards, I was under so much stress, because I did not want to accept what my doctor was saying about my disease. I refused to accept that it is incurable and that at some point in the future I would have to take

---

110 Klenner, FR. Response of Peripheral and Central Nerve Pathology to Mega-Doses of the Vitamin B-Complex and Other Metabolites. *Journal of Applied Nutrition*, 1973.

interferon, because of the relapses. I read that there are so many side-effects as far as interferon is concerned with minor improvement of the disease and I decided that I would never take it.

Then, despite my psychological stress and disappointment from doctors, I was motivated to find out whether there was another way to deal with my problem. I had a feeling that there must be a way to deal with it. I started searching the internet for an alternative. I started looking into the field of Natural Medicine and during the year 2005, I started taking natural supplements on my own, ordering them from the Internet. I changed my eating habits, I improved my nutrition and I felt slightly better. I also had gastroesophageal reflux and it was markedly improved after changing my eating habits.

From December 2006 until February 2007, I removed 9 amalgam fillings, but I used a recommended protocol with natural medicine supplements before I removed them. In April 2007, I experienced the third relapse. My spinal cord was now affecting me. I had complete numbness on my left hand. There was damage on the 5th cervical spinal nerve and osteophytes started to grow. The relapse persisted for a few months and I used cortisone three times until August 2007 where I again took 72 mg of cortisone and my hand was improved leaving some sensory loss.

I then first visited the Da Vinci Natural Health center in August 2007. I had an extensive series of tests called the IDEL Diagnostic program which is designed to identify and eliminate the causes of my health problems. After Dr Georgiou completed the testing procedure I was surprised to find plenty of problems that we had to deal with.

As I began the treatment protocol, beginning with a comprehensive detoxification programme, followed by the Candida protocol, I felt a huge difference. Using PAPIMI from the very first time I also felt a great deal of difference. My progression was interesting and I improved over time.

Because my job is very stressful, this is not very helpful. Since August 2007, my next relapse was June 2008 but not so severe. I did not use cortisone that time but I used PAPIMI instead to deal with the relapse. Whenever I feel my arm going numb and pain in my neck I now use the PAPIMI and I no longer need corticosteroids – this is an incredible finding as the side-effects of high-dose cortisone are many.

Following a few PAPIMI sessions the pain gradually goes away and I feel that I can live a normal life again without using any medication which would not really improve my disease and would cause a serious number of side-effects. My progression is promising since I have managed to stabilise my condition using basically three steps: change of eating habits following the recommendations of Dr Georgiou, taking food supplements, and using the PAPIMI whenever I feel I need it. I feel very energetic, less stressed and very positive because this works and I experience it every day. Thank you to the DaVinci Natural Health Center and Dr. Georgiou who have really helped to change my life and give me hope for a normal life, something that was not forthcoming from the medical profession.

Dr. Georgiou's final comments on Mr. P

Mr. P was really an excellent example of how high levels of toxicity, particularly from removal of mercury amalgams can cause havoc to the nervous system.

In addition, this has also been a test case for demonstrating the power of the Pulsing Electromagnetic Device called the PAPIMI in alleviating MS crises that would normally have required high-dose cortisone. In July 2008 he developed muscle weakness of the left arm, shoulder and neck due to high stress levels at work. After only 4-5 PAPIMI sessions all these symptoms had reduced to more or less zero in a period of less than 3 weeks. Under normal circumstances, crises like this would take much longer to overcome using high-dose cortisone with all its known side effects.

There are many causative factors involved in the pathogenesis of MS; the cocktail of heavy metals, including mercury which has a natural affinity for degenerating the neurofibrils of the nervous system – there is an excellent video made at the University of Calgary, Faculty of Medicine - Department of Physiology and Biophysics.[111]

It clearly shows how brain neurons growing in a petri dish in the laboratory can be destroyed so quickly when a very small amount of mercury is introduced - the brain cells literally disappear in front of your eyes!

---

111 http://movies.commons.ucalgary.ca/mercury

Digestive issues are also another major issue in the pathogenesis of any disease as the 40 or so vital nutrients required daily by the body are not available, so the body enters a downward spiral of deficiencies and biochemical imbalances that will over time lead to chronic, degenerative disease. Addressing the digestive issues is a crucial part of any restorative programme. The Klenner protocol using high-dose B-complex vitamins was also another important step in helping the myelin sheath to restore itself.

Mr. P is now generally well and stable even though he works in a high-stress job with lots of daily responsibilities. There have been no further crises for the last year, even though he maintains his health with an optimal diet and maintenance sessions on the PAPIMI every month.

Case No. 13, Mr. A, age 64 years

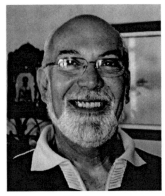

Main presenting problem: Diabetes Type II, Hypertension, High Uric Acid levels

Medical diagnosis

Diagnosed as diabetes mellitus type II about three years ago by his medical doctor as his blood glucose levels in January 2008 were 122 (80-100) and could reach levels of 160 or more. Mr. A. was not taking medication for diabetes. His hypertension reached levels of 170/95 and was diagnosed 12 years ago – he has been taking antihypertensive medication ever since. Uric acid levels have also been elevated for some time – a January 2008 blood analysis showed 7.86mg/dl, when the upper limit is 7.0.

Holistic diagnosis

Iridology showed deficiencies in minerals and vitamins, cervical and lumbar subluxations, blood sugar fluctuations, severe lymphatic congestion, liver congestion and irritation with a general toxic load.

VEGA food intolerance testing showed the following food intolerances that are all capable of causing inflammation: wheat, lactose and all dairy, pork, chicken, sugar, nightshade family of vegetables (potatoes, tomatoes, peppers and aubergines) and caffeine.

He was also found to have systemic Candidiasis after extensive abuse of antiobiotics over a number of years. When Candida is identified, all yeast-related products will aggravate this condition such as yeast, mushrooms, alcohol products and vinegar products.

Hair Tissue Mineral Analysis has shown a general deficiency of many minerals and trace elements such as potassium, copper, iron, manganese, chromium and cobalt. Many of these are critical for insulin production. There were also high levels of circulating arsenic, also known to destroy the pancreas, as well as mercury, cadmium and aluminium.

Testing using Professor Rothbart's protocol showed that he had a Primus Metatarsus Supinatus foot type, otherwise known as "Rothbart's foot."

This can cause gross disturbances in posture as well as causing spinal subluxations with all their neurological consequences. This was adjusted using patented proprioreceptor foot soles.

Holistic treatments

He began an alkaline detoxification diet with fruit, raw and cooked vegetables with vegetable juices and soups over a 15-day period. In the first month he lost 7 kg (15 lbs) and was feeling a lot more energetic with stamina – his morning blood pressure dropped from 170/95 to 140/85 during this period. His morning glucose levels had dropped from 120 to 100.

A month later his blood pressure had dropped to 120/65 and he decided that he was going to terminate his blood pressure medication, along with the aspirin, which was substituted with vitamin E and omega 3 fatty acids. This he did and his blood pressure remained completely stable throughout, even though he has been taking anti-hypertensives for 12 years consecutively. Probably the main reason for this is that the high levels of inflammation and free radicals and lipid peroxidation products decreased with the detoxification.

Celery seed tea has helped to alleviate the joint pains related to the high uric acid levels.

Shortly after the detox he began the DaVinci Candida protocol (see chapter 5) using a variety of different herbal, nutritional, homeopathic and isopathic remedies – this protocol lasted 3 months. At the end of the Candida treatment his glucose levels were averaging 110 without diabetic medication, which he stopped about a month prior.

Mr. A was given a formula that contained Goat's Rue, cinnamon (CinSulin®), bitter melon, quercetin and vanadyl sulfate - all have been studied for their ability to lower blood sugar, increase insulin sensitivity and protect against the damaging effects of high blood sugar.

Galega officinalis (Goat's rue) has been used with success as an insulin-controlling agent. Goat's rue is rich in guanidine, its hypoglycemic component. The guanidine in goat's rue improves insulin sensitivity and is used to support the health of type 1 and 2 diabetics. Galega officinalis (20% guanylhydrazine) – is a botanical source for the life extension drug metformin (GlucoPhage – the drug that he was previously taking) which can decrease the formation of advanced glycosylation end products.

Goat's rue causes a long-lasting reduction of blood sugar content in rats and an increase in carbohydrate tolerance. This herb lowers blood sugar in both normal and diabetic humans.[112]

Cinnamon is another blood-sugar supporting nutrient that improves insulin sensitivity during in vitro, animal and human studies. Cinnamon reduces mean fasting serum glucose by 18-29 percent in subjects with type 2 diabetes after 40 days of daily consumption of 1-6 grams of cinnamon. Furthermore, subjects with the metabolic syndrome who consume cinnamon have been shown to have improved fasting blood glucose, systolic blood pressure, percentage body fat and increased lean body mass compared with the placebo group.[113]

Cinnamon works especially well when combined with chromium, a mineral that has been found to improve insulin sensitivity (see footnote 111 below). Chromium also is helpful in reducing carbohydrate cravings.

Bitter melon is another botanical that has reduced insulin resistance in animals, partly through its ability to improve the function of insulin receptors in the liver. It also has been widely researched in animal studies for its ability to improve glucose and insulin tolerance.[114]

Quercetin, another important component of any blood-sugar supporting formula, is a flavonoid - recent research is unveiling additional properties of quercetin, including its ability to protect against oxidative stress in rodents with experimental diabetes and to prevent damage to the insulin-producing beta cells of the pancreas.[115,116] It also strongly inhibits aldose

---

[112] Petricic J, Kalodera Z. Galegin in the goats rue herb: its toxicity, antidiabetic activity and content determination. Acta Pharm Jugosl. 32(3):219-23, 1982.

[113] Anderson RA. Chromium and polyphenols from cinnamon improve insulin sensitivity. Proc Nutr Soc. 67(1):48-53, Feb 2008.

114 Nerurkar PV, Lee YK, Motosue M, Adeli K, Nerurkar VR. Momordica charantia (bitter melon) reduces plasma apolipoprotein B-100 and increases hepatic insulin receptor substrate and phosphoinositide-3 kinase interactions. Br J Nutr. 5;1-9, Mar 2008.

[115] Kim EK, Kwon KB, Song MY, Han MJ, Lee JH, Lee YR, Lee JH, Ryu DG, Park BH, Park JW. Flavonoids protect against cytokine-induced pancreatic beta-cell damage through suppression of nuclear factor kappaB activation. *Pancreas.* 35(4):e1-9, Nov 2007.

[116] Coskun O, Kanter M, Korkmaz A, Oter S. Quercetin, a flavonoid antioxidant, prevents and protects streptozotocin-induced oxidative stress and beta-cell damage in rat pancreas. *Pharmacol Res.* 51(2):117-23, Feb 2005.

reductase, an enzyme which converts blood glucose into sorbitol, which is strongly implicated in the complications of diabetes. Quercetin also protects insulin-producing cells in the pancreas by blocking the genetic expression of cytokines and enzymes that are important mediators of inflammatory responses.[117]

Vanadyl Sulfate can work with goat's rue, bitter melon, and quercetin to help support healthy blood sugar levels. In one of the newest studies on this mineral, it protected against damaging changes that occurred in the aortas of rats with experimental diabetes.[118] In obese humans with diabetes, vanadyl sulfate may improve a defect in insulin signaling specific to type 2 diabetes.[119]

Bitter Melon extract (Momordica charantia) can lower blood glucose without increasing insulin. In one study, bitter melon significantly improved glucose tolerance in diabetics by almost 54%.[120] Also added was Pyridoxine (Vitamin B-6) as it protects against the development of diabetic neuropathy and other complications of diabetes by inhibiting the glycosylation of proteins.

N-acetyl cysteine (NAC) - is a derivative of the sulfhydryl amino acid cysteine. Cysteine is converted into the important antioxidant, glutathione. Cysteine, in fact, is considered the rate-limiting factor in the production of glutathione. NAC has both cytoprotective and antioxidant effects and prevents complications of diabetes. NAC also inhibits the activation of a key pro-inflammatory molecule called nuclear factor-kappa beta.[121] In addition, animal studies show that NAC inhibits the blood glucose surge

117 Zunino SJ, Storms DH, Stephensen CB. Diets rich in polyphenols and vitamin A inhibit the development of type I autoimmune diabetes in nonobese diabetic mice. *J Nutr.* 137(5):1216-21, May 2007.

[118] Akgün-Dar K, Bolkent S, Yanardag R, Tunali S. Vanadyl sulfate protects against streptozotocin-induced morphological and biochemical changes in rat aorta. *Cell Biochem Funct.* 25(6):603-9, Nov-Dec 2007.

[119] Halberstam M, Cohen N, Shlimovich P, Rossetti L, Shamoon H. Oral vanadyl sulfate improves insulin sensitivity in NIDDM but not in obese nondiabetic subjects. *Diabetes.* 1996.

120 Welihinda J, Karunanayake EH, Sheriff MH, Jayasinghe KS. Effect of Momordica charantia on the glucose tolerance in maturity onset diabetes. *J Ethnopharmacol.* 17(3):277-82, Sept 1986.

[121] Ho E, Chen G, Bray TM. Supplementation of N-acetylcysteine inhibits NFkappaB activation and protects against alloxan-induced diabetes in CD-1 mice. *FASEB J.* 13(13):1845-54, 1999.

and weight gain that occurs after consuming a sucrose-rich diet,[122] while also protecting against oxidative stress, a major factor in diabetic complications.

Vitamin E - is the major fat-soluble antioxidant that improves insulin action and helps prevent long-term complications of diabetes, especially cardiovascular disease. Studies reveal a strong independent association between low vitamin E status before follow-up and an excess risk of diabetes at four years. For Type 2 diabetics vitamin E supplements reduce oxidative stress, improve membrane physical characteristics and improve glucose sensitivity and transport.

Vitamin C (ascorbic acid & ascorbyl palmitate) - inhibits sorbitol accumulation and glycosylation of proteins that cause any complications of diabetes. According to a large study of nearly 6,500 people aged 45-74 years, a vitamin C deficiency increased HbA1c, a measure of long-term blood sugar control that indicates how much glycation is occurring in the body. This study found that plasma vitamin C levels were significantly higher in subjects with HbA1c less than 7 percent compared with those whose HbA1c levels were 7 percent or more. The researchers concluded, "dietary measures to increase plasma vitamin C may be an important health strategy for reducing the prevalence of diabetes."[123]

Human studies have demonstrated that vitamin C supplements may help lower blood glucose levels in diabetics. Vitamin C may also produce additional reductions in low-density lipoprotein (LDL) and plasma free radicals.[124] A recent study of nearly 22,000 non-diabetic patients found that those whose plasma vitamin C levels were in the top 20 percent had a 62 percent lower risk of developing diabetes than those in the lowest fifth.[125] Vitamin C also inhibits sorbitol accumulation and glycation of proteins that cause diabetic complications.

---

122 Diniz YS, Rocha KK, Souza GA, et al. Effects of N-acetylcysteine on sucrose-rich diet-induced hyperglycaemia, dyslipidemia and oxidative stress in rats. *Eur J Pharmacol.* 543(1-3):151-7, Aug 2006.
123 Sargeant LA, Wareham NJ, Bingham S, et al. Vitamin C and hyperglycemia in the European Prospective Investigation into Cancer--Norfolk (EPIC-Norfolk) study: a population-based study. *Diabetes Care.* 23(6):726-32, June 2000.
124 Afkhami-Ardekani M, Shojaoddiny-Ardekani A. Effect of vitamin C on blood glucose, serum lipids & serum insulin in type 2 diabetes patients. Indian J Med Res. 126(5):471-4, Nov 2007.
125 Harding AH, Wareham NJ, Bingham SA, et al. Plasma vitamin C level, fruit and vegetable consumption, and the risk of new-onset type 2 diabetes mellitus: the European

All these ingredients help to improve glucose tolerance, inhibit the evolution of hyperglycemia and a life-long exposure to even normal blood sugar levels and prevent hyperglycemia by:

❖ improving hepatic and peripheral insulin sensitivity;
❖ enhancing insulin-mediated uptake of glucose into cells and glycogen synthesis;
❖ increasing glucose oxidation and glycogen synthesis;
❖ increasing insulin sensitivity by enhancing cell receptor binding of insulin.

These actions combine to reduce plasma glucose levels without abnormal and excessive insulin secretion, while simultaneously decreasing insulin requirements. These actions also inhibit the development of diabetes and its complications, including cardiopathy, angiopathy, neuropathy, retinopathy, nephropathy and other disorders of hyperglycemia. This is exactly what was achieved with Mr. A.

Patient's own account

My main problem was eating too much without thinking of the consequences. Eventually, I gained weight, my sugar and cholesterol levels went straight up and for the past 15 years I have hypertension. The cardiologist prescribed antihypertensive pills which I still took until four months ago. My blood pressure reached 180/110 mm Hg. I continued eating unhealthy, and my sugar levels remained high and my doctor suggested starting taking anti-diabetic pills too.

I also had palpitations, I felt a heavy feeling in my head, tiredness, very low energy levels and by evening I was too exhausted to do anything. All I wanted was to sleep more hours. My knees started to be painful. The stress at my work was making me feel weaker and weaker. Added to this I was a smoker too. I could not fit into any of my clothes and because of food allergies I had also stomach distention and felt uncomfortable. After my doctor told me to start taking anti-diabetic pills I reacted. I didn't want to hear anymore about this. I refused and I tried to find solutions on my own when a close friend told me about the Da Vinci Natural Health Center. I thought I had nothing to lose since I couldn't find any medical solution to my problem apart from taking more and more pills.

prospective investigation of cancer—Norfolk prospective study. *Arch Intern Med.* 28;168(14):1493-9, Jul 2008.

I booked an appointment and after a series of tests we were able to identify and eliminate all the possible causes of my health problems. Starting with the detox diet and eventually with the Candida protocol (I had taken many antibiotics in the past) things started to return back to normal for me.

It's been 4 months since I began treatment and my health has dramatically improved. I lost 15 kg (33 lbs), I completely changed my eating habits and my mood and memory even though I am 65 years old, have greatly improved. I feel very much alive with excellent energy levels and the most important of all my sugar level are now back to normal as well as my blood pressure! I threw away the antihypertensive pills as well as the diabetic medication and my stress levels have diminished a lot. I stopped taking my blood pressure medication a month ago and my knee pains have also disappeared, probably a side-effect of the pills.

My progression was so obvious and I was very happy about it. Thanks to the guidance of the Da Vinci Natural Health Center I feel completely healthy again and have every intention to maintain it.

Dr Georgiou's final comments

This is another pretty typical bread-and-butter case where all the symptoms presenting in this patient were suppressed using drugs without really understanding the causative factors underlying these symptoms. For example, blood pressure can be caused by inflammatory chemicals such as cytokinines and COX-2 chemicals that can also cause a constriction of internal blood vessels, hence elevating blood pressure. Food intolerances usually involve Immunoglobulin G (IgG) which can linger in the body for many months, sometimes up to a year. This IgG can bind to food proteins or lipids and become implanted in tissues in the form of 'immune complexes' which can cause many inflammatory disease processes.

Toxicity levels in the body from heavy metals and xenobiotics can also cause inflammatory responses as well as many other health issues – these 'invisible' toxins not seen by the usual technology used by medical doctors seem to be completely ignored. Toxins accumulate in the body over time causing 'additive effects' as well as 'synergistic effects' where mixing toxins greatly magnifies the sum of their parts – let's say toxin A has a toxic value of 2 and toxin B a value of 5 – if they react synergistically the total may be 23. The older we get the more the toxic load in our bodies, so learning the art of detoxification is akin to learning how to clean our houses – this man had not cleaned his 'house' for over 60 years when I first met him in clinical practice the first time!

In addition, nutritional deficiencies in minerals, trace elements and vitamins, as well as fatty acids can cause serious free radical activity that damage cells and tissues over time. Spinal subluxations are also a cause of many symptoms depending on which spinal nerve is being impinged. Body posture is also important and many people have a Primus Metatarsus Supinatus (PMS) or Rothbart's foot which grossly affects body posture and spinal positioning – this can easily be adjusted using Rothbart's proprioreceptive insoles, as were fitted in the case of this patient and his knee pain subsided in less than a month.

It never ceases to amaze me how a patient like this, after all their health improvements, and coming off all medications that he had been on for more than a decade, can sit and talk to their medical doctor about all these positive health changes and the only response that they get is: "Dr. Georgiou is not a medical doctor." But how do they explain the fact that a non-medical doctor can achieve these results, or is the issue not one of medical vs non-medical but one of self-interests?

What further disturbs me is even if they see the evidence first hand, and hear from their own patients, they dismiss these attempts without even trying to understand how the patient improves. This particular patient became so disoriented with this polemic reaction from the medical fraternity that he has vowed never to return to a medical practitioner for as long as he lives!

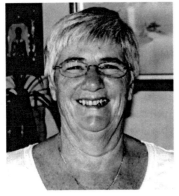

Case 14, Mrs. S, aged 64

Main presenting problem: Hiatus hernia with reflux, pain in stomach, bloating, frequent defecation with slushy stools, back problems with pain, sciatica, knee pain, headaches.

Medical diagnosis:

Mrs. S was a chronic patient with many of her symptoms spanning more than 30 years. In 2006 she had a gastroscopy which diagnosed gastro-esophageal reflux disorder (GERD), as well as gastritis and hiatus hernia. She was defecating at least 6 times a day with pain and the stools were slushy.

She also had degenerative changes of the spine and had previously undergone 3 spine operations with fusion of 4 lumbar discs which had degenerated. There was sciatica of 30 years standing with pain in the knees which made it very difficult climbing stairs. Her feet were also diagnosed as being out of alignment, but nothing further was done about this. She also had frequent headaches and was on the borderline of depression, worrying about her deteriorating health and the restrictions this would impose on her active lifestyle.

Indeed, one of the medical reports written by her orthopaedic surgeon in the UK in 2000 said:

"The MRI of two years ago showed no surgically remediable disease and this matches my clinical findings today (degenerative osteoarthritis). I think the sensible way forward is to speak to the DHSS and confirm that Mrs. S is indeed disabled and unable to work so that she gets reasonable compensation and to refer her to the local pain clinic. If we can treat Mrs. S's pain effectively she can then get on with her life with much greater happiness and much more confidence than she can at the moment. This doesn't solve her problem but I think is our best way of mitigating her problems."

Further blood test just before coming to the DaVinci Holistic Health Centre showed elevated uric acid at 6.5 mg/dl (2.6-6.0) and elevated total cholesterol at 218 mg/dl (100-200) with an elevated risk factor index of 3.9

(<3.3 is preferable). Her ESR levels, an indication of inflammation in the body were high at 22 mm/hr.

Holistic diagnosis:

VEGA food intolerance testing showed that she was intolerant to a number of foods such as wheat, lactose and milk products, eggs, chicken, pork, apples, sugar, caffeine and the onion family.

Further VEGA and ART testing showed that she had systemic Candidiasis.

Iris analysis showed that she had a chronic and severe case of hypochlorhydria (low hydrochloric acid secretion) – unfortunately she had been taking H-proton inhibitors for many years which depress further the already deficient production of hydrochloric acid by the stomach. This is a typical scenario that I have seen in hundreds of other cases of GERD. When the stomach reduces its production of hydrochloric acid, this results in protein concentrates spending a lot more time in the stomach in its attempt to digest this food.

This leads to fermentation of the food, with bloating of the stomach and pressure being applied to the cardiac and pyloric sphincter muscles – this results in the gastroesophageal reflex - that is triggered when the stomach is over distended. When it occurs, it causes a special ring of muscle located at the lower end of the oesophagus (cardiac sphincter) to relax. This allows acid to erupt back into the lower oesophagus. Normally, when the food enters the stomach from the oesophagus, this valve is closed. Unlike the stomach, the oesophagus lacks a layer of protective mucus and therefore the refluxed acid can burn the tissue. If this occurs often enough, heartburn, belching and a sensation of fullness can result - a condition doctors call dyspepsia. Over time this hypochlorhydria will lead to the hiatus hernia developing.

The iris analysis also found a weakened pancreas which resulted in a deficiency of digestive enzymes which led to further bloating and distension in the gut. There was a thyroid marking which later was found to be subclinical hypothyroidism based on the Barnes's Basal Temperature Test. There were also indications of toxicity judging from the murky iris colour in a lymphatic constitution. There was also a subluxation in the lower lumber region of the spine.

561

Hair Tissue Mineral Analysis showed very low levels of certain minerals and trace elements such as potassium, manganese, boron and molybdenum. Many of these are crucial for bone development, thyroid functioning and enzyme production. There was also some circulating mercury, uranium, arsenic and cadmium.

Holistic treatments:

First, Mrs. S began with an alkaline detoxification diet for 15 days with fruit, steamed vegetables, salads, vegetable juices and herbal teas. She was also given nutritional supplements such as a multivitamin, a multimineral, omega 3,6 and 9 fatty acids for the inflammation, betaine HCl and pepsin to improve the stomach digestion and hypochlorhydria, as well as pancreatic enzymes to help improve the gut digestion. In addition, she was given glucosamine sulphate (2,000 mg daily), calcium with magnesium, aloe vera juice and a herbal drainage formula called Organic Lavage (see chapter 7).

In addition, she was checked and found to have a Rothbart's foot or a Primus Metatarsus Supinatus[126] foot type which can greatly aggravate the spine and misalign the body posture,[127] also putting pressure on the knees.[128] She was fitted with 6mm proprioreceptor insoles[129] in order to adjust the Rothbart's foot.

Two weeks into the detoxification and supplement protocol, she had lost 8 lbs in weight, most of which must have been oedematous fluid as her bloating also disappeared; there were no further pains in the stomach and no reflux. The pains in her knees had also improved tremendously. There was a point when she felt light-headed, lethargic and weak – VEGA testing showed that she was reacting to the betaine HCl as her body was not accepting this supplement, probably because of the existing irritation of the stomach lining. When she was asked to rate her improvement as a

---

126 Rothbart BA, Medial Column Foot Systems: An Innovative Tool for Improving Posture. *Journal of Bodywork and Movement Therapies* (6)1:37-46, 2002.
127 Rothbart BA, Liley P, Hansen, el al. Resolving Chronic Low Back Pain. The Foot Connection. *The Pain Practitioner* (formerly American Journal of Pain Management) 5(3): 84-89, 1995.
128 Rothbart BA, Yerratt M. An Innovative Mechanical Approach to Treating Chronic Knee Pain: A BioImplosion Model. *The Pain Practitioner* (formerly American Journal of Pain Management) 4(3): 13-18, 1994.
129 Rothbart BA. Proprioceptive Insoles. From a Podiatric Point of View. Health and Healing Wisdom (*Price-Pottinger Nutrition Foundation Journal*) Vol 29(3):11, 2005.

percentage, she said that she had improved by 95% from the point of starting two weeks ago.

This quick response of the body with a huge percentage improvement in a matter of weeks I have seen on many occasions. Probably the main factor behind this rapid healing response is that the alkaline detoxification diet helps to bring back the body's pH to an alkaline level, therefore removing much of the inflammation related to an acidic milieu. The removal of many toxic deposits from tissues and organs also helps to accelerate the healing response and anti-inflammatory effect. The addition of the various orthomolecular substances that the body is lacking in further helps to accelerate the healing process.

On the 16.9.08, 10 weeks into her therapy, she had lost 28 lbs or about 14 kilos. Her reflux had now completely gone, stools were forming much better and her back pain, sciatica and knee pain was much better after fitting the proprioreceptor insoles. She had just returned from a vacation with her son in the UK and had walked around Leed's Castle, a feat that greatly impressed her son who would normally see his mother in pain when trying lesser feats. Indeed, the 8 tablets of Colderol analgesics that she had been taking every day for the last 8 years has now been stopped completely, with no more pain! She was highly elated over this achievement and I rejoiced with her – the stomach would now have a much better chance of healing properly.

By the time she had completed the DaVinci Candida protocol (see chapter 5) she was functioning very well. Her son had commented that this was the best that he had seen her in over 10 years. Most of her symptoms had now abated completely, with weight stable and taking no more medicinal drugs, something that she had been taking for over 20 years of her life. She is now thoroughly enjoying life and is active on many fronts.

The only issue that requires more work is the stomach which sometimes plays up and causes discomfort, particularly if she eats or drinks something that upsets her. She has not been able to tolerate the betaine HCl and pepsin which is crucial to helping the stomach digest concentrated proteins, something that she is unable to do due to the hypochlorhydria. It may require a new approach with some healing herbs for the stomach, along with digital homeopathics and some PAPIMI treatments to facilitate the healing.

Betaine hydrochloride (HCl) is a nutritional supplement that has been used for over 100 years to safely restore normal gastric acidity and to support healthy gut function. Pepsin also has a long history of medicinal use and is considered very safe when administered to assist digestion, typically in conjunction with hydrochloric acid.

Patient's own account:

As far as I remember, my problems started 52 years ago at the age of 12. Things got progressively worse with time. My stomach problems became unbearable a couple of years ago. I had a terrible abdominal distention, gastroesophageal reflux, multiple diarrheas, sometimes more than six times per day for six consecutive months, felt easily tired and on the verge of depression. I was a very active person and I became apathic.

I was diagnosed with hiatus hernia and in addition to this; I have also arthritis, problems with my spine which I operated 3 times and knee pain, which was serious enough to stop working at the age of 50, because I couldn't walk.

I visited my family doctor and he gave me analgesics for my knee pain and at the same time he recommended a gastroenterologist for my stomach. I was using analgesics for over 20 years! I visited a podiatrist who said that it was my back problem and therefore I had a bad alignment of my feet and gave me more analgesics. When I visited the gastroenterologist, he insisted to go for a stomach biopsy and I wasn't really fond of the idea. Actually, I refused, even though he insisted and his words were definitely not encouraging as they threw me into a deeper and deeper depression.

In June 2008, a friend of mine recommended to pay a visit to the DaVinci Natural Health Center. I had nothing to lose. The environment was so friendly and I immediately felt positive. I went through certain tests at the Centre and based upon these results we started the detoxification programme and eventually the Candida protocol.

I could never imagine my progress being so fast and positive. First of all my stomach reflux has completely gone, as well as the bloating. I don't have any slushy stools, I lost 14 kg and I feel more relaxed and energetic. I can walk now without any significant pain in my knees. The pain has now gone and my son is really amazed to see me walking again without the expression of pain on my face. I can climb the stairs now effortlessly with no pain. I feel like I am reborn! My nutritional habits improved and I don't take analgesics anymore for the pain. I have to admit that I have a 90% improvement as far as I am concerned thanks to Dr. Georgiou and the DaVinci Natural Health Center.

Dr Georgiou's final comments on Mrs. S:

Mrs. S was an example of a patient who had entered the downward spiral of chronic, degenerative disease but the only attempts to better these conditions was to use a variety of drugs for symptom suppression. Analgesics for the pain without addressing the causes of the pain are simply "symptom suppression."

There were many aetiological factors identified in Mrs. S's case – one important issue was the digestive problems such as hypochlorhydria in the stomach.

Numerous studies have shown that hydrochloric acid secretion declines with advancing age. In one study US researchers found that over 30 percent of men and women past the age of 60 suffer from atrophic gastritis, a condition marked by little or no acid secretion.[130] A second study found that up to 40% of postmenopausal women have no basal gastric acid secretions.[131]

In a second study involving 3,484 subjects, researchers found that among both males and females, 27% suffered from achlorhydria, with the greatest incidence (39.8%) occurring in females aged 80 to 89 years.[132]

Researchers in Japan have also measured a similar age-related drop in gastric acidity in elderly Japanese subjects. In 1984 researchers found that 60 percent of Japanese men and women over 50 years age suffered from achlorhydria. New research based on data collected from 1989 to 1999 continued to substantiate a substantial age-related decrease in stomach acid

---

130 Krasinski SD, Russell RM, Samloff IM, Jacob RA, Dallal GE, McGandy RB, Hartz SC. Fundic atrophic gastritis in an elderly population. Effect on hemoglobin and several serum nutritional indicators. *J Am Geriatr Soc.* 34(11):800-6, Nov 1986.
131 Grossman MI, Kirsner JB, Gillespie IE. Basal and histalog-stimulated gastric secretion in control subjects and in patients with peptic ulcer or gastric cancer. *Gastroenterology* 45:15-26, 1963.
132 Sharp GS, Fister HW. The diagnosis and treatment of achlorhydria: ten-year study. *J Amer Ger Soc* 15:786-791, 1967.

production, though the total percentage of achlorhydric subjects dropped from 60 percent to 40 percent.[133]

Hydrochloric acid (HCl) initiates the digestion of protein in the stomach by converting pepsinogen into the proteolytic enzyme, pepsin. Once formed, pepsin acts to break proteins into smaller peptides that can be absorbed by the small intestine. Without adequate gastric secretions, incompletely digested macromolecules can be absorbed into the systemic circulation.

HCl supports the digestion and absorption of carbohydrates, fats, and vitamins A and E by stimulating the release of pancreatic enzymes and bile into the small intestine.

HCl also aids in the absorption and assimilation of vitamins and minerals such as folic acid, ascorbic acid, beta-carotene and iron, by increasing their bioavailability and effecting their release from food. Jonathan Wright MD, Medical Director of the Tahoma Clinic, reports observing that a number of minerals and micro-trace elements are poorly absorbed in cases of low stomach acid, including calcium, magnesium, zinc, copper, chromium, selenium, manganese, vanadium, molybdenum and cobalt.[134]

Other factors in Mrs. S's case were mineral and vitamin deficiencies, Rothbart's foot affecting the body posture, spine and knees, heavy metals facilitating the degeneration due to free radical damage, food intolerance causing further inflammation and systemic Candidiasis releasing 79 toxins which further aggravated these conditions. On top of all this was the worry that her body was degenerating and there was not much that she could do to stop this, even though she was trying hard to get the help that she desperately needed.

All these causative factors and more cannot simply disappear with the use of medication – they need to be identified and off-loaded, then the body can be helped to repair and rebuild – this is the essence of the holistic approach to healing that is demonstrated here.

---

133 Young DG. A stain for demonstrating Helicobacter pylori in gastric biopsies. *Biotech Histochem* 76(1):31-4, Jan 2001.
134 Wright JV. Treatment of childhood asthma with parenteral vitamin B12, gastric re-acidification, and attention to food allergy, magnesium and pyridoxine. Three case reports with background and an integrated hypothesis. *J Nutr Med* 1:277-282, 1990.

Case No. 15, Mrs. G, Age: 66

Main presenting problem:

Parasthesia after stroke, speech impediment, dizziness, chronic fatigue, poor concentration and depression, high cholesterol levels, high glucose levels, high blood pressure, tachycardia.

Medical diagnosis:

CVA, Hypercholesteremia, Hypertension, Supraventricular tachycardia, Diabetes, Atherosclerosis of carotids, Sick Sinus Syndrome.

Mrs. G had a history of five operations within a 4-year period – two of these were for ovarian cysts and the third was for a total hysterectomy due to fibroids. She also had a history of abusing pain killers for many years for painful period pains and other pains, as well as being on diuretics for over 20 years.

In 2005 she had a CVA with dysarthria and right sided paraesthesia. She underwent a triplex examination of the carotid arteries that indicated atheromatous plaques of both arteries without significant stenosis (soft plaque in the right internal carotid artery. She was prescribed Medostatin 20mg daily, Perstantin (75mg x 3), Teveten (75mg daily) and Aspirin (75 mg daily).

Complaints of episodes of palpitations and shortness of breath led her to go to a cardiologist. Heart Echo did not show any remarkable abnormal findings. A 24hr ambulatory ECG device was used that recorded short episodes of supraventricular tachycardia (P waves were differing from the regular sinus ones) with just 100ppm that were followed by almost 2s sinus pause. It was recommended that she have an electrophysiological study for Sick Sinus Syndrome.

Cholesterol levels were 285 and glucose 115.

Holistic diagnosis:

Mrs. G initially came to the DaVinci Natural Health Centre in 2006 as she was interested in finding out the reasons behind her stroke and she was desperate to come off the Statin drugs and other medications that she was taking for many years, due to suspected side effects. She underwent a series of tests which are part of the IDEL Diagnostic Programme in order to determine the underlying causes of her health problems. VEGA testing showed a number of food intolerances including wheat, lactose and all milk products, pork, chicken, sugar and caffeine.

VEGA testing of the organs showed organ weaknesses such as thyroid, auditory canals (there was considerable hearing loss), auditory ossicle, coronary artery, left breast, aorta and pancreas. Oxyuren (pinworms) were also detected with resonance testing.

Autonomic Response Testing showed that the primary factor blocking her regulation or ANS was lactose. There were also organ weaknesses in the ascending colon, thyroid, pancreas, teeth, breasts and the primary organ was the right hemisphere of the brain. ART also showed a scar focus on one portion of her hysterectomy scar. In addition, there were 6 tooth foci detected, teeth 5 (large intestine meridian), 14, 20 and 21 (all stomach meridian), 31 (large intestine meridian) and 32 (small intestine meridian).

Iridology indicated a lumbar subluxation, thyroid irritation, a large lacuna in the liver and gallbladder region indicating hereditary weaknesses of these organs as well as irritation – there was also an overall murky appearance in a blue, lymphatic constitution that is an indication of chronic accumulation of toxins. There were also indications of chronic hypochlorhydria (low levels of hydrochloric acid production).

Examination of living blood under darkfield microscopy showed that there was a rather congested picture with plenty of rouleau (stickiness in the red blood cells) as well as protein linkage, fibrinogen indicating liver toxicity and generally the white blood cells were sluggish. There were also a number of large parasites seen in the blood picture.

Biological Terrain Analysis which is an examination of urine, saliva and blood and measures pH, resistivity and redox potential of these three fluids. This test showed that there was incomplete digestion related to a deficiency of hydrochloric acid and pancreatic enzymes. There was also indication of lymphatic and liver congestion. Malabsorption was also detected with low levels of minerals as well as low ATP production related to nutrient deficiencies (coenzyme Q10, zinc, carnitine) in the electron transport pathways.

Thermography showed a discrete bilateral hyperthermia over the ethmoid sinuses indicating a developing sinusitis. Hyperthermic patterns encircling the buccal cavity possibly indicate an oral (dental or periodontal) pathology. There was hyperthermia over the platysma related to muscular tension in the neck. There was slight diffuse hyperthermia in the upper back and between the scapulas indicating myofascial involvement of the trapezius and rhomboid muscles. There was a central type periumbilical hypothermia that may indicate a developing visceral involvement of the colon.

Heart Rate Variability (HRV) testing produced a relatively good score for her overall fitness level of 5.5 (1.1 is the best physical fitness; 13.7 is the worst). This is probably reflecting more functional problems rather than chronic degenerative conditions.

Holistic treatments:

The first stages of therapy consisted of detoxifying her using ozone sauna, matrix regeneration therapy, infrared sauna, alkaline detoxification diet for two weeks using fruit, salads, steamed vegetables, vegetable juices and herbal teas. She also completed a gallbladder flush and removed a considerable number of stones. She also began a supplement programme using multivitamins, organic flaxseed oil, vitamin c, digestive enzymes and betaine HCl to improve gut and stomach digestion respectively, coenzyme Q10 (myocardial biopsies of patients with various cardiac diseases showed a CoQ10 deficiency in up to 75% of cases)[135], vitamin E[136] and magnesium (transdermal application of magnesium oil)[137,138] and hawthorn[139] to stabilize the heartbeat and arrhythmias. Taurine was also another important addition.

135 Folkers K., Vadhanavikit S., Mortensen S.A. (1985) Biochemical rationale and myocardial tissue data on the effective therapy of cardiomyopathy with coenzyme Q10. In: Proc. Natl. Acad. Sci., U.S.A., vol. 82(3), pp 901-904.
136 Murray, Michael T. The Encyclopedia of Nutritional Supplements: the essential guide for improving your health naturally. Prima Publishing, Rocklin, California, USA. 1996:48.
137 McLean, R. M. Magnesium and its therapeutic uses: a review. American Journal of Medicine. 96(1):63-76, 1994.
138 Sjogren, A., et al. Magnesium deficiency in coronary artery disease and cardiac arrhythmias. Journal of Internal Medicine. 226:213-222, 1989.
139 Miller, A. L. Botanical influences on cardiovascular disease. Alt Med Rev. 3(6):422-431, 1998.

The Sanum remedy Mucokehl was given from day one to help with the rouleau seen in the live blood picture. Also silymarin and polycosonol for her elevated cholesterol levels. In three studies,[140,141,142] Polycosonol was compared with statin drugs. Polycosonol typically did as well, or much better, than the statins in raising HDL and lowering total and LDL cholesterol and triglycerides.

Taurine modulates the activity of cyclic adenosine monophosphate (cAMP), which belongs to a class of substances known as "second messengers," and is one of the most important cell-regulating compounds. Among its many roles, cAMP activates numerous enzymes involved in diverse cellular functions. Through its cAMP-modulating activity, taurine affects enzymes in heart muscle that contribute to contractility. Taurine also plays a role in calcium metabolism and may affect entry of calcium into heart muscle cells where it is essential in the generation and transmission of nerve impulses.[143]

Research shows that taurine may prevent arrhythmogenesis by limiting cardiac hypertrophy and calcium overload of the myocardium.[144] Taurine also protects the heart against reperfusion-induced arrhythmias via its properties as a membrane stabilizer and as an oxygen free radical scavenger.[145]

She had also decided to stop her Statins and had began reducing the dosage over time with the help of her cardiologist – she had completely stopped all her medications including the statins, the antihypertensives, diuretics and aspirin within a three month period.

In addition, her tooth and scar foci were treated with Low Intensity Lazer Therapy (LILT). Interesting, after the third treatment for her hysterectomy

---

140 Crespo, N. et al. Comparative study of the efficacy and tolerability of policosanol and lovastatin. Int J Clin Pharm Res, 19:117-27, 1999.
141 Ortensi, G. et al. Policosanol vs. simvistatin. Curr Ther Res, 58: 390-401, 1997.
142 Castano, G. et al. Effects of policosanol and pravastatin on lipid profile in older hypercholesterolemic patients. Int J Clin Pharm Res, 19: 105-116, 1999.
143 Sebring, LA. and Huxtable, RJ. Sulfur Amino Acids: Biochemical & Clinical Aspects, 1983.
144 Hernández J, Artillo S., Serrano MI, and Serrano JS. Res Commun Chem Patho Pharma. 43(2):343-346, 1984.
145 Bousquet P, Feldman J, Bloch R, and Schwartz J. Eur. J. Pharmacol. 98:269-273, 1984.

scar focus she had regained considerable sensation and strength in her right leg which was very numb and weak.

Within two months her dizziness had disappeared, her speech impediment had gone (very soon after she stopped the Statin drugs completely), her legs were much stronger and it was easier for her to sit up in the bath and did not require the use of the banisters to climb the stairs – in fact, she could now run up the stairs to the utter surprise of her husband who used to push her along. Sensations had returned in the right side of her body – she could now drink tea holding the cup with only one hand instead of two, the sensitivity to hot and cold had returned and she would no longer burn her hand without realizing and was breaking far fewer glasses in the kitchen. Her writing had much improved and so have her finer movements – she reported an 85% improvement in the function of her hands and feet at this stage.

Her blood pressure was stable at 120/70 without antihypertensive medication, probably because the detoxification protocols had removed a considerable amount of inflammation from the body, one of the prime causes of high blood pressure. Her total cholesterol levels still remained high, but her good cholesterol (HDL) had increased and her bad cholesterol (LDL) had decreased – risk factor had dropped from 5.4 to 2.8. By the third month she had regained pain sensation in both her arm and leg as well as her hip, with a very significant strengthening of the muscles.

It was decided to try to use bioresonance therapy using the BICOM device to try to regenerate further her nervous system (nerve regeneration programme using the gold probe). Shortly after 3-4 such treatments she noticed a significant improvement in her tongue muscles and her stuttering had more or less gone – one friend who had not seen her for a few weeks commented that her speech had greatly improved to the point where she could now understand everything she was saying.

Patient's own account:

I first went to the DaVinci Natural Health Center on 12th January 2006 after having a Coronary Vascular Accident (CVA) or stroke about one year before this in February 2005. I am presently 66 years old. I had a considerable number of symptoms including:

- ❖ Numbness on the right side of my body – paraesthesia.
- ❖ Speech impediment – had difficulty thinking the words.
- ❖ Suffered from dizziness.
- ❖ Suffered from apathy, depression, poor concentration, anxiety, exhaustion after light exercise, tender and sore muscles, insomnia, breast pain and cold hands.
- ❖ Chronically fatigued.
- ❖ Hypertension diagnosed in 2003 – 220/100 – placed on Medostatin & Aspirin 75mg x 1 and Persantin 75mg x 3.
- ❖ Supraventricular tachycardia, with shortness of breath – placed on Teveten 600 1x1.
- ❖ High Cholesterol Levels – 285 levels.
- ❖ Blood glucose levels high at 115.
- ❖ In March 2005 underwent a triplex examination of the carotid arteries that found atheromatous plaque in both arteries.

At the DaVinci Natural Health Center I went through a full diagnostic programme which discovered a number of causative factors such as:

- ❖ Food intolerances such as wheat, lactose, pork, chicken, sugar and caffeine.
- ❖ Live Blood Analysis showed a lot of rouleau – red blood cells sticking together and preventing the normal oxygenation of the blood.
- ❖ Parasite load – small pin worms.
- ❖ Tooth foci.
- ❖ Scar foci.
- ❖ Congested lymphatic system.
- ❖ Weakened physiological systems.
- ❖ Digestive problems – low hydrochloric acid and pancreatic enzyme production.

I began a bespoke treatment protocol based upon the diagnostic information that was gathered at the DaVinci Center. This included a detoxification programme using an alkaline detoxification diet, liver and gall bladder cleanse, ozone sauna, MRT and lymphatic drainage, neutralization of tooth and scar foci with laser therapy and a supplement programme that included, amongst other things, a multivitamin formula, flaxseed oil, Vitamin C, Vitamin E, Co Enzyme Q10, Magnesium, Betaine HCL and Pancreatic Enzymes taken with food.

My progression was interesting and I would like to point out how I improved over time.

About a month into the treatment my legs are feeling a lot stronger and I find it a lot easier to sit up in the bath. I also find that I do not need to use the banisters when climbing stairs. I decided to reduce my Statin drugs by 50% and was finding that my speech was rapidly improving. I was also noticing that I could feel more in my right side.

A couple of months into the treatment and I could now run up the stairs without holding onto the banisters. I could also drink my cup of tea with only one hand, without requiring need to pull myself up anymore, I was just rising normally. I also found that my writing had drastically improved. I estimate that I have now recovered about 85% of my functioning and feel much more optimistic about my health. At this stage my depression, apathy, cold hands, fatigue, anxiety, dizziness, poor concentration, tiredness after exercise, insomnia, speech impediment and my general parasthesia on the right side of my body had more or less disappeared.

Third month into treatment my blood pressure is now 120/65 - I have decided to wean myself off the antihypertensive medication gradually. I also did a gall bladder cleanse for the first time and found that I eliminated a large number of stones. My cholesterol levels were still quite high at 263 so I was given some herbal remedies for the liver. Towards the end of the third month, my blood pressure is now stable at 120/70 without any anti-hypertensive medication - I stopped taking all medication for blood pressure about one week ago. I also began at this time to feel pain in both my arm and leg on the right side of my body, something that I could not feel before. About a month after I am feeling itchiness in my right foot which was amazing given that this foot was completely paralyzed before.

About 6 months into treatment and I am now feeling the cotton thread on my fingers when I sow, something that was impossible before. I can also turn the meat in the pan with tongs without dropping it and burning myself.

Generally, I can say that after the diagnosis I really thought that this was the end of my life, as I knew it, I was afraid that I would deteriorate quickly and have another stroke, which would be devastating. I was also afraid of staying on all the drugs that I was on as I knew that these were no good for me.

It was a true blessing that I managed to find the DaVinci Natural Health Center and Dr. Georgiou who helped me along the path to health that is described above. As he puts it: "It is not I that have cured you, but Mother Nature that is inside all of us. This innate intelligence, when given the right resources has the power of healing anything, but we must understand its intent and not suppress its voice with drugs. Listen to the symptoms; they are the body's way of talking to us. Try to understand how they develop – follow their pathway all the way back to the beginning. Begin off-loading superfluous loads and give the body what it requires to heal – it really as simple as this!"

Dr Georgiou's final comments on Mrs. G:

This is an interesting case where presenting symptoms over time were treated by polypharmacy – simply suppressing symptoms instead of identifying their causes. Many of these drugs, including the anti-arrhythmic drugs[146] and diuretics can have very serious side-effects. Being on diuretics for 20 years certainly caused an imbalance in the potassium flow in and out of cardiac muscle cells, thereby adversely affecting the electrical excitability of the cell membranes of cardiac muscle. Diuretics have been shown in research studies to increase the excretion and loss of calcium, they cause magnesium loss into the urine by inhibiting the reabsorption of magnesium in the kidneys.[147]

Magnesium plays an important part in the how blood vessels process the natural chemicals around them, known as endothelial function. That's because the endothelial cell lining of blood vessels constitutes the "brains" of the vessel. Abnormalities in such function are the first stages of an impending heart attack or stroke.[148]

Diuretics also deplete the levels of iodine, potassium and zinc as well as coenzyme Q10[149,150] - all these nutrients are crucial for cardiovascular

146 Podrid PJ, Lampert S, Graboys TB, Blatt CM, Lown B. Aggravation of arrhythmia by antiarrhythmic drugs - incidence and predictors. *Am J Cardiol* 59:38E-44E, 1987.
147 Saris, NEL., et al. Magnesium: an update on physiological, clinical and analytical aspects. *Clinica Chimica Acta.* 294:1-26, 2000.
148 Saris, NEL., et al. Magnesium: an update on physiological, clinical and analytical aspects. *Clinica Chimica Acta.* 294:1-26, 2000.
149 Pelton, Ross et al. Drug-Induced Nutrient Depletion Handbook. Lexi-Comp. 1999.

functioning and was probably one of the main causes of her arrhythmias and Sick Sinus Syndrome, which she had to have a pacemaker fitted in 2007. It was also interesting to note that her blood pressure normalized after she came off a number of medications, including the anti-hypertensives, diuretics and aspirin, but also after undergoing a thorough detoxification programme that certainly helps to lower the level of inflammatory chemicals in the body.

Over the years a lot of emphasis has been given to using Statin drugs to lower cholesterol levels, as if cholesterol is the enemy that needs to be attacked viciously. However, it is the inflammation that oxidizes the cholesterol (and other fats) that leads to the arterial "crud" associated with atherosclerosis. Likewise, oxidized LDL-cholesterol and other oxidized fats also damage brain cells. These oxidized lipids consist of omega-6 oils such as corn, sunflower, peanut, safflower, and canola and soybean oils. The irony is that it is these vegetable oils that are recommended by the American Heart Association and other heart associations around the world, as well as by many dieticians giving diets to heart patients.

When scientists measure inflammation in large groups of people, they find that high levels of inflammatory markers (such as TNF-alpha, IL-6, CRP, and IL-1) predict more accurately who is at a greater risk of a stroke or heart attack than cholesterol levels.

In fact, in those with advanced atherosclerosis, all the lipids in the artery are oxidized, meaning that it is not a cholesterol problem but an inflammation problem. High blood sugar stimulates the growth of visceral fat. The increased amounts of fat trigger the release of high levels of inflammatory cytokines, which worsen the inflammation.

Finally, chronically high sugar levels in the blood and tissues generate destructive elements called AGEs that accelerate the damage. Within tissues and organs, sugar in excess amounts interacts with proteins and amino acids by a chemical process called glycation. Over time they form even more complex chemicals called advanced glycation end products, also called AGEs.

---

150 Folkers K., Vadhanavikit S., Mortensen S.A. Biochemical rationale and myocardial tissue data on the effective therapy of cardiomyopathy with coenzyme Q10. *In: Proc. Natl. Acad. Sci.*, U.S.A., vol. 82(3), pp 901-904, 1985.

Appendix A

PARASITE QUESTIONNAIRE

There are many causes for each symptom listed below. Assign points to each symptom and see if a pattern develops.

A = Symptom never occurs
B = Symptom occurs occasionally
C = Symptom occurs frequently
D = Symptom occurs regularly

	QUESTIONS	A	B	C	D
1	Restless sleep – (tossing & turning, waking often)	0	1	2	3
2	Skin problems, rashes, itches	0	1	2	3
3	Increased appetite, hungry after meals	0	1	2	3
4	Frequent diarrhoea, loose stools	0	1	2	3
5	Grinding of teeth when asleep	0	1	2	3
6	Variable, changeable consistency of stools	0	1	2	3
7	Picking of nose, boring nose with finger	0	1	2	3
8	Abdominal pains	0	1	2	3
9	Vertical wrinkles around mouth	0	1	2	3
10	Rectal, anal itching	0	1	2	3
11	Parallel lines (tracks) in soles of feet	0	1	2	3
12	Intestinal cramps, burning	0	1	2	3
13	Irritabilaty (no apparent reason)	0	1	2	3
14	Feeling bloated, gaseous – no known reason	0	1	2	3
15	Diarrhoea alternating with constipation	0	1	2	3
16	Bowel urgency, occasional accidents	0	1	2	3
17	Hyperactive tendency (nervous)	0	1	2	3
18	Dark circles under eyes	0	1	2	3
19	Need for extra sleep, waking unrefreshed	0	1	2	3
20	Allergies, food sensitivities	0	1	2	3
21	Fevers of unknown origin	0	1	2	3
22	Night sweats (not menopausal)	0	1	2	3
23	Kissing pets, allowing them to lick your face	0	1	2	3
24	Anaemia	0	1	2	3
25	Frequent colds, flu, sore throat	0	1	2	3

	QUESTIONS	A	B	C	D
26	Going barefoot in parks, public streets	0	2	3	4
27	Travelling in 3rd world countries	0	2	3	4
28	Eating lightly cooked pork products	0	2	3	4
29	Eating sushi, sashimi	0	2	3	4
30	Sleeping with pets on bed	0	2	3	4
31	Bed wetting	0	1	2	3
32	Men: sexual dysfunction	0	1	2	3
33	Forgetfulness	0	1	2	3
34	Slow reflexes	0	1	2	3
35	Loss of appetite	0	1	2	3
36	Yellowish face	0	1	2	3
37	Heart beat rapid	0	1	2	3
38	Heart pain	0	1	2	3
39	Pain in the umbilicus	0	1	2	3
40	Blurry, unclear face	0	1	2	3
41	Pain: back, thighs, shoulders	0	1	2	3
42	Lethargy, apathy	0	1	2	3
43	Numbness, tingling in hands, feet	0	1	2	3
44	Burning pains in the stomach, intestines	0	1	2	3
45	Menstrual problems	0	1	2	3
46	Dry lips during day, damp at night	0	1	2	3
47	Drooling while asleep	0	1	2	3
48	Occult blood in stool (shown from lab test)	0	1	2	3
49	History of giardia, pin worms, other worms	0	1	2	3
50	Swimming in creeks, rivers, lakes	0	1	2	3

TOTAL SCORE:
10-14 POINTS = MAYBE PARASITE INFESTATION
15-20 POINTS = SUSPECT PARASITES
22-25 POINTS = LIKELY – (FURTHER TESTING HELPFUL)
25 OR MORE = PARASITES INVOLVEMENT HIGH LIKELY

Appendix B
Dr. Crooks Candida Questionnaire

If you would like to know if your health problems are yeast-related take this comprehensive test. Questions in Section A focus on your medical history-factors that promote the growth of Candida albicansan and that are frequently found people with yeast-related health problems. In Section B you will find a list of 23 symptoms that are often present in patients with yeast-related health problems. Section C consists of 33 other symptoms that are sometimes seen in people with yeast-related problems – yet they may also be found in people with other disorders.

Fill out and score the questionnaire should help you, and your physician, evaluate the possible role that candida albicans plays in your health problems.

SECTION A: HISTORY

- Have you ever taken tetracycline, or other antibiotics, for acne for one month or longer? (points 35)
- Have you, at any time in your life , taken broad-spectrum antibiotics or other antibacterial medication for respiratory, urinary or other infections for two months or longer, or in shorter courses four or more times in a one-year period? (Points 35).
- Have you taken a broad-spectrum antibiotic drug even in a single dose? (points 6)
- Have you at any time in your life been bothered by persistent prostatitis, vaginitis or other problems affecting your reproductive organs? (points 25)
- Are you bothered by memory or concentration problems do you some times feel spaced out? (points 20)
- Do you feel "sick all over", yet despite visits to many different physicians the cause has not been found? (points 20)
- Have you been pregnant two or more times? (points 5)
- One time? (points 3)
- Have you taken birth control pills for more than two years? (points 15)
- For six months to two years? (points 8)
- Have you taken steroids orally, by injection or inhalation for more than two weeks? (points 15)
- For two weeks or less? (points 6)
- Does exposure to perfume, insecticides, fabric shop odors and other chemicals provoke symptoms? Moderate to severe (points 20); Mild (points 5)
- Does tobacco smoke really bother you? (points 10)
- Are your symptoms worse on damp, muggy days or in moldy places? (points 20)
- Have you had athlete's foot, ring worm, jock itch or other chronic fun-gal infections of the skin or nails? Severe or persistent (points 20); Mild to moderate (points 10)
- Do you have crave sugar? (points 10)

Total Score, Section A _____

SECTION B: MAJOR SYMPTOMS

For each of your symptoms, enter the appropriate figure in the pint score column.

1.	If a symptom is occasional or mild		**3 points**
2.	If a symptom is frequent and/ or moderately severe		**6 points**
3.	If a symptom is severe and/ or disabling		**9 points**

Add total score and record it at the end of this section.

- Fatigue or lethargy _____
- Feeling of being "drained" _____
- Depression or manic depression _____
- Numbness, burning or tingling _____
- Headache _____
- Muscle aches _____
- Muscle weakness or paralysis _____
- Paint and/ or swelling in joints _____
- Abdominal pain _____
- Constipation and/ or diarrhea _____
- Bloating, belching or intestinal gas _____
- Troublesome vaginal burning, itching or discharge _____
- Prostatitis _____
- Impotence _____
- Loss of sexual desire or feeling _____
- Endometriosis or infertility _____
- Cramps and/ or other menstrual irregularities _____
- Premenstrual tension _____
- Attacks of anxiety or crying _____
- Cold hands or feet, low bode temperature _____
- Hypothyroidism _____
- Shaking or irritable when hungry _____
- Cystitis or interstitial cystitis _____

TOTAL SCORE, SECTION B _____

SECTION C: OTHER SYMPTOMS

For each of your symptoms, enter the appropriate figure in the point score column.

1.	If a symptom is occasional or mild	**3 points**
2.	If a symptom is frequent and/ or moderately severe	**6 points**
3.	If a symptom is severe and/ or disabling	**9 points**

Add total score and record it at the end of his section.

- Drowsiness, including inappropriate drowsiness   _____
- Irritability   _____
- In coordination   _____
- Frequent mood swings   _____
- Insomnia   _____
- Dizziness/ loss of balance   _____
- Pressure above ears, tenderness of forehead/cheek   _____
- Tendency to bruise easily   _____
- Eczema, itching eyes   _____
- Psoriasis   _____
- Chronic hives (urticaria)   _____
- Indigestion or heartburn   _____
- Sensitivity to milk, wheat or other common foods   _____
- Mucus in stools   _____
- Rectal itching   _____
- Dry mouth or throat   _____
- Mouth rashes, including "white" tongue   _____
- Bad breath   _____
- Foot, hair or body odor not relieved by washing   _____
- Nasal congestion or postnasal drip   _____
- Nasal itching   _____
- Sore throat   _____
- Laryngitis, loss of voice   _____
- Cough or recurrent bronchitis   _____
- Pain or tightness in chest   _____
- Wheezing or shortness of breath   _____
- Urinary frequency or urgency   _____
- Burning on urination   _____
- Spots in front of eyes or erratic vision   _____
- Burning or tearing eyes   _____
- Recurrent infections or fluid in ears   _____
- Ear pain or deafness   _____

TOTAL SCORE, SECTION C   _____

GRAND TOTAL (SECTION A, B AND C)   _____

The **Grand Total Score** will help you and your physician decide if your health problems are yeast-connected. Scores in women will run higher, as seven items in the questionnaire apply to women, while only two apply exclusively to men.

- Yeast –connected health problems are almost certainly present in women with scores of **more than 180,** and in men with of **more than 140.**
- Yeast-connected health problems are probably present in women with scores of **more than 120,** and in men with scores **more than 90.**
- Yeast-connected health problems are possibly present in women with scores of **more than 60,** and in me of **more than 40.**
- With scores of less than 60 in women and 40 in men, yeasts are less likely to be the cause of health problems.

Score of **60-99** yeast a possible cause of health problems
Score of **100-139** yeast a probable cause of health problems.
Score of **140 or more** yeast **almost certainly** a cause of health problems.

Summary and Concluding Remarks

Modern medicine has become a dictatorial, monopolistic endeavour that attempts to eradicate disease without understanding the body's attempts to self-heal. It appears that disease is something we have no control of and that new drugs are the answer to all of man's ailments. This is the biomedical model of disease that has completely missed what the Father of Medicine, Hippocrates taught over 2,500 years ago. Ironically, all doctors take the Hippocratic oath when they qualify.

The social control of the population by the medical industry reinforces a morbid society, with its principle economic and profit making activities. These economic motivating factors are what prevent man from mobilizing his self-healing powers as turning the patient into a drug-dependent customer is far more important. It's as if the disease can be controlled by the routine prescription. This fostering of a drug-dependent culture with its principles of "symptom suppression" leads to moral degeneration and prevents disease from being cured.

Medical treatments have become the suppression of the natural survival mechanisms that are so vital at protecting the body against all types of disease.

The Holistic Model of health does not want to suppress symptoms; to the contrary, the symptoms are an important part of unravelling and understanding where the body has lost its balance and why. Once this is determined, then on the one hand it's a simple case of giving the body what it requires to regain the balance, on the other hand, taking away what may have caused the imbalance in the first place.

Listening to the body was an art that was admired many years ago before technological medicine came in and doctors were taught to pay more attention to the blood tests and scans, while literally ignoring the important information that is being shared by the patient. What often occurs is that the medical tests do not indicate pathological parameters and the doctor simply says: "it's all in your head, or it could be genetic." Meanwhile the patient is feeling as sick as a dog and they are told that it is all in their head and there is really not a lot that can be done. A tranquilizer is usually given to placate the patient who now goes home and gradually deteriorates as they are left in a helpless and hopeless state. This is very soul-destroying and demoralizing.

It is my hope that this book will help these patients to understand some of the possible underlying causes of their symptoms and ways that they can help themselves regain balance.

In no way is this an exhaustive account of all the causative factors of disease – there are many causative factors and treatments that have not been discussed due to space restrictions, these would include the issues of Lyme's disease, adrenal exhaustion, hypoglycaemia, syndrome X, chemical hypersensitivity, environmental illnesses, vaccination stress and more.

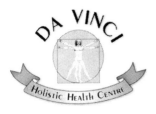

Clinical Consultations

To book appointments to see Dr. Georgiou at the DaVinci Holistic Medicine Centre simply call his secretary or email:

Tel: (+357) 24-823322
Fax: (+357) 24-823321
Email: admin@docgeorge.com
Web: www.docgeorge.com

DaVinci College of Holistic Medicine (DCHM)

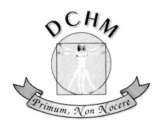

Anyone interested in completing their studies in Holistic Medicine can apply to take a Bachelors of Science in Holistic Medicine - BSc (HM) – or a Doctor of Science in Holistic Medicine – DSc (HM).

Tel: (+357) 24-823322
Fax: (+357) 24-823321
Email: admin@collegenaturalmedicine.com
Web: www.collegenaturalmedicine.com

584

ABOUT THE AUTHOR

Dr. George John Georgiou was born 14th December 1956 and is presently a clinical practitioner in Holistic Medicine specialising in the treatment of chronic diseases. He is also an active researcher and author.

He has been educating himself for over 25 years and has been awarded a number of degrees and diplomas such as a Bachelor of Science (B.Sc) honours degree in Biology/Psychology from Oxford Brook's University, Oxford, England, a Master's of Science degree (M.Sc) in Clinical Psychology from the University of Surrey, Guildford, England, a Doctor of Philosophy degree (Ph.D). in Clinical Sexology from The Institute for Advanced Study of Human Sexuality, San Francisco, USA. He also holds a Doctor of Science (D.Sc) degree in Alternative Medicine from the International Open University of Alternative Medicine - his main research interests at present are studying the use of natural compounds in the detoxification of heavy metals.

He also has diplomas and degrees (all with distinction) in Clinical Nutrition (Dip.ION) from the Institute of Optimum Nutrition (ION), London, England; diplomas in Naturopathy, Medical Herbalism (M.H.) and Iridology (R.Ir.,MRNI) from the Holistic Health College, London, UK; and a Diploma in Electronic Impulse Therapy (Dip.E.I.Th) from the Euro College of Complementary Medicine, UK. He has also been awarded a Diploma in Homeopathic Medicine (DIHom.) from the British Institute of Homeopathy, Middlesex, England. He has a Licentiate Diploma in Chinese Acupuncture (L.Dip.Ac.,aM.A.C.Ac.-TCMI) from the College of Oriental Medicine, UK and the Cyprus Acupuncture Institute; and is a qualified Su Jok Acupuncturist. He is also a qualified Hellinger Family Constellations practitioner conducting 'soul healing' groups and individual sessions in clinical practice.

Dr. Georgiou has also been a clinician most of his life and is the Director of the DaVinci Natural Health Centre in Larnaca, Cyprus which specializes in many aspects of Holistic Medicine such as naturopathy, herbal medicine, orthomolecular nutrition, homeopathy, thermography, iridology, VEGA allergy testing, Live Blood Analysis, colon hydrotherapy, Bio-resonance therapy, Biological Terrain Analysis, Rife technology, PAPIMI, Hyperthermia, Infrared and ozone sauna, MRT,

HRV, ART, Orgone Accumulator, Psychotherapy and Naturopathic Sexology – see www.docgeorge.com.

The DaVinci Natural Health Centre specializes in the treatment of chronic diseases, heavy metal toxicity and Candidiasis, along with many other health problems. His patients come from all walks of life including Presidents, Prime Ministers, Sheiks, CEOs, to the humble family person - he treats all with a healthy respect and a real interest in helping each one optimize their health.

On the research front, which is one of his loves, he has been the Principal Investigator for the World Health Organization in studies on AIDS and Drug Use, as well as other research involving alcoholism, drug abuse and sexual dysfunctions. He is also the Director and Founder of the DaVinci LifeSciences Research Centre, equipped with a PE 3000XL Inductively Coupled Plasma Optical Emission Spectrometer (ICP-OES) and a PSA Mercury Analyzer for research in heavy metal toxicity and detoxification. His research has led him to develop a unique, natural heavy metal detox agent that has been thoroughly tested using a double-blind, placebo-controlled trial with 350 people – he is the owner of a worldwide patent-pending for this discovery which is called HMD™ (www.detoxmetals.com).

He has lectured to Masters students in Psychology at an external campus for Indiana University, USA, and has been a prolific writer of health articles for the general public. He has written 4 books and had his own radio program for 2 years entitled Human Sexuality on the island of Cyprus, and is the Editor for the chapter on Cyprus in the International Encyclopedia of Sexuality, Volume 4.

This wealth of knowledge and clinical experience is now being transformed into the DaVinci College of Holistic Medicine - www.collegenaturalmedicine.com, of which Dr. Georgiou is the Academic Director. This has developed into awarding accredited degrees and diplomas – Bachelor of Science in Holistic Medicine and Doctor of Science in Holistic Medicine.

Wearing other hats, he has also been an Aviation Consultant/Human Factors (Aeronautical Medicine) and Crew Resource Management Program Developer and Facilitator Trainer (Crew safety) for a number of years to Cyprus Airways and EuroCypria Airlines, given that he is also a keen Private Pilot himself.

On a professional front, he is a Member of the following Associations/Institutes:

- ❖ The Institute of Biology, UK (MIBiol.)
- ❖ Chartered Biologist, UK (C. Biol)
- ❖ The Royal Microscopy Society, UK
- ❖ The General Council and Register of Naturopaths, UK (GCRN)
- ❖ The Register of Naturopathic Iridologists, UK (M.R.N.I.)
- ❖ The British Association of Nutritional Therapists, UK (BANT)
- ❖ The Association of Master Herbalists, UK. (AMH)
- ❖ Fellow of the British Institute of Homeopathy, UK (FBIH)
- ❖ The American College of Clinical Thermology, USA
- ❖ The International Su Jok Therapy Association, Russia
- ❖ The British Holistic Medical Association, UK (BHMA)
- ❖ The Institute of Complementary Medicine, UK (ICM)
- ❖ The National Iridology Research Association, USA (NIRA)
- ❖ Associate Fellow of the British Psychological Society, UK
- ❖ Chartered Psychologist, UK, BPS (C.Psychol)
- ❖ Diplomate of the American Board of Sexology, USA (ABS)
- ❖ Registered Sex Therapist with ABS, USA
- ❖ The American College of Sexologists, USA (ACS)
- ❖ Fellow of the American Academy of Clinical Sexologists, USA
- ❖ The World Association for Sexology (WAS), USA

His hobbies and interests include flying a private plane, water skiing, horse riding, classic antique motorbike and car restoration, antique furniture restoration, model making, web master, travelling and a family life.

Dr. Georgiou is also a Knight of Honour, diplomatic Cultural Attaché in Cyprus of one of the oldest charity organizations in the world, the Sovereign Medical Order of the Knights Hospitaller, St. John of Jerusalem - http://smokh.org.

The aims and objectives of the Order are:

- ❖ To establish, equip, staff and maintain humanitarian relief and medical treatment centres and hospitals.

587

❖ To promote and participate in all phases of education of physicians, therapists, nursing staff, paramedical and nutritional care personnel.

❖ To raise funds for all these humanitarian, organizational, and medical needs.

❖ To promote peace and prosperity, by diplomacy, cooperation and consensus; and not by confrontation.

❖ To cooperate with IGO's (Intergovernmental Organizations), NGO's (Non-governmental Organizations), and Governmental Organizations for purposes humanitarian and medical needs.

NOTES

NOTES

Breinigsville, PA USA
15 November 2009
227585BV00001B/71/P